D0049581

Statistical Methods for Biostatistics and Related Fields

Wolfgang Härdle · Yuichi Mori
Philippe Vieu

Statistical Methods for Biostatistics and Related Fields

With 91 Figures and 57 Tables

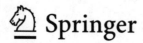 Springer

Professor Wolfgang Härdle
CASE - Center for Applied Statistics and Economics
Institute for Statistics and Econometrics
School of Business and Economics
Humboldt Universität zu Berlin
Spandauer Str. 1
10178 Berlin
haerdle@wiwi.hu-berlin.de

Professor Yuichi Mori
Department of Socio-information
Okayama University of Sciences
1-l Ridai-cho
700-0005 Okayama
mori@soci.ous.ac.jp

Professor Philippe Vieu
Laboratoire de Statistique et Probabilités
Université Paul Sabatier
118 route de Narbonne
31062 Toulouse Cedex
vieu@cict.fr

Library of Congress Control Number: 2006934207

ISBN-13 978-3-540-32690-8 Springer Berlin Heidelberg New York

Springer is part of Springer Science+Business Media

springer.com

© Springer-Verlag Berlin Heidelberg 2007

Production: LE-TEX Jelonek, Schmidt & Vöckler GbR, Leipzig
Cover-design: Erich Kirchner, Heidelberg

SPIN 11681021   154/3100YL - 5 4 3 2 1 0   Printed on acid-free paper

Preface

Biostatistics is one of the scientific fields for which the developments during the last decades of the 20th century have been the most important. Biostatistics is a pluri-disciplinary area combining statistics and biology, but also agronomics, medicine or health sciences. It needs a good knowledge of the mathematical background inherent in statistical methodology, in order to understand the various fields of applications. The idea of this book is to present a variety of research papers on the state of art in modern biostatistics.

Biostatistics is interacting with many scientific fields. To highlight this wide *diversity*, we deliberately put these interactions at the center of our project. Our book is therefore divided into two parts. Part I is presenting several statistical models and methods for different biologic applications, while Part II will be concerned with problems and statistical methods coming from other related scientific fields.

This book intends to provide a basis for many people interested in biostatistics and related sciences. Students, teachers and academic researchers will find an overview on modelling and statistical analysis of biological data. Also, the book is meant for practicioners involved in research organisations (pharmacologic industry, medicine, food industry,..) for which statistics is an indispensable tool.

Biology is a science which has always been in permanent interaction with many other fields such as medicine, physics, environmetrics, chemistry, mathematics, probability, statistics .... On the other hand, statistics is interacting with many other fields of mathematics as with almost all other scientific disciplines, including biology. For all these reasons, biostatistics is strongly dependent on other scientific fields, and in order to provide a wide angle overview we present here a rich *diversity* of applied problems.

Each contribution of this book presents one (or more) real problem. The variation ranges from biological problems (see Chapter 1 and 10), medical contributions (see Chapters 2, 4, 5, 8, 9 or 11) and genomics contributions (see Chapters 3 and 7), to applications coming from other scientific areas, such as environmetrics (see Chapters 12), chemometrics (see Chapter 13), geophysics (see Chapters 17 and 18) or image analysis (see Chapter 18). Because all these disciplines are continuously taking benefits one from each other, this choice highlights as well how each biostatistical method and modelling is helpful in other areas and vice versa.

A good illustration of such a duality is provided by hazard analysis, which is originally a medical survival problem (see Chapters 4, 9 or 11) but which leads to substancial interest in many other fields (see e.g. the microearthquakes analysis presented in Chapter 17). Another example is furnished by spatial statistics (see Chapters 15 or 18) or food industry problems (see Chapter 13), which are apparently far from medical purposes but whose developments have obvious (and strong) consequences in medical image analysis and in biochemical studies.

Due to the variety of applied biostatistical problems, the scope of methods is also very large. We adress therefore the *diversity* of these statistical approaches by presenting recent developments in descriptive statistics (see Chapters 7, 9, 14 and 19), parametric modelling (see Chapters 1, 2, 6 and 18) nonparametric estimation (see Chapters 3, 4, 11, 15 and 17) and semi-parametrics (see Chapters 5, 8 and 10). An important place is devoted to methods for analyzing functional data (see Chapters 12, 13, 16), which is currently an active field of modern statistics.

An important feature of biostatistics is to have to deal with rather large statistical sample sizes. This is particular true for genomics applications (see Chapters 3 and 7) and for functional data modelling (see Chapters 12, 13 and 16). The computational issues linked with the methodologies presented in this book are carried out thanks to the capacities of the XploRe environment. Most of the methodological contributions are accompanied with automatic and/or interactive XploRe quantlets.

We would like to express our gratitude to all the contributors. We are confident that the scope of papers will insure a large impact of this book on future research lines and/or on applications in biostatistics and related fields. We would also like to express our sincere gratitude to all the researchers that we had the opportunity to meet in the past years. It would be tedious (and hardly exhaustive) to name all of them expressely here but specific thanks have to be adressed to our respective teams, will special mention to Anton Andriyashin in Berlin and to the participants of the STAPH working group in Toulouse.

July 2006   *Wolfgang Härdle, Yuichi Mori*
Berlin, Okoyama, Toulouse   and *Philippe Vieu*

Contents

I   Biostatistics   **1**

1   Discriminant Analysis Based on Continuous and Discrete Variables   3

Avner Bar-Hen and Jean-Jacques Daudin

   1.1   Introduction   3

   1.2   Generalisation of the Mahalanobis Distance   4

        1.2.1   Introduction   4

        1.2.2   Kullback–Leibler Divergence   5

        1.2.3   Asymptotic Distribution of Matusita Distance   10

        1.2.4   Simulations   12

   1.3   Methods and Stopping Rules for Selecting Variables   13

   1.4   Reject Option   15

        1.4.1   Distributional Result   15

        1.4.2   Derivation of the Preliminary Test   18

   1.5   Example   22

        1.5.1   Location Model   22

        1.5.2   Comparison with the Linear Discriminant Analysis . .   24

        1.5.3   Conclusion   24

   Bibliography   25

2 Longitudinal Data Analysis with Linear Regression   29

Jörg Breitung, Rémy Slama and Axel Werwatz

2.1   Introduction   29

2.2   Theoretical Aspects   32

    2.2.1   The Fixed-effect Model   32

    2.2.2   The Random Effects Model   36

2.3   Computing Fixed and Random-effect Models   37

    2.3.1   Data Preparation   37

    2.3.2   Fixed and Random-effect Linear Regression   38

    2.3.3   Options for `panfix`   38

    2.3.4   Options for `panrand`   39

2.4   Application   40

    2.4.1   Results   41

Bibliography   43

3 A Kernel Method Used for the Analysis of Replicated Micro-array Experiments   45

Ali Gannoun, Beno Liquetît, Jérôme Saracco and Wolfgang Urfer

3.1   Introduction   45

3.2   Statistical Model and Some Existing Methods   46

    3.2.1   The Basic Model   47

    3.2.2   The T-test   47

    3.2.3   The Mixture Model Approach   48

3.3   A Fully Nonparametric Approach   49

    3.3.1   Kernel Estimation of f_0 and f   50

    3.3.2   The Reflection Approach in Kernel Estimation   50

    3.3.3   Implementation of the Nonparametric Method   51

3.4   Data Analysis   52

    3.4.1   Results Obtained with the Normal Mixture Model . .   53

        3.4.2   Results Obtained with the Nonparametric Approach .   53

        3.4.3   A Simulation Study   56

    3.5   Discussion and Concluding Remarks   58

    Bibliography   59

4   Kernel Estimates of Hazard Functions for Biomedical Data Sets   63

Ivana Horová and Jiří Zelinka

    4.1   Introduction   63

    4.2   Kernel Estimate of the Hazard Function and Its Derivatives .   64

    4.3   Choosing the Shape of the Kernel   68

    4.4   Choosing the Bandwidth   69

    4.5   Description of the Procedure   74

    4.6   Application   75

    Bibliography   83

5   Partially Linear Models   87

Wolfgang Härdle and Hua Liang

    5.1   Introduction   87

    5.2   Estimation and Nonparametric Fits   89

        5.2.1   Kernel Regression   89

        5.2.2   Local Polynomial   90

        5.2.3   Piecewise Polynomial   93

        5.2.4   Least Square Spline   96

    5.3   Heteroscedastic Cases   97

        5.3.1   Variance Is a Function of Exogenous Variables   98

        5.3.2   Variance Is an Unknown Function of T   99

        5.3.3   Variance Is a Function of the Mean   99

    5.4   Real Data Examples 100

    Bibliography 102

6   Analysis of Contingency Tables   **105**

Masahiro Kuroda

6.1   Introduction   105

6.2   Log-linear Models   105

   6.2.1   Log-linear Models for Two-way Contingency Tables   .   106

   6.2.2   Log-linear Models for Three-way Contingency Tables .   107

   6.2.3   Generalized Linear Models   109

   6.2.4   Fitting to Log-linear Models   111

6.3   Inference for Log-linear Models Using XploRe   113

   6.3.1   Estimation of the Parameter Vector λ   113

   6.3.2   Computing Statistics for the Log-linear Models   113

   6.3.3   Model Comparison and Selection   114

6.4   Numerical Analysis of Contingency Tables   115

   6.4.1   Testing Independence   115

   6.4.2   Model Comparison   119

Bibliography   124

7   Identifying Coexpressed Genes   **125**

Qihua Wang

7.1   Introduction   125

7.2   Methodology and Implementation   127

   7.2.1   Weighting Adjustment   128

   7.2.2   Clustering   132

7.3   Concluding Remarks   142

Bibliography   144

8 Bootstrap Methods for Testing Interactions in GAMs 147

Javier Roca-Pardiñas, Carmen Cadarso-Suárez
and Wenceslao González-Manteiga

8.1 Introduction 147

8.2 Logistic GAM with Interactions 149

    8.2.1 Estimation: the Local Scoring Algorithm 150

8.3 Bootstrap-based Testing for Interactions 152

    8.3.1 Likelihood Ratio-based Test 153

    8.3.2 Direct Test 153

    8.3.3 Bootstrap Approximation 153

8.4 Simulation Study 154

8.5 Application to Real Data Sets 156

    8.5.1 Neural Basis of Decision Making 156

    8.5.2 Risk of Post-operative Infection 159

8.6 Discussion 162

8.7 Appendix 163

Bibliography 165

9 Survival Trees 167

Carmela Cappelli and Heping Zhang

9.1 Introduction 167

9.2 Methodology 170

    9.2.1 Splitting Criteria 170

    9.2.2 Pruning 173

9.3 The Quantlet stree 174

    9.3.1 Syntax 174

    9.3.2 Example 175

Bibliography 179

10 A Semiparametric Reference Curves Estimation   **181**

Saracco Jérôme, Gannoun Ali, Guinot Christiane and Liquet Benoît

  10.1 Introduction 181

  10.2 Kernel Estimation of Reference Curves 184

  10.3 A Semiparametric Approach Via Sliced Inverse Regression . . 187

     10.3.1 Dimension Reduction Context 187

     10.3.2 Estimation Procedure 191

     10.3.3 Asymptotic Property 192

     10.3.4 A Simulated Example 193

  10.4 Case Study on Biophysical Properties of the Skin 195

     10.4.1 Overview of the Variables 196

     10.4.2 Methodological Procedure 197

     10.4.3 Results and Interpretation 198

  10.5 Conclusion 200

  Bibliography 201

11 Survival Analysis   **207**

Makoto Tomita

  11.1 Introduction 207

  11.2 Data Sets 208

  11.3 Data on the Period up to Sympton Recurrence 208

     11.3.1 Kaplan-Meier Estimate 208

     11.3.2 log-rank Test 210

  11.4 Data for Aseptic Necrosis 211

     11.4.1 Kaplan-Meier Estimate 214

     11.4.2 log-rank Test 214

     11.4.3 Cox's Regression 215

  Bibliography 217

II Related Sciences   219

12 Ozone Pollution Forecasting   221

Hervé Cardot, Christophe Crambes and Pascal Sarda

12.1 Introduction 221

12.2 A Brief Analysis of the Data 222

    12.2.1 Description of the Data 222

    12.2.2 Principal Component Analysis 224

    12.2.3 Functional Principal Component Analysis 225

12.3 Functional Linear Model 226

    12.3.1 Spline Estimation of α 227

    12.3.2 Selection of the Parameters 228

    12.3.3 Multiple Functional Linear Model 229

12.4 Functional Linear Regression for Conditional Quantiles Estimation 231

    12.4.1 Spline Estimator of Ψ_α 232

    12.4.2 Multiple Conditional Quantiles 234

12.5 Application to Ozone Prediction 235

    12.5.1 Prediction of the Conditional Mean 236

    12.5.2 Prediction of the Conditional Median 236

    12.5.3 Analysis of the Results 238

Bibliography 242

13 Nonparametric Functional Chemometric Analysis   245

Frédéric Ferraty, Aldo Goia and Philippe Vieu

13.1 Introduction 245

13.2 General Considerations 246

    13.2.1 Introduction to Spectrometric Data 246

    13.2.2 Introduction to Nonparametric Statistics for Curves . 248

  13.2.3 Notion of Proximity Between Curves 249

  13.2.4 XploRe Quantlets for Proximity Between Curves . . . 251

 13.3 Functional Nonparametric Regression 252

  13.3.1 The Statistical Problem 252

  13.3.2 The Nonparametric Functional Estimate 253

  13.3.3 Prediction of Fat Percentage from Continuous
     Spectrum 254

  13.3.4 The XploRe Quantlet 255

  13.3.5 Comments on Bandwidth Choice 256

 13.4 Nonparametric Curves Discrimination 257

  13.4.1 The Statistical Problem 257

  13.4.2 A Nonparametric Curves Discrimination Method . . . 258

  13.4.3 Discrimination of Spectrometric Curves 260

  13.4.4 The XploRe Quantlet 261

 13.5 Concluding Comments 262

 Bibliography 263

14 Variable Selection in Principal Component Analysis   265

Yuichi Mori, Masaya Iizuka, Tomoyuki Tarumi and Yutaka Tanaka

 14.1 Introduction 265

 14.2 Variable Selection in PCA 267

 14.3 Modified PCA 268

 14.4 Selection Procedures 269

 14.5 Quantlet 272

 14.6 Examples 273

  14.6.1 Artificial Data 273

  14.6.2 Application Data 279

 Bibliography 282

15 Spatial Statistics   285

Pavel Čížek, Wolfgang Härdle and Jürgen Symanzik

15.1 Introduction 285

15.2 Analysis of Geostatistical Data 287

    15.2.1 Trend Surfaces 288

    15.2.2 Kriging 290

    15.2.3 Correlogram and Variogram 292

15.3 Spatial Point Process Analysis 297

15.4 Discussion 303

15.5 Acknowledgements 303

Bibliography 303

16 Functional Data Analysis   305

Michal Benko

16.1 Introduction 305

16.2 Functional Basis Expansion 307

    16.2.1 Fourier Basis 308

    16.2.2 Polynomial Basis 309

    16.2.3 B-Spline Basis 309

    16.2.4 Data Set as Basis 309

16.3 Approximation and Coefficient Estimation 310

    16.3.1 Software Implementation 312

    16.3.2 Temperature Example 313

16.4 Functional Principal Components 314

    16.4.1 Implementation 317

    16.4.2 Data Set as Basis 319

16.5 Smoothed Principal Components Analysis 321

    16.5.1 Implementation Using Basis Expansion 323

    16.5.2 Temperature Example 323

Bibliography 326

17 Analysis of Failure Time with Microearthquakes Applications   329

Graciela Estévez-Pérez and Alejandro Quintela del Rio

17.1 Introduction 329

17.2 Kernel Estimation of Hazard Function 330

17.3 An Application to Real Data 336

    17.3.1 The Occurrence Process of Earthquakes 336

    17.3.2 Galicia Earthquakes Data 337

17.4 Conclusions 342

Bibliography 343

18 Landcover Prediction   347

Frédéric Ferraty, Martin Paegelow and Pascal Sarda

18.1 Introduction 347

18.2 Presentation of the Data 348

    18.2.1 The Area: the Garrotxes 348

    18.2.2 The Data Set 348

18.3 The Multilogit Regression Model 349

18.4 Penalized Log-likelihood Estimation 351

18.5 Polychotomous Regression in Action 352

18.6 Results and Interpretation 353

Bibliography 356

19 The Application of Fuzzy Clustering to Satellite Images Data   357

Hizir Sofyan, Muzailin Affan and Khaled Bawahidi

19.1 Introduction 357

19.2 Remote Sensing 358

19.3 Fuzzy C-means Method 359

19.3.1 Data and Methods 361

19.4 Results and Discussions 362

Bibliography 366

Index **367**

Part I

Biostatistics

1 Discriminant Analysis Based on Continuous and Discrete Variables

Avner Bar-Hen and Jean-Jacques Daudin

1.1 Introduction

In discrimination, as in many multivariate techniques, computation of a distance between two populations is often useful. For example in taxonomy, one can be interested not only in discriminating between two populations but in having an idea of how far apart the populations are. Mahalanobis' Δ^2 has become the standard measure of distance when the observations are quantitative and Hotelling derived its distribution for normal populations. The aim of this chapter is to adapt these results to the case where the observed characteristics are a mixture of quantitative and qualitative variables.

A problem frequently encountered by the practitioner in Discriminant Analysis is how to select the best variables. In mixed discriminant analysis (MDA), i.e., discriminant analysis with both continuous and discrete variables, the problem is more difficult because of the different nature of the variables. Various methods have been proposed in recent years for selecting variables in MDA. Here we use two versions of a generalized Mahalanobis distance between populations based on the Kullback-Leibler divergence for the first and on the Hellinger-Matusita distance for the second. Stopping rules are established from distributional results.

1.2   Generalisation of the Mahalanobis Distance

1.2.1   Introduction

Following Krzanowski (1983) the various distances proposed in the literature can be broadly classified in two categories:

1. Measures based on ideas from information theory (like Kullback-Leibler measures of information for example)

2. Measures related to Bhattacharya's measure of affinity (like Matusita's distance for example)

A review of theses distance measures can be found, for example, in Adhikari and Joshi (1956).

Mixture of continuous and discrete variables is frequently encountered in discriminant analysis. The location model (Olkin and Tate, 1961; Krzanowski, 1990) is one possible way to deal with these data. Gower (1966) proposed a formula for converting similarity to distance. Since this transformation corresponds to the transformation of Bhattacharya's measure of affinity to Matusita's distance, Krzanowski (1983) studied the properties of Matusita's distance in the framework of the location model. Since no distributional properties were obtained, Krzanowski (1984), proposed to use Monte Carlo procedures to obtain percentage points. This distance was also proposed as a tool of selection of variables (Krzanowski, 1983). Distributional results for Matusita will be presented in Section 1.2.3. At first we present another generalization of the Mahalanobis distance, J, based on the Kullback-Leibler divergence.

One of the aims of discriminant analysis is the allocation of unknown entities to populations that are known *a priori*. A preliminary matter for consideration before an outright or probabilistic allocation is made for an unclassified entity X is to test the assumption that X belongs to one of the predefined groups π_i $(i = 1, 2, \ldots, n)$. One way of approaching this question is to test if the smallest distance between X and π_i is null or not. Most of the results were obtained in the case of linear discriminant analysis where the probability distribution function of the populations is assumed to be normal and with a commom variance–covariance matrix Σ (McLachlan, 1992). Generally, the squared Mahalanobis distance is computed between X and each population π_i. X will be assessed as atypical if the smallest distance is bigger than a given threshold. Formally a preliminary test is of the form:

$$H_0 : \min_i d(X, \pi_i) = 0 \qquad \text{versus} \qquad H_1 : \min_i d(X, \pi_i) > 0$$

In practical case, the assumption of normality can be unrealistic. For example in taxonomy or in medicine, discrete and continuous measurements are taken. We propose a preliminary test to the general parametric case

1.2.2   Kullback–Leibler Divergence

The idea of using distance to discriminate between population using both continuous and categorical variables was studied by various authors, see Cuadras (1989), Morales, Pardo and Zografos (1998), Nakanishi (1996), Núñez, Villarroya and Oller (2003). We generalise the Mahalanobis distance using the divergence defined by Kullback-Leibler (Kullback, 1959) between two generalised probability densities $f_1(X)$ and $f_2(X)$:

$$
\begin{aligned}
J &= J\{f_1(X)\,;\,f_2(X)\} \\
&= \int \{f_1(X) - f_2(X)\} \log \frac{f_1(X)}{f_2(X)} d\lambda
\end{aligned}
$$

where λ , μ_1 and μ_2 are three probability measures absolutely continuous with respect to each other and f_i is the Radon–Nikodym derivative of μ_i with respect to λ.

Except the triangular inequality, the Kullback-Leibler distance has the properties of a distance. Moreover, if f_1 and f_2 are multivariate normal distributions with common variance-covariance matrix then $J(f_1; f_2)$ is equal to the Mahalanobis distance.

Application to the Location Model

Suppose that q continuous variables $X = (X_1 , \ldots , X_q)^\top$ and d discrete variables $Y = (Y_1,\ldots,Y_d)^\top$ are measured on each unit and that the units are drawn from the population π_1 or the population π_2.

Moreover suppose that the condition of the location model (Krzanowski, 1990) holds. This means that:

- The d discrete variables define a multinomial vector Z containing c possible states. The probability of observing state m in the population π_i is:

$$
p_{im} > 0 \quad (m = 1,\ldots,c) \qquad \text{and} \qquad \sum_{m=1}^{c} p_{im} = 1 \ , \ (i = 1, 2)
$$

- Conditionally on $Z = m$ and π_i, the q continuous variables X follow a multivariate normal distribution with mean $\mu_i^{(m)}$, variance–covariance matrix $\Sigma_i^{(m)}$ and density:

$$f_{i,m}(X) = f(X \mid Z = m, \pi_i)$$

- For the sake of simplicity, we assume $\Sigma_1^{(m)} = \Sigma_2^{(m)} = \Sigma$.

Since the aim is to compute the distance between π_1 and π_2 on the basis of the measurement made on X and Z, the joint density of X and Z given π_i is needed:

$$
\begin{aligned}
f_i(x, z) &= \sum_{m=1}^{c} f_{i,m}(x)p(Z = m \mid \pi_i)\boldsymbol{I}(z = m) \\
&= \sum_{m=1}^{c} f_{i,m}(x)p_{im}\boldsymbol{I}(z = m)
\end{aligned}
$$

This model was extended by some authors. Liu and Rubin (1998) relaxed the normality assumption. Bedrick,, Lapidus and Powell (2000) considered the inverse conditioning and end up with a probit model and de Leon and Carrière (2004) generalize the Krzanowski and Bedrick approach.

PROPOSITION 1.1 By applying the Kullback–Leibler measure of distance to the location model, we obtain:

$$J = J_1 + J_2 \tag{1.1}$$

with

$$J_1 = \sum_m (p_{1m} - p_{2m}) \log \frac{p_{1m}}{p_{2m}}$$

and

$$J_2 = \frac{1}{2} \sum_m (p_{1m} + p_{2m})(\mu_1^{(m)} - \mu_2^{(m)})^{\top} \Sigma^{-1}(\mu_1^{(m)} - \mu_2^{(m)})$$

The proof is straightforward.

Remark: This expression is meaningless if $p_{im} = 0$.

COROLLARY 1.1 *If the continuous variables are independent of the discrete variables then:*

$$\mu_1^{(m)} = \mu_1 \qquad and \qquad \mu_2^{(m)} = \mu_2 \qquad for\ all\ m$$

and

$$J = \sum_m (p_{1m} - p_{2m}) \log \frac{p_{1m}}{p_{2m}} + (\mu_1 - \mu_2)^\top \Sigma^{-1} (\mu_1 - \mu_2)$$

which means that the Kullback-Leibler distance is equal to the sum of the contribution of the continuous and the discrete variables. This result is logical since J_1 represents the information based on Z, and J_2 the information based on X knowing Z.

Asymptotic Distribution of the Kullback-Leibler Distance in the Location Model

Generally the p_{im}, μ_{im} and Σ are unknown and have to be estimated from a sample using a model. Consider that we have two samples of size n_1 and n_2 respectively available from the population π_1 and π_2 and let n_{im} be the number of individuals, in the sample drawn from π_i, occupying the state m of the multinomial variable Z. In the model, there are two kinds of parameters: those which depend on the populations, and noisy parameters which are independent from the populations. They can be considered as noisy parameters since this category of parameters is not involved in the distance J. For example, if the mean is modelled with an analysis of variance model:

$$\mu_{im} = \mu + \alpha_i + \beta_m$$

where α is the population effect and β the discrete state effect. The expression of the distance is:

$$\mu_{1m} - \mu_{2m} = \alpha_1 - \alpha_2$$

So the β_m can be considered to be noisy parameters since they are not involved in the distance.

Let p be the vector of probability associated to the multinomial state of Z then

$$\hat{p} = p(\hat{\eta}) \tag{1.2}$$

where $\eta = (\eta_a, \eta_{ib})$; η_a is the set of noisy parameters and η_{ib} is the set of parameters used to discriminate between two populations.

Let r be the cardinal of η_{ib}. In the case of the location model, the p_{im} are generally estimated through a log-linear model.

Let μ be the vector of the mean of the continuous variables for the different states of Z then:

$$\hat{\mu} = \mu(\hat{\xi}) \tag{1.3}$$

where $\xi = (\xi_a, \xi_{ib})$; ξ_a is the set of noisy parameters and ξ_{ib} is the set of parameters used to discriminate between two populations.

Let s be the cardinal of ξ_{ib}. In the case of the location model, the μ_{im} are generally estimated through an analysis of variance model. Asparoukhov and Krzanowski (2000) also studied the smoothing of the location model parameters.

The aim of this section is to study the distributional property of both parts of the distance to obtain a test and a confidence interval for the classical hypothesis. Formally the following hypothesis are tested:

$$
\begin{array}{lll}
H_{01} : J_1 = 0 & \text{versus} & H_{11} : J_1 > 0 \\
H_{02} : J_2 = 0 & \text{versus} & H_{12} : J_2 > 0 \\
H_0 : J = 0 \;\; (H_{01} \cap H_{02}) & \text{versus} & H_1 : J > 0 \;\; (H_{11} \cup H_{12})
\end{array}
$$

Asymptotic Results

Let $\theta_i = (\eta_a, \xi_a, \eta_{ib}, \xi_{ib}) = (\theta_a, \theta_{ib})$ for $i = 1, 2$ where $\eta_a, \xi_a, \eta_{ib}, \xi_{ib}$ are defined in (1.2) and (1.3). The following regularity conditions are assumed:

- θ_i is a point of the parameter space Θ, which is assumed to be an open convex set in a $(r + s)$-dimensional Euclidean space.

- $f(x, \theta_i)$ has continuous second–order partial derivatives with respect to the θ_i's in Θ,

- $\hat{\theta}_i$ is the maximum likelihood estimator of $\hat{\theta}_i$

- For all $\theta_i \in \Theta$,

$$\int \frac{\partial f(x, \theta_i)}{\partial \theta_i} d\lambda(x) = \int \frac{\partial^2 f(x, \theta_i)}{\partial^2 \theta_i} d\lambda(x) = 0 \quad i = 1, 2$$

- The integrals

$$c(\theta_i) = \int \left\{ \frac{\partial \log f(x, \theta_i)}{\partial \theta_i} \right\}^2 f(x, \theta_i) d\lambda(x) \quad i = 1, 2$$

are positive and finite for all $\theta_i \in \Theta$.

It is obvious that the location model satisfies these conditions. Let $\hat{J} = J(\hat{\theta})$ be an estimator of J.

PROPOSITION 1.2 *Under H_0: $\theta_1 = \theta_2 = \theta_0$, when $n_1 \to \infty$, $n_2 \to \infty$ and $\frac{n_1}{n_2} \to u$:*

$$\frac{n_1 n_2}{n_1 + n_2} \hat{J} \sim \chi^2(r + s) \tag{1.4}$$

where r are s are the dimension of the space generated by η_{ib} and ξ_{ib}

Proof:

$$\hat{J} = \int \left\{ f(x, \hat{\theta}_1) - f(x, \hat{\theta}_2) \right\} \log \left\{ \frac{f(x, \hat{\theta}_1)}{f(x, \hat{\theta}_2)} \right\} d\lambda(x) \tag{1.5}$$

Since $p_{im} > 0$, the regularity conditions are satisfied. Therefore, Under H_0: $\theta_1 = \theta_2 = \theta_0$ a Taylor expansion of first order of $f(x, \hat{\theta}_1)$ and $f(x, \hat{\theta}_2)$ at the neighbourhood of θ_0 can be used:

$$
\begin{aligned}
\hat{J} =\ & J + (\hat{\theta}_1 - \theta_1)^{\mathsf{T}} \frac{\partial J}{\partial \theta_1} + (\hat{\theta}_2 - \theta_2)^{\mathsf{T}} \frac{\partial J}{\partial \theta_2} \\
& + \frac{1}{2}(\hat{\theta}_1 - \theta_1)^{\mathsf{T}} \frac{\partial^2 J}{\partial \theta_1^2}(\hat{\theta}_1 - \theta_1) + \frac{1}{2}(\hat{\theta}_2 - \theta_2)^{\mathsf{T}} \frac{\partial^2 J}{\partial \theta_2^2}(\hat{\theta}_2 - \theta_2) \\
& + (\hat{\theta}_2 - \theta_2)^{\mathsf{T}} \frac{\partial^2 J}{\partial \theta_1 \partial \theta_2}(\hat{\theta}_1 - \theta_1) + \sigma(\hat{\theta}_1 - \theta_1) + \sigma(\hat{\theta}_2 - \theta_2)
\end{aligned}
$$

Under H_0:

$$\frac{\partial J}{\partial \theta_1} = \int \left[\frac{\partial f(x, \theta_1)}{\partial \theta_1} \log \left\{ \frac{f(x, \theta_1)}{f(x, \theta_2)} \right\} - \frac{\partial f(x, \theta_1)}{\partial \theta_1} \frac{f(x, \theta_2)}{f(x, \theta_1)} \right] d\lambda(x) = 0$$

since $\theta_1 = \theta_2 = \theta_0$ and $\int \frac{\partial f(x, \theta_1)}{\partial \theta_1} = 0$. For the same reason $\frac{\partial J}{\partial \theta_2} = 0$

For all $i, j = 1, 2$:

$$
\begin{aligned}
\frac{\partial^2 J}{\partial \theta_i \partial \theta_j} &= (\hat{\theta}_i - \theta_i)^{\mathsf{T}} \int \frac{f'^2(x, \theta_0)}{f(x, \theta_0)} d\lambda(x)(\hat{\theta}_j - \theta_j) \\
&= (\hat{\theta}_i - \theta_i)^{\mathsf{T}} I(\theta_0)(\hat{\theta}_j - \theta_j)
\end{aligned}
$$

where $I(\theta_0)$ represents the information matrix of Fisher.

Asymptotically, under H_0, (1.5) becomes:

$$
\begin{aligned}
\hat{J} &= \frac{1}{2}(\hat{\theta}_1 - \theta_0)^\top I(\theta_0)(\hat{\theta}_1 - \theta_0) + \frac{1}{2}(\hat{\theta}_2 - \theta_0)^\top I(\theta_0)(\hat{\theta}_2 - \theta_0) \\
&\quad + (\hat{\theta}_1 - \theta_0)^\top I(\theta_0)(\hat{\theta}_2 - \theta_0) \\
&= (\hat{\theta}_1 - \hat{\theta}_2)^\top I(\theta_0)(\hat{\theta}_1 - \hat{\theta}_2)
\end{aligned}
$$

Since $\hat{\theta}_i$ is the maximum likelihood estimator of θ_0 (Rao, 1973):
$\sqrt{n_i}(\hat{\theta}_i - \theta_0) \sim N_p\left\{0, I^{-1}(\theta_0)\right\}$ $(i = 1, 2)$ Then:

$$
\begin{aligned}
\sqrt{\frac{n_1 n_2}{n_1 + n_2}}(\hat{\theta}_1 - \theta_0) &\sim N_p\left\{0, \frac{1}{1+u}I^{-1}(\theta_0)\right\} \\
\sqrt{\frac{n_1 n_2}{n_1 + n_2}}(\hat{\theta}_2 - \theta_0) &\sim N_p\left\{0, \frac{u}{1+u}I^{-1}(\theta_0)\right\}
\end{aligned}
$$

Then

$$
\sqrt{\frac{n_1 n_2}{n_1 + n_2}}I(\theta_0)^{\frac{1}{2}}\left(\hat{\theta}_1 - \hat{\theta}_2\right) \sim N_p(0, 1)
$$

Finally,

$$
\frac{n_1 n_2}{n_1 + n_2}\left(\hat{\theta}_1 - \hat{\theta}_2\right)^\top I(\theta_0)\left(\hat{\theta}_1 - \hat{\theta}_2\right) \sim \chi^2(r + s)
$$

COROLLARY 1.2 *Under H_{01}:*

$$
\frac{n_1 n_2}{n_1 + n_2}\hat{J}_1 \sim \chi^2(r) \qquad \text{when } n_1 \to \infty, \ n_2 \to \infty \text{ and } \frac{n_1}{n_2} \to u
$$

Proof: It is enough to apply the proposition 1.2 with $q = 0$, which means the absence of continuous variables.

PROPOSITION 1.3 *Under H_{02}:*

$$
\frac{n_1 n_2}{n_1 + n_2}\hat{J}_2 \sim \chi^2(s) \qquad \text{when } n_1 \to \infty, \ n_2 \to \infty \text{ and } \frac{n_1}{n_2} \to u
$$

Proof: The proof is very similar to the proof of the proposition 1.2.

1.2.3   Asymptotic Distribution of Matusita Distance

Krzanowski (1983) used Bhattacharya's affinity measure:

$$
\rho = \int f^{\frac{1}{2}}(x, \theta_1)f^{\frac{1}{2}}(x, \theta_2)d\lambda(x)
$$

to define the distance:

$$\Delta = \int \left\{ f^{\frac{1}{2}}(x,\theta_1) - f^{\frac{1}{2}}(x,\theta_2) \right\}^2 d\lambda(x)$$
$$= 2 - 2\rho$$

This distance is also known as the Hellinger distance. In the location model context Krzanowski has obtained:

$$K = 2 - 2\sum_m (p_{1m}p_{2m})^{\frac{1}{2}} \exp\{-\frac{1}{8}(\mu_{1,m} - \mu_{2,m})^{\top}\Sigma^{-1}(\mu_{1,m} - \mu_{2,m})\}$$

Let $\theta_i = (\eta_a, \xi_a, \eta_{bi}, \xi_{bi}) = (\theta_a, \theta_{bi})$ for $i = 1,2$. Under $H_0 = (\theta_1 = \theta_2)$, we have $\xi_{bi} = 0$ and $\eta_{bi} = 0$ for $i = 1,2$.

Under the usual regularity conditions, we prove the following result:

PROPOSITION 1.4 *Let* $u \in]0,1[$, $\hat{K} = K(\hat{\theta}_1, \hat{\theta}_2)$ *with*

$$\hat{K} = 2 - 2\sum_m (\hat{p}_{1m}\hat{p}_{2m})^{\frac{1}{2}} \exp\{-\frac{1}{8}(\hat{\mu}_{1,m} - \hat{\mu}_{2,m})^{\top}\hat{\Sigma}^{-1}(\hat{\mu}_{1,m} - \hat{\mu}_{2,m})\}$$

Assume that H_0: $\theta_1 = \theta_2 = \theta_0$ *is true and that* $\hat{\theta}_1$ *and* $\hat{\theta}_2$ *are independent asymptotically efficient estimates of* θ_0. *Then for* $n_1 \to \infty$, $n_2 \to \infty$, $n_1/n_2 \to u$

$$\frac{4n_1 n_2}{(n_1 + n_2)} K(\hat{\theta}_1, \hat{\theta}_2) \sim \chi^2(r + s)$$

Proof

Under H_0: $\theta_1 = \theta_2 = \theta_0$, we obtain:

$$K(\theta_0) = 0$$

$$\frac{\partial K}{\partial \theta_1} = \frac{\partial K}{\partial \theta_2} = 0$$

and

$$\frac{\partial^2 K}{\partial \theta_1^2} = \frac{\partial^2 K}{\partial \theta_2^2} = -\frac{\partial^2 K}{\partial \theta_1 \partial \theta_2} = \frac{1}{2}\int \frac{f'^2(x,\theta_0)}{f(x,\theta_0)}d\lambda(x) = \frac{1}{2}I(\theta_0)$$

where $I(\theta_0)$ is the information matrix of Fisher. Under usual regularity conditions (Bar-Hen and Daudin, 1995), the Taylor expansion of the affinity at the neighborhood of θ_0 can be derived and using the previous result we have, under H_0:

$$K(\hat{\theta}_1, \hat{\theta}_2) \approx \frac{1}{4}(\hat{\theta}_1 - \hat{\theta}_2)^{\top} I(\theta_0)(\hat{\theta}_1 - \hat{\theta}_2)$$

Since $\hat{\theta}_i$ are independent asymptotically efficient estimator of θ_0, $n_i^{\frac{1}{2}}(\hat{\theta}_i - \theta_0) \sim N_p\left(0, I^{-1}(\theta_0)\right)$ $(i = 1, 2)$. Then:

$$\left(\frac{n_1 n_2}{n_1 + n_2}\right)^{\frac{1}{2}} (\hat{\theta}_1 - \theta_0) \quad \sim \quad N_p\left\{0, \frac{1}{1 + u} I^{-1}(\theta_0)\right\}$$

$$\left(\frac{n_1 n_2}{n_1 + n_2}\right)^{\frac{1}{2}} (\hat{\theta}_2 - \theta_0) \quad \sim \quad N_p\left\{0, \frac{u}{1 + u} I^{-1}(\theta_0)\right\}$$

Then

$$\left(\frac{n_1 n_2}{n_1 + n_2}\right)^{\frac{1}{2}} I(\theta_0)^{\frac{1}{2}} \left(\hat{\theta}_1 - \hat{\theta}_2\right) \sim N_p(0, 1)$$

Additional results can be found in Bar-Hen and Daudin (1998).

1.2.4 Simulations

The level and the power of the test described in the previous section were evaluated through simulations. One continuous variable and two binary variables are considered. Hence the multinomial vector Z has 4 levels. The estimates of the means, the proportions and the variance are the maximum likelihood estimates. These estimates corresponds to saturated model and therefore the test of the distance has 7 degrees of freedom. It has to be noted that no correction factor for the case $p_{im} = 0$ and therefore empty cells are taken into account for the computation of the distance.

Four cases were studied:

1. no population effect for the discrete variables and no population effect for the continuous variables ($K = 0$);

2. no population effect for the discrete variables but a population effect for the continuous variables;

3. a population effect for the discrete variables but no population effect for the continuous variables;

4. a population effect for the discrete and the continuous variables.

For the continuous variables, the population effect is equal to the standard error:

$$\frac{\mu_{1,m} - \mu_{2,m}}{\sigma} = \begin{cases} 0 & \text{if population effect is present} \\ 1 & \text{if population effect is not present} \end{cases}$$

For the discrete variables:

$$\log \left(\frac{p_{1m}}{p_{2m}} \right) = \begin{cases} 0 & \text{if population effect is present} \\ 1 & \text{if population effect is not present} \end{cases}$$

Since the aim of these simulations is to estimate the rate of convergence of the asymptotic distributions, populations of size 20 and 100 were considered. This gives three new cases:

1. population π_1 of size 10 and population π_2 of size 10

2. population π_1 of size 30 and population π_2 of size 30

3. population π_1 of size 100 and population π_2 of size 100

There are 12 combinations of hypotheses and populations sizes. 1000 simulations were done for each combination. The table below presents the number of non–significant tests at the 5% level.

By using the property of the binomial distribution, one may expect to obtain $50 \pm 1.96 \times (1000 \times 0.5 \times 0.95)^{\frac{1}{2}} = 50 \pm 14$ tests to be non–significant if the null hypothesis is true.

From Table 1.1, we deduce that the level of the test is respected as soon as $n \geq 30$. This means 30/4 observations per cell. The power of the test tends to 1 but the convergence is slower for the discrete variables. This result is not surprising.

It has to be noted that these simulations are limited. The use of non-saturated model for the estimation of the parameters and the use of a correction factor for empty cell can probably alter the results.

1.3   Methods and Stopping Rules for Selecting Variables

As in the usual discriminant analysis with continuous variables, selection of variables is a problem of practical importance. In fact, in the location model

Table 1.1: Number of significant test at the 5% level for the various hypotheses

| population effect for | | size of population | | Hypothesis tested |
discrete var.	continuous var.	π_1	π_2	$K = 0$
no	no	10	10	68
no	no	30	30	60
no	no	100	100	60
no	yes	10	10	251
no	yes	30	30	798
no	yes	100	100	1000
yes	no	10	10	144
yes	no	30	30	255
yes	no	100	100	711
yes	yes	10	10	344
yes	yes	30	30	872
yes	yes	100	100	1000

context, the question is more precisely "which terms and which continuous variables must be included in the model?" where the models concerned are log-linear and MANOVA. Interest in this topic has been shown regularly since the paper published by Vlachnonikolis and Marriot (1982). Krzanowski (1983) used a Matusita-Hellinger distance between the populations, Daudin (1986) used a modified AIC method and Krusinska (1989), Krusinska (1990) used several methods based on the percentage of misclassification, Hotelling's T^2 and graphical models.

Based on Hellinger distance, Krzanowski (1983) proposed the use of a distance K to determine the most discriminative variables.

Our asymptotic results allow us to propose stopping rules based on the P-value of the test of $J = 0$ or $K = 0$. These two methods were then compared with a third, based on the Akaike Information Criterion (AIC) described by Daudin (1986): classically, AIC penalize the likelihood by the number of parameters. A direct use of AIC on MANOVA models (described in Section 1.2.2) will lead to noncomparable log-likelihood. Daudin (1986) proposed to eliminate the noisy parameters (noted β_m) and to penalize the log-likelihood by the number of parameters related to the population effect. It permits to judge whether the log-likelihood and the increase of AIC is only due to population factor terms in the ANOVA model and is not coming from noisy parameters.

Krzanowski (1983) used the distance K to select variables. It should be noted that $\hat{K}$ increases when the location model contains more variables without guaranteeing that this increase is effective: it is therefore necessary to discount any slight increase that may be caused by chance. We propose to include a new discriminant variable or a new term in the location model if it increases the evidence that H_0 ($K = 0$) is false as measured by the P-value of the test of the null hypothesis, using the asymptotic distribution of $\hat{K}$.

It would be interesting to test whether the increase of K due to a new term in the model is positive. Unfortunately when K is positive (H_0 false) the asymptotic distribution of the increase in $\hat{K}$ due to a new term is not easily tractable under the hypothesis that the new parameter is null.

An alternative criterion is an Akaike-like one: $K - AIC = 4\frac{n_1 n_2}{n_1 + n_2}\hat{K} - 2(r+s)$. According to this method, the best model is that which maximizes $K - AIC$.

It is also possible to use $\hat{J}$ with the same methods: we can use the P-value of the chi-square test of $J = 0$ or alternatively $J - AIC = \frac{n_1 n_2}{n_1 + n_2}\hat{J} - 2(r+s)$

Based on simulations, Daudin and Bar-Hen (1999) showed that all three competing methods (two distances and Daudin-AIC) gave good overall performances (nearly 85% correct selection). The K-method has weak power with discrete variables when sample sizes are small but is a good choice when a simple model is requested. The J-method possesses an interesting decomposition property of $J = J_1 + J_2$ between the discrete and continuous variables. The K-AIC and J-AIC methods select models that have more parameters than the P-value methods. For distance, the K-AIC method may be used with small samples, but the J-AIC method is not interesting for it increases the overparametrization of the $J - P$ method. The Daudin-AIC method gives good overall performance with a known tendency toward overparametrization.

1.4 Reject Option

1.4.1 Distributional Result

Since the aim is to test the atypicality of X, we have to derive the distribution of the estimate of the divergence J between X and π_i under the hypothesis $J(X, \pi_i) > 0$. We don't make assumptions about the distribution of the populations but the same regularity conditions as before are assumed. Bar-Hen and Daudin (1997) and Bar-Hen (2001) considered the reject option for the case of normal populations.

PROPOSITION 1.5 *Under* $H_1 : J > 0$, $n_1 \to \infty$, $n_2 \to \infty$, $\frac{n_1}{n_2} \to u > 0$:

$$\sqrt{n_1 + n_2}(\hat{J} - J) \xrightarrow{\mathcal{L}} N(0, V)$$

with

$$V = (1 + u^{-1}) \left(\frac{\partial J}{\partial \theta_1} \right)^\top I^{-1}(\theta_1) \left(\frac{\partial J}{\partial \theta_1} \right) + (u + 1) \left(\frac{\partial J}{\partial \theta_2} \right)^\top I^{-1}(\theta_2) \left(\frac{\partial J}{\partial \theta_2} \right)$$
(1.6)

where $I(\theta_i)$ *represents the Fisher information matrix based on* θ_i.

The proof can be found in Bar-Hen (1996).

Remark : From this proposition one may construct confidence intervals for $\hat{J}$.

COROLLARY 1.3 *Let* J_i *be the divergence between* X *and* π_i $(i = 1, \dots, n)$. *Let assume that the parameters of each population are estimated with independent samples. Let* n_i *be the sample size of the sample coming from* π_i *and* n_x *the sample size of the sample coming from* X.
If X *is not coming from any* π_i, *then , asymptotically, the joint probability distribution function of* $\sqrt{n_i + n_x}(\hat{J}_i - J_i)$ *is a multivariate normal probability distribution function.*

Proof: Every $\sqrt{n_i + n_x}(\hat{J}_i - J_i)$ is distributed as a normal probability distribution function. Therefore it has to be proved that every linear combination of the $\sqrt{n_i + n_x}(\hat{J}_i - J_i)$ is also distributed as a normal probability distribution function.

$$\sum_i a_i \sqrt{n_i + n_x}(\hat{J}_i - J_i)$$
(1.7)

$$\approx \sum_i a_i \sqrt{n_i + n_x} \left\{ (\hat{\theta}_i - \theta_i)^\top \frac{\partial J_i}{\partial \theta_i} + (\hat{\theta}_x - \theta_x)^\top \frac{\partial J_i}{\partial \theta_x} \right\}$$

$$= \sum_i a_i \sqrt{n_i + n_x} (\hat{\theta}_x - \theta_x)^\top \frac{\partial J_i}{\partial \theta_x}$$

$$+ \sum_i a_i \sqrt{n_i + n_x} (\hat{\theta}_i - \theta_i)^\top \frac{\partial J_i}{\partial \theta_i}$$
(1.8)

Since the samples used to estimate the parameter of the populations are independent, asymptotically, (1.8) corresponds to a weighted sum of independent normal probability distribution functions. Then (1.8) is distributed as a normal probability distribution function (Rao, 1973).

The asymptotic mean and variance of $\sqrt{n_i + n_x}(\hat{J}_i - J_i)$ had been obtained in the proposition 1.5. To characterize the joint probability distribution function $\hat{J}_i$, we have to compute the covariance between the divergence.

COROLLARY 1.4 *Let $\pi_1, \ldots, \pi_m$ be m distinct populations. Let assume that the distribution of the populations has the previous regularity conditions. Assume that $\hat{\theta}_1, \ldots, \hat{\theta}_m$ are estimated with independent samples of size $n_1, \ldots, n_m$ respectively. Let $\hat{J}_{ij}$ be the estimator of the divergence between the population π_i and π_j $(i, j = 1, \ldots, m)$ then if*

$$n_k \to \infty, \ n_j \to \infty, \ n_i \to \infty, \ \frac{n_j}{n_i} \to u > 0 \ , \ \frac{n_k}{n_i} \to v > 0 :$$

$$\mathrm{Cov}\left(\sqrt{n_j + n_i}(\hat{J}_{ij} - J_{ij}), \sqrt{n_i + n_k}(\hat{J}_{ik} - J_{jk})\right)$$

$$= \ \sqrt{(1+u)(1+v)} \left(\frac{\partial J_{ij}}{\partial \theta_i}\right)^{\top} I^{-1}(\theta_i) \left(\frac{\partial J_{ik}}{\partial \theta_i}\right)$$

where $I(\theta_i)$ represent the Fisher information matrix based on θ_i

and

$$\mathrm{Cov}\left(\sqrt{n_j + n_i}(\hat{J}_{ij} - J_{ij}), \sqrt{n_l + n_k}(\hat{J}_{lk} - J_{lk})\right) = 0$$
$$\forall i \neq k, i \neq l, j \neq k, j \neq l$$

Proof:

$$\mathrm{Cov}\left\{\sqrt{n_j + n_i}(\hat{J}_{ij} - J_{ij}), \sqrt{n_i + n_k}(\hat{J}_{ik} - J_{ik})\right\} \approx$$

$$\mathrm{Cov}\left[\sqrt{n_j + n_i}\left\{(\hat{\theta}_i - \theta_i)^{\top}\frac{\partial J_{ij}}{\partial \theta_i} + (\hat{\theta}_j - \theta_j)^{\top}\frac{\partial J_{ij}}{\partial \theta_j}\right\}^{\top} \right.$$

$$\left. \sqrt{n_i + n_k}\left\{(\hat{\theta}_i - \theta_i)^{\top}\frac{\partial J_{ik}}{\partial \theta_i} + (\hat{\theta}_k - \theta_k)^{\top}\frac{\partial J_{ij}}{\partial \theta_k}\right\}\right]$$

$$= \ \sqrt{n_i + n_k}\sqrt{n_j + n_i}\left(\frac{\partial J_{ij}}{\partial \theta_i}\right)^{\top} Var(\hat{\theta}_i - \theta_i) \left(\frac{\partial J_{ik}}{\partial \theta_i}\right)$$

$$= \ \sqrt{\frac{(n_i + n_k)(n_j + n_i)}{n_i^2}}\left(\frac{\partial J_{ij}}{\partial \theta_i}\right)^{\top} I^{-1}(\theta_i) \left(\frac{\partial J_{ik}}{\partial \theta_i}\right)$$

Moreover

$$\mathrm{Cov}\left\{\sqrt{n_j + n_i}(\hat{J}_{ij} - J_{ij}), \sqrt{n_l + n_k}(\hat{J}_{lk} - J_{lk})\right\} = 0$$
$$\forall i \neq k, i \neq l, j \neq k, j \neq l$$

because the estimates of J_{ij} and J_{lk} are independent.

1.4.2   Derivation of the Preliminary Test

Suppose that X iscoming from any of the predefined population π_i. In this case, the estimator of the divergence between X and π_i is asymptotically distributed as a normal probability distribution function. If there are n predefined populations, we obtain n estimates of the divergence and each of them is distributed as a normal probability distribution function. Since the observations coming from X are used in the computation of the estimate of each of the divergences, the resulting normal probability distribution functions are not independent.

For a given level of confidence, X will be considered as atypical if the hypothesis that the smallest divergence between X and π_i is greater than zero is not rejected.

To test this hypothesis we have to obtain the probability distribution function of the minimum of correlated normal probability distribution functions.

The following proposition is an extension of the result of Dunnett and Sobel (1955)

PROPOSITION 1.6 Let $Z_1, \ldots, Z_n$ be $N(\mu_i, \sigma_i^2)$ random variable such that $Cov(Z_i, Z_j) = b_i b_j \ \forall i \neq j \ (i, j = 1, \ldots, n)$ and $\sigma_i^2 - b_i^2 > 0 \ \forall i = 1, \ldots, n$. Then:

$$P(\min_{i \geq 1} Z_i < \bar{u}) = 1 - \int \prod_{i=1}^{n} P(X_i \geq \bar{u} - b_i x) \varphi(x) dx$$

when

$$X_i \sim N(\mu_i, \sigma_i^2 - b_i^2) \quad independent \quad \forall i = 1, \ldots, n$$

Proof: Let $X_0, X_1, \ldots, X_n$ be $n + 1$ independent normal probability distribution functions such that

$$X_0 \sim N(0, 1) \qquad and \qquad X_i \sim N(\mu_i, \sigma_i^2 - b_i^2)$$

Let

$$Z_i = b_i X_0 + X_i \quad i = 1, \ldots, n$$

It is easy to see that:

$$\begin{aligned} Cov(Z_i, Z_j) &= b_i b_j \\ Var(Z_i) &= \sigma_i^2 \\ E(Z_i) &= \mu_i \end{aligned}$$

Thus:

$$
\begin{aligned}
P(\min_{i\geq 1} Z_i < \bar{u}) &= 1 - P(\min_{i\geq 1} Z_i \geq \bar{u}) \\
&= 1 - P(\bigcap_{i=1}^{n}(Z_i \geq \bar{u})) \\
&= 1 - P\left\{\bigcap_{i=1}^{n}(b_i X_0 + X_i \geq \bar{u})\right\} \\
&= 1 - P(\bigcap_{i=1}^{n} X_i \geq \bar{u} - b_i X_0) \\
&= 1 - \int P(\bigcap_{i=1}^{n} X_i \geq \bar{u} - b_i x | X_0 = x) \times \\
&\quad \times \; \varphi(x)dx \\
&= 1 - \int P(\bigcap_{i=1}^{n} X_i \geq \bar{u} - b_i x)\varphi(x)dx
\end{aligned}
$$

since X_0 is independent of X_i

$$
P(\min_{i\geq 1} Z_i < \bar{u}) = 1 - \int \prod_{i=1}^{n} P(X_i \geq \bar{u} - b_i x)\varphi(x)dx \quad (1.9)
$$

For the derivation of the preliminary test, we will also need the following proposition.

PROPOSITION 1.7 $H(\bar{u}) = \int \prod_{i=1}^{n} P(X_i \geq \bar{u} - b_i x)\varphi(x)dx$ *is a monotone function of* $\bar{u}$

Proof:

$$
\begin{aligned}
H(\bar{u}) &= \int \prod_{i=1}^{n} P(X_i \geq \bar{u} - b_i x)\varphi(x)dx \\
&= \int \prod_{i=1}^{n} \Phi\left(\frac{b_i x + \mu_{0i} - \bar{u}}{\sqrt{\sigma_i^2 - b_i^2}}\right)\varphi(x)dx
\end{aligned}
$$

$$\frac{\partial H(\bar{u})}{\partial \bar{u}} = \sum_{j=1}^{n} \frac{1}{\sqrt{\sigma_j^2 - b_j^2}} \int \prod_{\substack{i=1 \\ j \neq i}}^{n} \Phi\left(\frac{b_i x + \mu_{0i} - \bar{u}}{\sqrt{\sigma_i^2 - b_i^2}}\right) \times$$

$$\times \varphi\left(\frac{b_j x + \mu_{0j} - \bar{u}}{\sqrt{\sigma_j^2 - b_j^2}}\right) \varphi(x) dx$$

Therefore $\frac{\partial H(\bar{u})}{\partial \bar{u}} > 0$. So $H(\bar{u})$ is a monotone function of $\bar{u}$.

Various approximations of the integral (1.9) had been proposed but many mathematical packages allow this kind of computation in reasonable time.

Decision Rule for the Preliminary Test

Let $\pi_1, \ldots, \pi_m$ be m populations and let X be an unclassified observation. The regularity conditions are assumed. The parameters θ_i $(i = 1, \ldots, m)$ are estimated with independent samples of size n_i respectively. The parameter θ_x of X is estimated with a sample of size n_x. Let $\hat{J}_i$ be the estimator of J_i, the divergence between X and π_i.

Under the hypothesis that X is coming from any of the predefined population π_i, all the J_i are positive and, asymptotically, the joint probability distribution function of $\sqrt{n_i + n_x}(\hat{J}_i - J_i)$ is a multidimensional centered normal probability distribution function with a variance covariance matrix $V = (v_{ij})$ (V is defined in equation (1.6) and in the corollary 1.4).

A decision rule should permit to choose between:

$$H_0 \quad : \quad \exists i \text{ such that } J_i \leq J_{i0}$$
$$H_1 \quad : \quad \forall i , J_i > J_{i0}$$

This decision rule will be like:

$$\min_i \hat{J}_i < \alpha \quad \text{ then } H_0$$

The $\alpha > 0$ of this decision rule has to be such that, if $J_i = J_{i0}$ with J_{i0} known and different from zero then:

$$P(\text{wrong decision of } H_0) = \beta \quad \quad \beta \text{ given}$$

It means that in this decision rule, the type III error is controlled. Therefore the test controls the risk of not detecting that X is not coming from one of the predefined population.

Since zero is a boundary of the parameter space J_{i0} cannot be null but for many practical purposes this limitation is not so strong. For example, in taxonomy, a variety will be considered as a new variety if this new variety is enough far from the known ones. Therefore the value of J_{i0} has to be fixed by the user.

The joint probability distribution function of $\hat{J}_i$ is asymptotically a normal probability distribution function. Let consider that the sample sizes are large enough to allow this approximation. In this case:

$$\hat{J} = (\hat{J}_1, \ldots, \hat{J}_n) \sim N_n(J, \Sigma)$$

with $\Sigma = (\sigma_{ij})$ and

$$\sigma_{ii} = n_i \left(\frac{\partial J_i}{\partial \theta_i}\right)^\top I^{-1}(\theta_i) \left(\frac{\partial J_i}{\partial \theta_i}\right) + n_x \left(\frac{\partial J_i}{\partial \theta_x}\right)^\top I^{-1}(\theta_x) \left(\frac{\partial J_i}{\partial \theta_x}\right)$$

$$\sigma_{ij} = n_x \left(\frac{\partial J_i}{\partial \theta_x}\right)^\top I^{-1}(\theta_x) \left(\frac{\partial J_j}{\partial \theta_x}\right)$$

Then $\bar{u}$ will be determined by:

$$1 - \int \prod_{i=1}^n \mathrm{P}(X_i \geq \bar{u} - b_i x)\varphi(x)dx = \beta \qquad \beta \text{ given}$$

where $f(x)$ is the density of a reduced and centered normal probability distribution function,

$$X_i \sim N\left\{J_{i0}, n_i \left(\frac{\partial J_i}{\partial \theta_i}\right)^\top I^{-1}(\theta_i) \left(\frac{\partial J_i}{\partial \theta_i}\right)\right\} \text{ independent} \quad \forall i = 1, \ldots, n$$

and

$$b_i = \sqrt{n_x} \frac{\partial J_i}{\partial \theta_x}^\top I^{-\frac{1}{2}}(\theta_x)$$

when the value of J_{Ii0} have been fixed, it is possible to determine α such that the probability of a wrong choice of H_0 is equal to β. The proposition 1.7 ensures the uniqueness of α. The decision rule is based on the comparison between α and the minimum of $\hat{J}_i$.

1.5   Example

We have used the kangaroos data set from Andrews et al. (Andrews and Hertzberg, 1985). The data are available at
http://lib.stat.cmu.edu/datasets/Andrews/. Three populations of kangaroos must be classified using one discrete variable (sex) and eighteen continuous skull measurements. 148 observations have known labels, and three are unknown. The sample is well balanced as it can be seen from Table 1.2. Therefore, the sex cannot be useful for classification by its own. However, it

Table 1.2: Contingency table of sex and populations

population	males	females
1	25	25
2	23	25
3	25	25

may help to discriminate if it is combined with the skull measurements.

1.5.1   Location Model

The multinomial vector Z contains 2 states (male, female), and the continuous variables are analyzed using an ANOVA model with two factors (sex and population) with interaction. The selection procedure has been made using DAIC. The results are given in Table 1.3. After step 6 no variable can be suppressed. At each step, the possibility of elimination of the interaction between sex and population in the MANOVA model is tested and rejected. For example, if we suppress at the last step the interaction sex*population, the DAIC decreases from 253.7 to 245.34. This indicates that the sex is useful for discriminating between the populations.

The posterior probabilities have been computed using the selected model and the classification performance obtained by crossvalidation is given in Table 1.4. The overall estimated rate of missclassification is equal to 16.9%. The posterior probabilities computed for the unlabelled kangaroos are given in Table 1.5 and the generalized squared Mahalanobis distances in Table 1.6.

It is interesting to check if the third unlabelled kangaroo really pertains to one of the three group. Actually it seems to be far from the nearest population. It is possible to test this hypothesis using the asymptotic distribution of the Kullback-Liebler distance.

Table 1.3: Result of the selection procedure

step	model	DAIC
1	complete model (all continuous variables and interaction sex*population)	229.89
2	variable 4 suppressed	235.66
3	variable 16 suppressed	240.83
4	variable 7 suppressed	245.49
5	variable 11 suppressed	249.97
6	variable 14 suppressed	253.17

Q XCSBackwardDAICSelection.xpl

Table 1.4: Classification performance of the location model

true population	classified in 1	classified in 2	classified in 3	total
1	41	8	1	50
2	11	35	2	48
3	1	2	47	50
total	53	45	50	148

Q XCSCrossValidation.xpl

Under the hypothesis H_0 that the third unlabelled kangaroo pertains to population i, $\frac{n_i}{n_i+1}\widehat{J(x,\pi_i)}$ (where x stands for one observation and π_i for population i) is distributed as a chisquare with 26 degrees of freedom. The number of degrees of freedom is the number of parameters useful for discriminating purpose, with 13 continuous variables, the factor population and the interaction sex*population. Using the distances of Table 1.6, the $p-value$ associated with this test for each population are respectively 0.00025 0.000063 and 0.0010. Therefore there is a strong suspicion that the third unlabelled kangaroo does not pertain to any of the three populations. Note that no correction for multiple testing is necessary for an observation cannot pertain simultaneously to two populations. Therefore the null hypothesis is true at most only one time.

The reject option analysis give a similar conclusion (result not shown).

Table 1.5: Posterior probabilities for the unlabelled kangaroos

kangaroo	population 1	population 2	population 3
149	0.929	0.070	0.001
150	0.000	0.000	1
151	0.086	0.009	0.905

Q XCSPosteriorProbabilities.xpl

Table 1.6: Generalized Mahalanobis Distances for the unlabelled kangaroos

kangaroo	population 1	population 2	population 3
149	28.7	33.8	42.0
150	33.0	29.7	10.9
151	58.7	63.1	54.0

Q XCSDistances.xpl

1.5.2   Comparison with the Linear Discriminant Analysis

The extended Linear Discriminant Analysis of Vlachonikolis and Marriot (Vlachnonikolis and Marriot, 1982) has been applied on this data set. However, as a result of the selection procedure, no interaction between sex and any continuous variable has been introduced, so that the method resolves to a simple Linear Discriminant Analysis without the sex contribution. The descendant selection procedure eliminated the following variables : 1, 4, 7, 14 and 17. The performance of the classification rule,estimated by cross-validation, is given in Table 1.7. The overall misclassification rate is 19,7%, which is 2.8 points more than the location model. The posterior probabilities of the unlabelled kangaroos are similar to the results given by the location model. However the strength of evidence that kangaroo 151 pertains to the population 3 is greater from LDA than from the location model results.

1.5.3   Conclusion

In summary, the location model takes into account the importance of the discrete variable to discriminate between the populations. On the opposite, the Extended Linear Discriminant Analysis cannot catch its discriminating

Table 1.7: Classification performance of the Linear Discriminant Analysis

true population	classified in 1	classified in 2	classified in 3	total
1	38	11	1	50
2	11	35	2	48
3	1	3	46	50
total	50	49	49	148

Table 1.8: Posterior probabilities for the unlabelled kangaroos using LDA

kangaroo	population 1	population 2	population 3
149	0.882	0.117	0.001
150	0.001	0.001	0.998
151	0.000	0.000	1

power, which in turn lead to a lower performance. This example indicates that the location model is a better choice, but this point should be well assessed by other similar studies. The possibility (given by the reject option) of testing that an observation does not pertain to any population is often very useful. The Xplore routine given in the annexes should help the researchers to use it. It contains a routine for computing the parameters of the model, the posterior probabilities and the distances between the populations, one for the classification of training or tests samples and a routine for the selection of variables. These routines are suited to the kangaroo's example but it is not difficult to extend them to any data set. The only difficult task is to include the loglinear model in the actual routines.

Bibliography

Adhikari, B. P. and Joshi, D. D. (1956). Distance - discrimination et résumé exhaustif. *Publ. Inst. Statist. Univ. Paris 5*, 57–74.

Andrews, D. and Hertzberg, A. (1985). *DATA: A Collection of Problems from Many Fields for the Student and Research Worker*. New York: Springer-Verlag

Asparoukhov, O. and Krzanowski, W.J. (1985). Non-parametric smoothing of the location model in mixed variable discrimination. *Statistics and Computing*, **10**, 285-293.

Bar-Hen, A. (2001). Preliminary tests in discriminant analysis. *Statistica*, **61**, 585-594

Bar-Hen, A. and Daudin, J. J. (1998). Asymptotic distribution of Matusita's distance in the case of the location model. *Biometrika*, **85**, 477-481

Bar-Hen, A. and Daudin, J. J. (1997). A Test of a Special Case of Typicality in Linear Discriminant Analysis. *Biometrics*, **53**, 39–48

Bar-Hen, A. (1996). A preliminary test in discriminant analysis. *Journal of Multivariate Analysis*, **57**, 266–276

Bar-Hen, A. and Daudin, J. J. (1995). Generalisation of the Mahalanobis distance in the mixed case. *Journal of Multivariate Analysis*, **53:2**, 332–342

Bedrick, E.J., Lapidus, J. and Powell, J.F. (1997). Estimating the Mahalanobis distance from mixed continuous and discrete data. *Biometrics*, **56**, 394401

Cuadras, C. M. (1989). Distance analysis of discrimination and classification using both continuous and categorical variables. In *Statistical Data Analysis and Inference* , Y. Dodge (ed), 459-473. Amsterdam: Elsevier Science

Daudin, J. J. (1986). Selection of Variables in Mixed–Variable Discriminant Analysis *Biometrics*, **42**, 473–481.

Daudin, J. J. and Bar-Hen, A. (1999). Selection in discriminant analysis with continuous and discrete variables. *Computational Statistics and Data Analysis*, **32**, 161-175.

de Leon, A. R. and Carrière, K. C. (2004). A generalized Mahalanobis distance for mixed data. To appear in *Journal of Multivariate Analysis* doi:10.1016/j.jmva.2003.08.006

Dunett, C. W. and Sobel, M. (1955). Approximations to the probability integral and certain percentage points of a multivariate analogue of Student's *t*-distribution, *Biometrika*, **42**, 258–260.

Gower, J. C. (1966). Some distance properties of latent root and vector methods used in multivariate analysis. *Biometrika*, **53**, 325–338.

Krusińska, E. (1989). New procedure for selection of variables in location model for mixed variable discrimination. *Biom. J.*, 31(5):511–523.

Krusińska, E. (1990) Suitable location model selection in the terminology of graphical models. *Biom. J.*, **32**, 817–826.

Krzanowski, W. J. (1990). Mixture of continuous and categorical variables in discriminant analysis. *Biometrics*, **36**, 486–499.

Krzanowski, W. J. (1983). Distance between populations using mixed continuous and categorical variables. *Biometrika*, **70**, 235–243.

Krzanowski, W. J. (1983). Stepwise location model choice in mixed-variable discrimination. *Appl. Statist.*, **32**, 260–266.

Krzanowski, W. J. (1984). On the null distribution of distance between two groups, using mixed continuous and categorical variables. *Journal of Classification*, **1**, 243–253.

Kullback, S. (1959). *Information Theory and Statistics*. New-York: Dover.

Liu, C. and Rubin, D. B. (1988). Ellipsoidally Symmetric Extensions of the General Location Model for Mixed Categorical and Continuous Data. *Biometrika*, **85**, 673-688.

McLachlan, G. J. (1992). *Discriminant Analysis and Statistical Pattern Recognition*. New-York: Wiley.

Morales, D., Pardo, L. and Zografos, K. (1988). Informational distances and related statistics in mixed continuous and categorical variables. *Journal of Statistical Planning and Inference*, **75**, 47-63.

Nakanishi, H. (1996). Distance between populations in a mixture of categorical and continuous variables. *J. Japan Statist. Soc.*, **26**, 221230.

Núñez, M., Villarroya, A. and Oller, J. M. (1996). Minimum Distance Probability Discriminant Analysis for Mixed Variables. *Biometrics*, **59**, 248-253.

Olkin, I. and Tate, R. F. (1961). Multivariate correlation models with mixed discrete and continuous variables. *Ann. Math. Statist.*, **32**, 448–465. correction in **36**, 343-344.

Rao, C. R. (1973). *Linear Statistical Inference and its Applications*, 2nd ed. New-York: Wiley.

Vlachonikolis, I. G. and Marriot, F. H. C. (1982). Discrimination with mixed binary and continuous data. *Appl. Statist.*, **31**, 23–31.

2 Longitudinal Data Analysis with Linear Regression

Jörg Breitung, Rémy Slama and Axel Werwatz

2.1 Introduction

It has become common in economics and in epidemiology to make studies in which subjects are followed over time (longitudinal data) or the observations are structured into groups sharing common unmeasured characteristics (hierarchical data). These studies may be more informative than simple cross-sectional data, but they need an appropriate statistical modeling, since the 'classical' regression models of the GLM family Fahrmeir and Tutz (1994) assume statistical independence between the data, which is not the case when the data are grouped or when some subjects contribute for two or more observations.

Hierarchical regression models allow to analyze such surveys. Their main difference with classical regression models consist in the introduction of a group specific variable that is constant within each group, but differs between groups. This variable can be either a fixed-effect (classical) variable, or a random effect variable. From a practical point of view, the fixed or random-effect variable may be regarded as allowing to a certain extent to take into account unobserved characteristics (genetic, behavioral, ...) shared by the observations belonging to a given group. From a statistical point a view, the introduction of the group-level variable 'absorbs' the correlation between the different observations of a given group, and allow the residuals of the model to remain uncorrelated.

We will present here the fixed- and random-effect models in the case of linear regression. A particular attention will be given to the case of unbalanced longitudinal data, that is studies in which the number of observations per

group is not the same for all groups. This is an important issue in that
the implementation of models adapted to such data needs some adaptation
compared to the balanced case and since the elimination of the groups with
only one observation could yield selection biases. The models will be applied
to an epidemiological study about reproductive health, where women were
asked to describe the birth of weight of all their children born in a given
calendar period.

EXAMPLE 2.1 *We want to describe the influence of tobacco consumption
by the woman during her pregnancy on the birth weight of her baby. We conducted a study among a cross-sectional sample of $N = 1,037$ women living
in 2 French areas and asked them to describe retrospectively all their pregnancies leading to a livebirth during the 15 years before interview, and, for
each baby, to indicate the number of cigarettes smoked during the first term
of pregnancy (exposure, noted x).*

The influence of cigarette exposure could be studied by linear regression on
birth weight (dependent variable, noted y). Given the amount of information
lying in the other pregnancies and the cost of data collection, it is tempting
to try to make use of all the available information. Using all the pregnancies
($N\bar{T}$, where $\bar{T}$ is the mean number of pregnancies per woman) in a linear
regression model may not be appropriate, since the estimation of the linear
regression model

$$y_j = \mu + x_j^\top \beta + u_j, \quad j = 1, \ldots, N\bar{T} \tag{2.1}$$

by the ordinary least squares (OLS) method makes the assumption that the
residuals u_j are independent random variables. Indeed, there may be correlation between the birth weights of the children of a given woman, since the
corresponding pregnancies may have been influenced by the genetic characteristics of the woman and some occupational or behavioral exposures remaining
constant over the woman's reproductive life.

A possible way to cope with this correlation is to use hierarchical modelling.
The 2-level structure of the data (woman or *group* level, and pregnancy or
observation level) must be made explicit in the model. If we index by i the
woman and t the pregnancies of a given woman, then a hierarchical linear
regression model for our data can be written:

$$y_{it} = \mu + x_{it}^\top \beta + \alpha_i + u_{it}, \quad i = 1, \ldots, N \quad t = 1, \ldots, T_i \tag{2.2}$$

where y_{it} is the birth weight of the pregnancy number t of woman i. The number of pregnancies described by the woman i is a value T_i between 1 and say 12 and can vary between women. Of course, x_{it}, the mean number of cigarettes smoked daily, can vary between women and between the various pregnancies of a woman. The main difference with (2.1) is that the model now contains the α_i variables $(i = 1, \ldots, N)$ defined at the group (or woman) level.

This technique allows to obtain the output shown in Table 2.1

Table 2.1: Tobacco consumption by the woman during the first term of pregnancy

Parameters	Estimate	SE	t-value	p-value
Tobacco	-9.8389	2.988	-3.292	0.001
Sex(Girl=1)	-157.22	18.18	-8.650	0.000
(...)Constant	3258.1	83.48	39.027	0.000
St.dev of a(i): 330.16		St.dev of e(i,t): 314.72		
R2(without): 0.2426				

Q panrand.xpl

The model was adjusted for other variables, like duration of pregnancy, mother's alcohol consumption, sex of the baby, which are not shown in this output. The random-effect model estimates that, on average, tobacco consumption by the woman during the first term of pregnancy is associated with a decrease by 9.8 grams (95% confidence interval: $[-15.7; -4.0]$) of the birth weight of the baby per cigarette smoked daily.

Definitions and Notations

The cross-section unit (e.g. individual, household, hospital, cluster etc.) will be denoted group and be indexed by i, whereas t indexes the different observations of the group i. The t index can correspond to time, if a subject is followed and observed at several occasions like in a cohort study, but it may also be a mere identifying variable, for instance in the case of therapeutical trial about a new drug, realized in several hospitals. In this case, it may be appropriate to use a hierarchical model, with i standing for the hospital, and t indexing each subject within the hospital.

We will use indifferently the terms of *panel* or preferably *longitudinal* data to design data sets with a hierarchical structure, whatever the sampling method (cross-sectional or cohort surveys) although the term of panel study is sometimes used exclusively in the case of cohort studies. The data set is said unbalanced when the number of observations T_i is not the same for all groups, $i = 1, 2, \ldots, N$, and balanced when $T_i = T$ for all i. The explained quantitative variable will be denoted y_i, which is a vector of dimension T_i. The average number of observations is denoted as $\bar{T} = N^{-1} \sum_{i=1}^{N} T_i$.

In the first section of this chapter, we will present the theoretical bases of the fixed and random effect models, and give explicit formulas for the parameters. We turn to the practical implementation amd in the last section discuss the tobacco consumption application in more detail.

2.2 Theoretical Aspects

2.2.1 The Fixed-effect Model

The Model

For individual (or groups) i at time t we have

$$y_{it} = \alpha_i + x_{it}^{\top} \beta + u_{it}, \quad i = 1, \ldots, N, \quad t = 1, \ldots, T \qquad (2.3)$$

This model is also called the *analysis of covariance model*. It is a *fixed effects* model in the sense that the individual specific intercepts α_i are assumed to be non-stochastic. The vector of explanatory variables x_{it} is assumed independent of the errors u_{it} for all i and t. The choice of the fixed-effect model (as opposed to a random effect model) implies that statistical inference is conditional on the individual effects α_i.

Writing (2.3) for each observation gives

$$
\begin{bmatrix} \boldsymbol{y}_1 \\ \boldsymbol{y}_2 \\ \vdots \\ \boldsymbol{y}_N \end{bmatrix}
= \underbrace{\begin{bmatrix} \mathbf{1}_{T_1} & \mathbf{0} & \cdots & \mathbf{0} \\ \mathbf{0} & \mathbf{1}_{T_2} & \cdots & \mathbf{0} \\ \vdots & \vdots & \cdots & \vdots \\ \mathbf{0} & \mathbf{0} & \cdots & \mathbf{1}_{T_N} \end{bmatrix}}_{NT \times N}
\underbrace{\begin{bmatrix} \alpha_1 \\ \alpha_2 \\ \vdots \\ \alpha_N \end{bmatrix}}_{N \times 1}
+ \underbrace{\begin{bmatrix} \boldsymbol{x}_1^\top \\ \boldsymbol{x}_2^\top \\ \vdots \\ \boldsymbol{x}_N^\top \end{bmatrix}}_{NT \times k} \beta
+ \underbrace{\begin{bmatrix} \boldsymbol{u}_1 \\ \boldsymbol{u}_2 \\ \vdots \\ \boldsymbol{u}_N \end{bmatrix}}_{NT \times 1}
$$

$$\underbrace{\phantom{\begin{bmatrix}\boldsymbol{y}_1\end{bmatrix}}}_{NT \times 1}$$

(2.4)

or, in matrix notation,

$$y = D_N \alpha + X\beta + u. \tag{2.5}$$

Parameter Estimation

The matrix D_N can be seen as a matrix of N dummy variables. Therefore, the least-squares estimation of (2.3) is often called "least-squares dummy-variables estimator" Hsiao (1986). The coefficient estimates results as:

$$\widehat{\beta}_{WG} = \left(X^\top W_n X \right)^{-1} X^\top W_n y \tag{2.6}$$

$$\widehat{\alpha} = (D_N^\top D_N)^{-1} D_N^\top (y - X\widehat{\beta}_{WG}) \tag{2.7}$$

$$= \begin{bmatrix} T_1^{-1} \sum\limits_{t=1}^{T} (y_{1t} - \boldsymbol{x}_{1t}^\top \widehat{\beta}_{WG}) \\ \vdots \\ T_N^{-1} \sum\limits_{t=1}^{T} (y_{Nt} - \boldsymbol{x}_{Nt}^\top \widehat{\beta}_{WG}) \end{bmatrix} \tag{2.8}$$

where

$$W_n = I_{NT} - D_N (D_N^\top D_N)^{-1} D_N^\top$$

transforms the regressors to the deviation-from-the-sample-means form. Accordingly, $\widehat{\beta}_{WG}$ can be written as the "Within-Group" (WG) estimator:

$$\widehat{\beta}_{WG} = \left\{ \sum_{i=1}^{N} \sum_{t=1}^{T} (\boldsymbol{x}_{it} - \bar{\boldsymbol{x}}_i)(\boldsymbol{x}_{it} - \bar{\boldsymbol{x}}_i)^\top \right\}^{-1} \left\{ \sum_{i=1}^{N} \sum_{t=1}^{T} (\boldsymbol{x}_{it} - \bar{\boldsymbol{x}}_i)(y_{it} - \bar{y}_i) \right\},$$

(2.9)

where the individual means are defined as

$$\bar{y}_i = \frac{1}{T_i} \sum_{t=1}^{T_i} y_{it} \ , \quad \bar{x}_i = \frac{1}{T_i} \sum_{t=1}^{T_i} x_{it}.$$

To estimate the average of the individual effects $\bar{\alpha} = N^{-1} \sum_{i=1}^{N} \alpha_i$, the individual means can be corrected by the sample means $\bar{y} = (N\bar{T})^{-1} \sum_{i=1}^{N} \sum_{t=1}^{T_i} y_{it}$ and $\bar{x}$ is defined accordingly. The least-squares estimates of β and $\bar{\alpha}$ is obtained from the equation

$$y_{it} - \bar{y}_i + \bar{y} = \bar{\alpha} + (x_{it} - \bar{x}_i + \bar{x}_i)^{\top} \beta + \tilde{u}_{it} \ . \tag{2.10}$$

It is important to notice, from (2.9), that cross section units with only one observation do not contribute to the estimation $\widehat{\beta}$ of the parameters associated to the explaining variables x; that is, the same estimate results if these cross section units would be excluded from the data set. The groups with $T_i = 1$ only play a role in the estimation of the mean intercept.

Adequation of the Model to the Data

In complement to the parameter estimation, the degree of explanation of the model and the variance of the error terms can be estimated. It is also possible to test if the introduction of a group-specific variable makes sense with the data used, by means of a F-statistic test presented below.

There are two different possibilities to compute the degree of explanation R^2. First, one may be interested in the fraction of the variance that is explained by the explanatory variables comprised in x_{it}. In this case R^2 is computed as the squared correlation between y_{it} and $x_{it}^{\top}\widehat{\beta}_{WG}$. On the other hand, one may be interested to assess the goodness of fit when the set of regressors is enhanced by the set of individual specific dummy variables. Accordingly, the R^2 is computed as the squared correlation between y_{it} and $x_{it}^{\top}\widehat{\beta}_{WG} + \widehat{\alpha}_i$.

In practical applications the individual specific constants may have similar size so that it is preferable to specify the model with the same constant for all groups. This assumption can be tested with an F statistic for the hypothesis $\alpha_1 = \alpha_2 = \cdots = \alpha_N$.

In order to assess the importance of the individual specific effects, their "variances" are estimated. Literally, it does not make much sense to compute a variance of α_i if we assume that these constants are deterministic. Nevertheless, the variance of α_i is a measure of the variability of the individual effect and can be compared to the variance of the error u_{it}. The formula for estimating the variance of the fixed effects is similar to the computation of variances in the random-effects model. However, the residuals are computed using the within-group estimator $\widehat{\beta}_{WG}$ Amemiya (1981).

Options for the Fixed-effects Model

a) Robust standard errors
Arelano and Bond (1987) suggests an estimator of the standard errors for $\widehat{\beta}_{WG}$ that is robust to heteroskedastic and autocorrelated errors u_{it}:

$$\widetilde{Var}(\widehat{\beta}_{WG}) = \left(\sum_{i=1}^{N} \widetilde{X}_i^\top \widetilde{X}_i \right)^{-1} \left(\sum_{i=1}^{N} \widetilde{X}_i^\top \widehat{u}_i \widehat{u}_i^\top \widetilde{X}_i \right) \left(\sum_{i=1}^{N} \widetilde{X}_i^\top \widetilde{X}_i \right)^{-1},$$

where

$$\widetilde{X}_i = \begin{bmatrix} x_{i1}^\top - \bar{x}_i^\top \\ x_{i2}^\top - \bar{x}_i^\top \\ \vdots \\ x_{iT}^\top - \bar{x}_i^\top \end{bmatrix} \quad \text{and} \quad \tilde{u}_i = \begin{bmatrix} y_{i1} - \bar{y}_i - (x_{i1} - \bar{x}_i)^\top \widehat{\beta}_{WG} \\ y_{i2} - \bar{y}_i - (x_{i2} - \bar{x}_i)^\top \widehat{\beta}_{WG} \\ \vdots \\ y_{iT} - \bar{y}_i - (x_{iT} - \bar{x}_i)^\top \widehat{\beta}_{WG} \end{bmatrix}.$$

It should be noted that the estimation of this covariance matrix requires two steps. In the first step the within-group estimator is used to estimate β. In the second step, the covariance matrix is computed by using the residuals of the fixed-effects model. Therefore, the computation time is roughly doubled.

b) Test for autocorrelation
The test for autocorrelation tests the null hypothesis: $H_0 : \mathrm{E}(u_{it}u_{i,t-1}) = 0$. Since the residuals of the estimated fixed-effect model are correlated, a test for autocorrelation has to adjust for a correlation that is due to the estimated individual effect. Define

$$\tilde{u}_{i,t-1} = y_{i,t-1} - x_{i,t-1}^\top \widehat{\beta}_{WG} - (T-1)^{-1} \sum_{s=1}^{T-1} y_{is} - x_{is}^\top \widehat{\beta}_{WG}.$$

It is not difficult to verify that under the null hypothesis

$$\mathrm{E}\left\{ (y_{it} - x_{it}^\top \widehat{\beta}_{WG}) \tilde{u}_{i,t-1} \right\} = -\sigma_u^2/(T-1),$$

where $\sigma_u^2 = \mathrm{E}(u_{it}^2)$. The test statistic is therefore constructed as

$$\tilde{\rho} = \frac{\sum\limits_{i=1}^{N}\sum\limits_{t=2}^{T}\left\{(y_{it} - \boldsymbol{x}_{it}^\top\widehat{\boldsymbol{\beta}}_{WG})\tilde{u}_{i,t-1}/\widehat{\sigma}_u^2 + 1/(T-1)\right\}}{\sqrt{\sum\limits_{i=1}^{N}\sum\limits_{t=2}^{T}\tilde{u}_{i,t-1}^2}}.$$

Under the null hypothesis, the limiting distribution has a standard normal limiting distribution.

c) Estimates of the individual effects
The mean intercept is estimated by:

$$\widehat{\mu} = \bar{y} - \widehat{\boldsymbol{\beta}}^\top\bar{\boldsymbol{x}}. \tag{2.11}$$

It is also possible to estimate the group variables α_i:

$$\widehat{\alpha}_i = \bar{y}_i - \widehat{\mu} - \widehat{\boldsymbol{\beta}}^\top\bar{\boldsymbol{x}}_i. \tag{2.12}$$

2.2.2   The Random Effects Model

The Model

For the random effects model it is assumed that the individual specific intercept α_i in the model

$$y_{it} = \boldsymbol{x}_{it}^\top\boldsymbol{\beta} + \alpha_i + u_{it}, \quad i = 1,\ldots,N, \quad t = 1,\ldots,T \tag{2.13}$$

is a random variable with $\mathrm{E}(\alpha_i) = 0$ and $\mathrm{E}(\alpha_i^2) = \sigma_\alpha^2$. Furthermore we assume that

$$\begin{aligned}\mathrm{E}(\alpha_i u_{it}) &= 0 \qquad \text{for all } i, t,\\ \mathrm{E}(\alpha_i \boldsymbol{x}_{it}) &= \boldsymbol{0} \qquad \text{for all } i, t.\end{aligned}$$

In general the vector $\boldsymbol{x}_{it}$ includes a constant term.

The composed error term is written as $v_{it} = \alpha_i + u_{it}$ and the model assumptions imply that the vector $\boldsymbol{v}_i = (v_{i1},\ldots,v_{iT})^\top$ has the covariance matrix

$$\mathrm{E}(\boldsymbol{v}_i\boldsymbol{v}_i^\top) = \boldsymbol{\Psi} .$$

The model (2.13) can be efficiently estimated by using the GLS estimator

$$\widehat{\boldsymbol{\beta}}_{GLS} = \left(\sum_{i=1}^{N}\boldsymbol{X}_i^\top\boldsymbol{\Psi}^{-1}\boldsymbol{X}_i\right)^{-1}\left(\sum_{i=1}^{N}\boldsymbol{X}_i^\top\boldsymbol{\Psi}^{-1}\boldsymbol{y}_i\right), \tag{2.14}$$

where $X_i = (x_{i1}, \ldots, x_{iT})^\top$ and $y_i = (y_{i1}, \ldots, y_{iT})^\top$. This estimator is equivalent to a least-squares estimator of the transformed model

$$y_{it} - \psi \bar{y}_i = (x_{it} - \psi \bar{x}_i)^\top \beta + e_{it} \; , \tag{2.15}$$

where

$$\psi = \sqrt{\frac{\sigma_u^2}{\sigma_u^2 + T\sigma_\alpha^2}} \tag{2.16}$$

and $e_{it} = v_{it} - \psi \bar{v}_i$.

In general, the variances σ_u^2 and σ_α^2 are unknown and must be replaced by estimates. To this end several different estimators were suggested Baltagi (1995). The `panrand` quantlet employs the estimator suggested by Swamy and Arora (1972), which is based on two different regressions. First, the model is estimated by using the within-group estimator. The estimated error variance (corrected by the degrees of freedom) is an unbiased estimator for σ_u^2. The second regression is based on the individual means of the data

$$\bar{y}_i = \bar{x}_i^\top \beta + \bar{v}_i \; . \tag{2.17}$$

Since $E(\bar{v}_i^2) = \sigma_\alpha^2 + \sigma_u^2/T$, an estimator for σ_α^2 is obtained from the estimated residual variance of (2.17). Let $\hat{\sigma}_1^2$ denote the estimated residual variance of the between-group regression (2.17), which results from dividing the residual sum of squares by $(N - K - 1)$. The estimated variance of the individual effect results as $\hat{\sigma}_\alpha^2 = (\hat{\sigma}_1 - \hat{\sigma}_u^2)/T$. A serious practical problem is that the resulting estimator of $\hat{\sigma}_\alpha^2$ may become negative. In this case $\hat{\sigma}_\alpha^2$ is set to zero.

2.3   Computing Fixed and Random-effect Models

2.3.1   Data Preparation

Suppose we want to regress a quantitative variable y over explanatory variables noted x. The variable indexing the group will be noted id. Table 2.3.1 shows how the data set should look like in the case of two x variables:

If you have a balanced data set (same number of observations per group) sorted by group, then the id variable is not necessary. You will have to give the number of observations per subject instead of the id vector, that XploRe will then build for you.

Table 2.2: Raw data structure for longitudinal data analysis

id	y	x_1	x_2
1	3409	38	0
1	3755	41	1
2	1900	32	1
3	4200	41	1
3	4050	40	0
3	4300	41	1
...	...	...	...
100	3000	39	0
100	2850	39	1

2.3.2   Fixed and Random-effect Linear Regression

The fixed-effect linear regression model can be estimated using the panfix
quantlet.   **Q** panfix.xpl

The random-effect linear regression model can be estimated using the panrand
quantlet.   **Q** panrand.xpl

2.3.3   Options for panfix

The options must be defined by the **panopt** quantlet according to the syntax:

opt=panopt(optname,optvalue)

where **optname** is the name of the option, and **optvalue** the value associated
to the option. The name of the option has to be given as a string. You may
define several options at the same time according to the following syntax:

opt=panopt(optname1,optvalue1,
    optname2,optvalue2,optname3,optvalue3)

The following options can be defined:

alpha: If equal to 1, asks for the individual effect parameter to be estimated
and stored. The estimation is done assuming that the sum of all alpha
parameters is zero.

autoco: If equal to 1, an autocorrelation test is performed (only if the
number of observations is at least 2 for each group). Default is no test
performed.

ci: If this parameter is set to the value pval, then the confidence intervals
will be given at the level (100-pval)%. By default, no ci are given.

notab: If this parameter is set to 1, then no table of results is displayed.

robust: The robust estimates of variance given in Arelano and Bond
(1987) are used. These should be more valid than the classical variance
estimates in the case of heteroscedasticity. Default is the standard
variance estimates.

xlabel: Label of the explanatory variables, to make the output table more
explicit. This option must be given as a vertical array of the k strings
corresponding to the labels (constant term excluded). Maximum label
length is 11 characters. $(k \times 1)$ vector.

For example, if x is a vector of 2 columns containing the independent variables
tobacco and alcohol consumption, you may type:

```
lab="tobacco"|"alcohol"
opt=panopt("xlabel",lab)
p=panfix(id,y,x,opt)
```

In the output table, the parameters associated to the first and second variables will be labelled by the indicated names. Unspecified options will be set
at their default value, and the order in which the options are given is not
important.

2.3.4   Options for panrand

The options must be defined by the **panopt** quantlet according to the syntax:

```
opt=panopt(optname,optvalue)
```

where `optname` is the name of the option, and `optvalue` the value associated to the option.

The following options can be defined:

opt.shf: Allows you to see the various steps of the estimation procedure.

opt.xlabel: Label of the explanatory variables, to make the output table more explicit. This option must be given as a vertical array of the k strings corresponding to the labels (constant term excluded). Maximum label length is 11 characters and $(k \times 1)$ vector.

2.4   Application

In this section, we illustrate estimations based on real data. The data come from an epidemiologic study about human reproductive life events. Briefly, a cross-sectional sample of 1089 women from Bretagne and Normandie were questioned during spring 2000 about the birth weight of all their children born between 1985 and 2000. We present here the association between the birth weight (dependent variable), the gestational length, the age, and the parity (previous history of livebirth, no/yes) of the mother (independent variables). There was a total of 1963 births in the study period (1.8 pregnancy per woman) and the data can be considered as longitudinal data with a hierarchical structure, the woman being the first level, and the pregnancy the second level.

The use of fixed or random effect models allows to take into account all the pregnancies who took place in the study period described by the woman. In such epidemiological studies about human reproduction, the exclusion of couples with only one pregnancy may give rise to selection bias, since the couples with only one pregnancy are more likely than those with two or more pregnancies to have difficulties in conceiving. Here is a brief description of the data set:

Table 2.3: Summary statistics of the tobacco/birth weight data set

Variable	Mean	Std Dev	$5 - 95^{th}$ percentiles
Birth weight (g)	3409	510	2610-4250
Gestational length (days)	283	11.8	261-294
Mother's age (years)	27.2	4.4	20.1-35.1
Proportion of parous women	0.60		
Sex of the offspring			
(proportion of boys)	0.50		

2.4.1 Results

First, we will describe briefly our data **Q** XCSpanfix01.xpl

The first column of z contains the identified variable, whereas the next columns contain the dependent variables, and then the independent variables. If the panel is balanced and sorted by group, the first argument id can be replaced by a scalar indicating the number of observations per group. We obtain the following output:

Table 2.4: Statistics of panel data

	Minimum	Maximum	Mean	Within Var.%	Std.Error
Variable 1	750	5300	3409	23.8	509.6
Variable 2	-98	21	-5.715	27.56	11.76
Variable 3	14.37	45.71	27.18	26.77	4.366
Variable 4	0	1	0.595	66.82	0.491
Variable 5	0	1	0.5028	45.7	0.5001

Q XCSpanfix01.xpl

The column Within Var.% gives the value of the variance of the residuals of the withing-group estimator, divided by the overall variance.

We can then estimate a fixed-effect regression model.

Table 2.5: Estimated fixed-effects model for tobacco/birthweight data

Parameters	Estimate	SE	t-value	p-value
beta[1]	18.548	1.17	15.8908	0.0000
beta[2]	7.964	4.61	1.7263	0.0843
beta[3]	75.239	25.97	2.8970	0.0038
beta[4]	-144.51	21.27	-6.7931	0.0000
Constant	3326.1	115.3	28.8350	0.0000
St.dev of a(i): 321.47			St.dev of e(i,t):318.47	
Log-Likelihood: 22627.617			R2(without) : 0.2203	
F(no eff.) p-val: 0.0000			R2(with eff) : 0.8272	

Q XCSpanfix02.xpl

Thus, on average, an increase in 1 day of the duration of pregnancy was associated with a gain of weight of 18.4 grams (`beta[1]`), and girls are 145 g lighter than boys at birth (`beta[4]`), with a 95% confidence interval of [-186;-103] g. Moreover, women who already had a child have a tendency to give birth to heavier babies (77 g on average). There is a non-significant tendency to an increase in birth weight with mother's age.

The R^2 value of 0.22 indicates that only a small fraction of the variability of the data is explained by the model, and that other variables should be included (for instance height and weight of the mother before pregnancy, information on health,...).

In this case, there are some groups with only one observation (cf. output above); we cannot therefore perform an autocorrelation-test, nor obtain robust confidence-intervals estimates. In the case of a data set with all groups having at least 2 observations, this can be obtained by **Q** XCSpanfix03.xpl

For the data, the a-priori choice between the fixed-effect and the random-effect model would be the random-effect model, because the included women were randomly selected from two French rural areas, and we wish to infer the model estimates on the women who conceived between 1985 and 2000 in the whole area.

We obtain the random-effect model estimates in Table 2.6.

Table 2.6: Estimated random-effects model for tobacco/birthweight data

Parameters	Estimate	SE	t-value	p-value	95% CI	
beta[1]	18.927	0.8286	22.844	0.000	17.3	20.55
beta[2]	4.5912	2.638	1.740	0.082	-0.58	9.76
beta[3]	88.389	18.89	4.678	0.000	51.36	125.4
beta[4]	-152.53	17.46	-8.735	0.000	-186.8	-118.3
Constant	3413.3	68.94	49.509	0.000	3278.0	3548.0
St.dev of a(i): 337.9		St.dev of e(i,t): 312.19				
R2(without): 0.2206						

Q XCSpanrand04.xpl

On the whole, these estimates are consistent with those of the fixed-effect model. You can notice that for variable [2] (mother's age), the estimates from the two models differ (7.8 with a standard error of 4.6 for the fixed-effect model, and 4.6 with a standard error of 2.6 for the random effect model). In such a case, where the number of observations is small for many units, it is not rare that both models yield different parameter estimates.

Bibliography

Amemiya, T. (1981). Qualitative response models: A survey, *Journal of Economic Literature* **19**: 1483-1536.

Arellano, M. and Bond, S.R. (1987). Computing robust standard errors for within-groups estimators, *Oxford Bulletin of Economics and Statistics* **49**: 431-434.

Baltagi B.H., (1995). *Econometrics analysis of panel data*, Wiley, Chichester.

Fahrmeir and Tutz, (1994). *Multivariate Statistical Modelling Based on Generalized Linear Models*, Springer Series in Statistics.

Hsiao, (1986). *Analysis of Panel data, Cambridge University Press*, Cambridge.

Swami, P.A. and Arora, S.S., (1972). The exact finite sample properties of the estimators of coefficients in the error components regression models, *Econometrica* **40**: 261-275.

3 A Kernel Method Used for the Analysis of Replicated Micro-array Experiments

Ali Gannoun, Beno Liquetît, Jérôme Saracco and Wolfgang Urfer

.

Microarrays are part of a new class of biotechnologies which allow the monitoring of expression levels of thousands of genes simultaneously. In microarray data analysis, the comparison of gene expression profiles with respect to different conditions and the selection of biologically interesting genes are crucial tasks. Multivariate statistical methods have been applied to analyze these large data sets. To identify genes with altered expression under two experimental conditions, we describe in this chapter a new nonparametric statistical approach. Specifically, we propose estimating the distributions of a t-type statistic and its null statistic, using kernel methods. A comparison of these two distributions by means of a likelihood ratio test can identify genes with significantly changed expressions. A method for the calculation of the cut-off point and the acceptance region is also derived. This methodology is applied to a leukemia data set containing expression levels of 7129 genes. The corresponding results are compared to the traditional t-test and the normal mixture model.

3.1 Introduction

Gene expression regulates the production of protein, the ultimate expression of the genetic information, which in turn governs many cellular processes in biological systems. The knowledge of gene expression has applications ranging from basic research on the mechanism of protein production diagnosing, staging, treating and preventing of diseases. Microarray technologies provide a way of analysing the RNA expression levels of thousands of genes simultaneously; see for example Brown and Botstein (1999), Lander (1999),

Quackenbush (2001). A common objective in such analyses is to determine which genes are differentially expressed under two experimental conditions, which may refer to samples drawn from two types of tissues, tumors or cell lines, or at two points of time during important biological processes. Also, It has been noted that data based on a single array are highly noisy and may not be reliable and efficient, see for instance Chen, Dougherty and Bittner (1997). One reason is that the statistical variability of the expression levels for each gene is not taken into account. Moreover, the need for independent replicates has been recognized, see for example Lee, Kuo, Whitmore and Sklar (2000), and several methods combining information from several arrays have been proposed. These methods assign a test score to each of the genes and then select those that are 'significant'. In addition, an emerging novel idea, is that with replicates of microarrays, one can estimate the distribution of random errors using nonparametric methods. This idea was first suggested in an empirical Bayesian approch by Efron, Tibshirani, Goss and Chu (2000) and Efron, Storey and Tibshirani (2001). In one development here, we use the mixture model method developed by Pan (2002) and Pan, Lin and Le (2004). However, we replace the mixture of normal distributions by kernel method to get more flexible and powerful estimates of the two distributions of the test and null statistics. We then use a likelihood ratio test to determine genes with differential expression.

This chapter is organized as follows. In Section 3.2, we describe the statistical model and two existing testing methods, the t-test and the normal mixture approach. In Section 3.3, we propose a kernel estimation procedure, and we give a new method to determine the cut-off point and the acceptance region. This nonparametric approach is illustrated in Section 3.4 using the leukemia data of Golub, Slonim, Tamayo, Huard, Gaasenbeek, Mesirov, Coller, Loh, Downing, Caligiuri, Bloomfield and Lander (1999). The performance of this method is compared to the normal mixture model approach of Pan, Lin and Le (2004). Section 3.5 is devoted to the conclusion, some remarks and an outlook for further activities.

3.2   Statistical Model and Some Existing Methods

In this section, we present the general statistical model from which we make the comparative studies. Then, we recall the construction of the t-test method and the mixture modeling approach.

3.2.1 The Basic Model

Various models are proposed to summarize multiple measurements of gene expression. For example, general surveys are given by Thomas, Olson, Tapscott and Zhao (2001).

We can consider a generic situation that, for each gene i, $i = 1, ..., n$, we have expression levels $Y_{i1}, Y_{i2}, ..., Y_{iJ_1}$ from J_1 microarrays under condition 1, possibly treatment, and $Y_{iJ_1+1}, Y_{iJ_1+2}, ..., Y_{iJ_1+J_2}$ from J_2 microarrays under condition 2, possibly control. We suppose that $J = J_1 + J_2$, and J_1 and J_2 are even. The expression level can refer to summary measure of relative red to green channel intensities in a fluorescence-labeled complementary DNA or cDNA array, a radioactive intensity of a radiolabeled cDNA array, or summary difference of the perfect match (PM) and mis-match (MM) scores from an oligonucleotide array, see Li and Wong (2001). We focus on the following general statistical model:

$$Y_{ij} = \beta_i + \mu_i x_j + \varepsilon_{ij} \tag{3.1}$$

where $x_j = 1$ for $1 \leq j \leq J_1$ and $x_j = 0$ for $J_1 + 1 \leq j \leq J_1 + J_2$, and ε_{ij} are independent random errors with mean 0. Hence $\beta_i + \mu_i$ and β_i are the mean expression levels of gene i under the two conditions respectively.

Determining whether a gene has differential expression is equivalent to testing the null hypothesis:

$$H_0 : \mu_i = 0 \quad \text{against} \quad H_1 : \mu_i \neq 0.$$

To focus on the main issue, we use $\alpha = 0.01$ as the genome-wide significance level, and Bonferroni adjustment to deal with multiple comparisons. Other possibly better adjustment methods for multiple comparisons can be found in the statistical literature, see for example Dudoit, Yang, Speed and Callow (2002) and Thomas, Olson, Tapscott and Zhao (2001). Hence the gene-specific significance level (for a two-sided test) is $\alpha^* = \alpha/(2n)$.

In the following, we review briefly two existing methods along this line.

3.2.2 The T-test

Because usually both J_1 and J_2 are small, and there is no evidence to support equal variances as it is mentioned in Thomas, Olson, Tapscott and Zhao (2001), we only give an overview on the t-test with two independant small normal samples with unequal variances. Let $\overline{Y}_{i(1)}$, $s^2_{i(1)}$, $\overline{Y}_{i(2)}$ and $s^2_{i(2)}$ denote the sample mean and variance sample of expression levels of gene i under the two conditions. We use a t-type score as test statistic:

$$Z_i = \frac{\overline{Y}_{i(1)} - \overline{Y}_{i(2)}}{\sqrt{\frac{s^2_{i(1)}}{J_1} + \frac{s^2_{i(2)}}{J_2}}},$$

It is approximately t-distributed with degree of freedom

$$d_i = \frac{(s^2_{i(1)}/J_1 + s^2_{i(2)}/J_2)^2}{(s^2_{i(1)}/J_1)^2/(J_1-1) + (s^2_{i(2)}/J_2)^2/(J_2-1)}.$$

Large absolute t-statistics suggest that the corresponding genes have different expression levels. However, the strong normality assumptions may be violated in practice.

3.2.3   The Mixture Model Approach

The mixture model. Instead of imposing a strong parametric assumptions on the null distribution of the statistic Z, the idea is to estimate it directly by a so-called null statistic z such the distribution of z is the same as the null distribution of Z. The problem with the above t-test is its restrictive assumptions. Following Pan (2002) and Pan, Lin and Le (2004) the null statistics is constructed as:

$$z_i = \frac{Y_{i(1)}u_i/J_1 - Y_{i(2)}v_i/J_2}{\sqrt{\frac{s^2_{i(1)}}{J_1} + \frac{s^2_{i(2)}}{J_2}}}$$

where $Y_{i(1)} = (Y_{i1}, Y_{i2}, ..., Y_{iJ_1})$, $Y_{i(2)} = (Y_{iJ_1+1}, Y_{iJ_1+2}, ..., Y_{iJ_1+J_2})$, u_i is a random permutation of a column vector containing $J_1/2$ 1's and -1's respectively, and v_i is a random permutation of a column vector containing $J_2/2$ 1's and -1's respectively.

We suppose that Z_i and z_i are distibuted with density f and f_0. If we assume that the random errors ε_{ij} in (3.1) are independent and their distribution is symmetric about zero, then under H_0, $f = f_0$.

In the absence of strong parametric assumptions, the functions f and f_0 are not identifiable, see Efron, Storey and Tibshirani (2001). Lee, Kuo, Whitmore and Sklar (2000) and Newton, Kendziorski, Richmond, Blattner and Tsui (2001) considered parametric approaches by assuming Normal or

Gamma distributions for f and f_0 respectively. Efron, Tibshirani, Goss and Chu (2000) avoided such parametric assumptions and considered a nonparametric empirical Bayesian approach.

Pan, Lin and Le (2004) used a finite normal mixture model to estimate f_0 (or f): $f_0(z, \Omega_{g_0}) = \sum_{r=1}^{g_0} \pi_r \varphi(z, \mu_r, V_r)$, where $\varphi(., \mu_r, V_r)$ denotes the normal density function with mean μ_r and variance V_r, and the π_r's are mixing proportions. The set Ω_{g_0} represents all unknown parameters in a g_0-component mixture model: $\{(\pi_r, \mu_r, V_r) : r = 1, \ldots, g_0\}$. They used the EMMIX, a stand-alone Fortran program, described in McLachlan and Peel (1999), to fit such a normal mixture model using the well-known expectation-maximization (EM) algorithm of Dempster, Laird and Rubin (1977) to obtain maximum likelihood estimates. The Akaike Information Criterion (AIC) or the Bayesian Information Criterion (BIC), see for instance Schwarz (1978), can be used as model selection criterion to determine the number of components g_0.

The test procedure. As discussed in Efron, Storey and Tibshirani (2001), for a given Z, if we want to test for the null hypothesis H_0, we can construct a likelihood ratio test based on the following statistic:

$$LR(Z) = f_0(Z)/f(Z). \tag{3.2}$$

A large value of $LR(Z)$ gives no evidence against H_0, whereas a too small value of $LR(Z)$ leads to rejecting H_0. For any given genome wide significance level α, we solve the following equation:

$$\frac{\alpha}{n} = \int_{LR(z)<c} f_0(z)dz \tag{3.3}$$

to obtain a cut-off point c and to construct the corresponding rejection region for H_0:

$$\{Z : LR(Z) < c\}.$$

REMARK 3.1 *With the normal mixture model in Pan, Lin and Le (2004), it is possible to numerically solve the equation (3.3) using the bisection method, see Press, Teukolsky, Vetterling and Flannery (1992).*

3.3 A Fully Nonparametric Approach

Using z_i's and Z_i's, we will nonparametrically estimate f_0 and f by a kernel method and develop a procedure to determine the rejection region from an approximation of (3.3).

3.3.1   Kernel Estimation of f_0 and f

The construction of a kernel estimator of the density functions f and f_0 requires a choice of a real (density) function K (called kernel), and bandwidths h_n and h_{0n} which are sequences of positive numbers tending to 0 as n tends to infinity.

From $\{Z_i,\ i = 1, ..., n\}$ and $\{z_i,\ i = 1, ..., n\}$, f and f_0 can be estimated nonparametrically by:

$$f_n(z) = \frac{1}{nh_n} \sum_{i=1}^{n} K\left(\frac{z - Z_i}{h_n}\right) \quad \text{and} \quad f_{0n}(z) = \frac{1}{nh_{0n}} \sum_{i=1}^{n} K\left(\frac{z - z_i}{h_{0n}}\right).$$

(3.4)

Well-known theoretical results show that the choice of a reasonable K does not seriously affect the quality of the estimators (3.4). In order to get smoother estimation, one can use a kernel K which is bounded, symmetric and satisfying $|z| K(z) \to 0$ as $|z| \to \infty$ and $\int z^2 K(z)dz < \infty$. On the contrary the choice of the bandwidths h_n and h_{0n} turns to be crucial for the accuracy of the estimators (3.4). Some indications about this choice are given in Bosq and Lecoutre (1987). For example, one can use

$$h_n = \hat{\sigma}_n n^{-1/5} \quad \text{and} \quad h_{0n} = \hat{\sigma}_{0n} n^{-1/5},$$

(3.5)

where $\hat{\sigma}_n$ and $\hat{\sigma}_{0n}$ denote the empirical standard deviation of the Z_i's and the z_i's. From a theoretical point of view, this choice minimizes some asymptotic mean square error, see Deheuvels (1977). In practice, this choice gives an idea of the amount of smoothing needed for the estimator. For the graphical aspect of the corresponding estimated density function curve, the user can choose to increase or decrease the value of the bandwidth in order to obtain the desired smoothing of the density estimators.

Note that it is well-known that the kernel density estimator does not perform well on the support edges of the distribution. In the following, we suggest a method for overcoming edge effect problems, and in doing so, make it possible to achieve a more efficient estimator of the LR function.

3.3.2   The Reflection Approach in Kernel Estimation

Reflection principles in density estimation have been described and studied by Schuster (1985), Silverman (1986) and Cline and Hart (1991). Here we present a slighty different version of the geometric approach for removing the edge effects proposed by Hall and Wehrly (1991).

Let $x_{(1)}, \ldots, x_{(n)}$ be the initial ordered data from which we will determine the estimator of the density function, say g. We add $\beta\%$ artificial observations in the two tails of the distribution using the following principle.

- In the left tail, the "new" observations are $\tilde{x}_{(i+1)} = x_{(1)} - \left(x_{(i+1)} - x_{(1)}\right)$ for $i = 1, \ldots, [\beta n/2]$, where $[m]$ is the integer part of m.

- In the right tail, the "new" observations are
  $\hat{x}_{(i+1)} = x_{(n)} + \left(x_{(n)} - x_{(n-i)}\right)$ for $i = 1, \ldots, [\beta n/2]$.

Finally we estimate g from the overall data set (i.e. from the union of the original data x_i and the pseudo-data $\tilde{x}_i$ and $\hat{x}_i$).

REMARK 3.2 *When the number n of observations is large, the adjusted estimator is very sensitive to the percentage β of artificial observations. Generally, it suffices to take a minute percentage (around 0.5%) to obtain a reasonable estimator.*

REMARK 3.3 *If there are not enough observations close to the extreme values $x_{(1)}$ and $x_{(n)}$, we can adapt the same outline described previously, by replacing $x_{(1)}$ and $x_{(n)}$ by some extreme empirical quantiles, such as the 1st and 99th centiles of the data.*

3.3.3 Implementation of the Nonparametric Method

Here we propose an empirical method to solve (3.3). This method works, even in Pan's approach and with any estimator of f and f_0.

For the purpose of this paper, the densities f and f_0 are replaced by their kernel estimators f_n and f_{0n} given in (3.4). We solve the modified equation:

$$\frac{\alpha}{n} = \int_{\widehat{LR}(z) < c} f_{0n}(z)dz, \tag{3.6}$$

where $\widehat{LR}(z) = f_{0n}(z)/f_n(z)$.

For a fixed value $c > 0$, let $A_c = \{z : T < c\}$ where $T = LR(z)$. We generate an ordered grid of N points $\{\tilde{z}_k, \ k = 1, \ldots, N\}$ covering the support of the Z_i's. Let $\widehat{T}_k = \widehat{LR}(\tilde{z}_k)$, $k = 1, \ldots, N$; $\widehat{A}_c = \left\{\tilde{z}_k : \widehat{T}_k < c, \ k = 1, \ldots, N\right\}$; and $\overline{\widehat{A}_c} = \left\{\tilde{z}_k : \widehat{T}_k \geq c, \ k = 1, \ldots, N\right\}$, the complement of $\widehat{A}_c$. We assume now that $\overline{\hat{A}_c}$ is a convex set (that is an interval). Let $\tilde{z}_{c,(1)}, \tilde{z}_{c,(2)}, \ldots, \tilde{z}_{c,(q)}$ be the q ordered values of $\overline{\hat{A}_c}$. Then

$$\int_{A_c} f_0(z)dz \approx \int_{\hat{A}_c} f_{0n}(z)dz \approx \int_{-\infty}^{\tilde{z}_{c,(1)}} f_{0n}(z)dz + \int_{\tilde{z}_{c,(q)}}^{+\infty} f_{0n}(z)dz$$

$$\approx \int_{\tilde{z}_1}^{\tilde{z}_{c,(1)}} f_{0n}(z)dz + \int_{\tilde{z}_{c,(q)}}^{\tilde{z}_N} f_{0n}(z)dz.$$

The left hand side integral can be evaluated by classical numerical integration method (trapezoidal quadrature). Now, the approximate cut-off point is the value c^* of the set $\{\frac{l}{N}, \ l = 0, 1, \ldots, N\}$ where N is chosen as large as possible, such that:

$$\frac{\alpha}{n} \approx \int_{\hat{A}_{c^*}} f_{0n}(z)dz.$$

From this cut-off point c^*, we can easily deduce the rejection region which is given by:

$$\{Z : Z < \tilde{z}_{c^*,(1)} \ \text{ or } \ Z > \tilde{z}_{c^*,(q)}\}.$$

3.4   Data Analysis

This section is devoted to the application of our proposed method. We describe the data and present the results on expression level study of genes. We take $\alpha = 1\%$ as the genome-wide significance level. Then, using simulation study, we check the efficiency of the kernel method against the "true" Normal Mixture model.

We apply the methods to the leukemia data of Golub, Slonim, Tamayo, Huard, Gaasenbeek, Mesirov, Coller, Loh, Downing, Caligiuri, Bloomfield and Lander (1999). Data have been generated for leukemic myeloid (AML) and lymphoblastic (ALL) cells taken from different individuals. There are 27 ALL samples and 11 AML samples. In each sample, there are $n = 7129$ genes to study. Here our goal is to find genes with differential expression between ALL and AML.

3.4.1 Results Obtained with the Normal Mixture Model

Using the normal mixture approach, Pan (2002) proposed the following estimators for the density function f_0 and f:

$$f_{0m}(z) = 0.479\varphi(z, -0.746, 0.697) + 0.521\varphi(z, 0.739, 0.641) \qquad (3.7)$$

and

$$f_m(z) = 0.518\varphi(z, -0.318, 1.803) + 0.482\varphi(z, 0.7781, 4.501), \qquad (3.8)$$

The cut-off point obtained by Pan (2002) is $c = 0.0003437$. The corresponding rejection region for H_0 is $\{Z : Z < -4.8877 \text{ or } Z > 4.4019\}$, which gives 187 genes with significant expression changes.

3.4.2 Results Obtained with the Nonparametric Approach

To estimate nonparametrically f and f_0, we used the Gaussian density as kernel K. For the bandwidths h_n and h_{0n}, we first used the formulas given in (3.5). We obtained the following values: $h_n = 0.313$ and $h_{0n} = 0.187$. The estimated densities f_n and f_{0n} defined respectively in (3.4) are evaluated. With this choice of bandwidths, the curves seem to be under-smoothed. The deviations from the smooth curves are due to background noises which are not informative. Smoothest curves can be obtained by broadening the bandwidths. This is done by multiplying them by a factor of 1.8 which seems to be the "optimal value" with regard to visual introspection. The corresponding bandwidths are $h_n^* = 0.563$ and $h_{0n}^* = 0.337$. Figure 3.1 and 3.2 present the histograms of the z_i's and the Z_i's, and the estimated densities f_{0n} and f_n. For comparison, the density functions f_{0m} and f_m given in (3.7) and (3.8)) are also plotted in Figure 3.1 and 3.2. The corresponding LR function is shown in Figure 3.3.

To solve the equation (3.3), we use the approximation presented in (3.6) and the implementation procedure described in Section 3.3.3. We get the cut-off point $c = 0.00070$, yielding a rejection region of $\{Z : Z < -4.248 \text{ or } Z > 4.327\}$ for H_0. It gives 220 genes with significant expression changes compared to the 187 obtained with the normal mixture model of Pan (2002). Note that the common rejection region between kernel and normal mixture approaches is $\{Z : Z < -4.887 \text{ or } Z > 4.402\}$, and therefore the common number of genes with significant expression changes is 187. With the nonparametric approach, we obtain 33 differentially expressed genes not detected by Pan's approach.

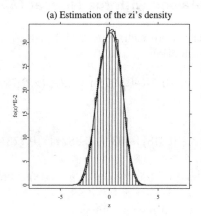

Figure 3.1: Estimation of the z_i's and Z_i's densities (blue dashed line: Pan estimators, red solid line: kernel estimators).

XCSGANLSUprog.xpl

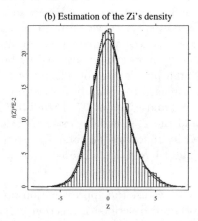

Figure 3.2: Estimation of the z_i's and Z_i's densities (blue dashed line: Pan estimators, red solid line: kernel estimators).

XCSGANLSUprog.xpl

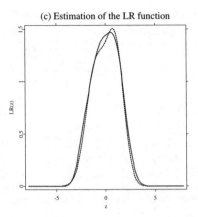

Figure 3.3: Estimation of the LR function.

Q XCSGANLSUprog.xpl

As we pointed out in Section 3.3, the kernel estimation method may be not very efficient in edges of the distribution. It may be one of the reasons why greater numbers of differentially expressed genes were detected by this non-parametric method compared to the normal mixture model. To improve the kernel estimator, we used the reflection method described in Section 3.3.2. The percentage β varies between 0% and 0.25%. Results are summarized in Table 3.1. For instance, with $\beta = 0.05\%$, our kernel approach find 178 genes with significant expression changes. The number of differentially expressed genes in common with the normal mixture model of Pan is 157. Then 21 differentially expressed genes have not been detected by Pan's approach; similarly 30 differentially expressed genes have been detected by the normal mixture model, but not with the nonparametric method.

The rejection region and the corresponding number of differentially expressed genes decrease as β increases. This phenomenom can be easily explained by the fact that the rejection techniques may artificially inflate the tail of the distribution if β is too large. In all cases, we observed that there were some differentially expressed genes detected by the proposed kernel approach which were not found by the normal mixture model of Pan (2002), and vice versa.

Table 3.1: Results obtained with the kernel method. (In the third column, the number in paranthesis is the number of differentially expressed genes in common with the normal mixture model of Pan.)

β	Rejection region of H_0	Number of differentially expressed genes
0%	$\{Z : Z < -4.248 \text{ or } Z > 4.327\}$	220 (187)
0.05%	$\{Z : Z < -4.327 \text{ or } Z > 4.645\}$	178 (157)
0.10%	$\{Z : Z < -4.327 \text{ or } Z > 4.724\}$	164 (143)
0.15%	$\{Z : Z < -4.407 \text{ or } Z > 4.883\}$	131 (115)
0.20%	$\{Z : Z < -4.486 \text{ or } Z > 4.962\}$	112 (102)
0.25%	$\{Z : Z < -4.560 \text{ or } Z > 4.962\}$	111 (102)

3.4.3 A Simulation Study

The aim of the simulation study is to validate the nonparametric computational approach to find the rejection region by solving the equation (3.3).

We consider the normal mixture model defined in (3.7) and (3.8) as the "true" model for f_0 and f. First, using our knowledge of f and f_0, we evaluate the "true" cut-off point and the corresponding "true" rejection region for H_0 by numerically solving (3.3) with $n = 7129$ (the sample size of our real data). We obtain $c = 0.000352$ and the rejection region $\{Z : Z < -4.804 \text{ or } Z > 4.327\}$, which are very close to those obtained by Pan (2002) with the bisection method.

Then, we generate $N = 200$ samples of size $n = 7129$ from this "true" normal mixture model. For each simulated sample, we estimate the cut-off point and the corresponding rejection region for H_0 by the kernel method described in Section 3.3, using the Gaussian kernel and the choice of the bandwidths described in Section 3.4.2. For each simulated sample, the lower and upper bounds of the rejection region are close to the "true" boundaries. Figure 3.4 shows the boxplots of these lower and upper bounds. The variations in the estimated bounds are due to the sampling fluctuations of the simulations, in particular those of the edge distributions.

Let n_k be the number of differentially expressed genes detected by the kernel approach, let n_t be the "true" number of differentially expressed genes, and let n_c be the number of differentially expressed genes in common. Let us now introduce the following efficiency measure: $\frac{n_c}{n_k + n_t - n_c}$. The closer this measure is to one, the better is the efficiency of the nonparametric approach.

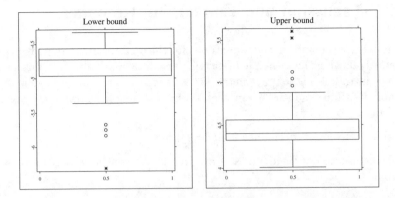

Figure 3.4: Boxplots of the lower and upper bounds of the rejection region
for H_0, for 200 simulated samples.

Figure 3.5 shows the boxplots of this measure over the 200 simulated samples.
One can observe that the efficiency measure is greater than 0.75 for most of
simulated samples.

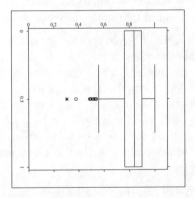

Figure 3.5: Boxplots of the efficiency measure, for 200 simulated samples.

3.5   Discussion and Concluding Remarks

We have reviewed and extended methods for the analysis of microarray experiments. Following the principle of "letting the data speak about themselves", we have introduced a nonparametric kernel method to estimate the density of the null distribution of the test null statistics. This method has four principal advantages.

1) An assumption of normality is not required.

2) The estimation of the degrees of freedom in the conventionally used t-test is avoided.

3) The proposed numerical method to estimate the cut-off point and the corresponding rejection region does not require a bootstrap approach.

4) A reflection method can be found to overcome the edge effect of the kernel estimators.

For microarray data, small sample sizes are very common. Thus the asymptotic justification for the t-test is not applicable, and its validity depends on normality assumptions. Alternatives have been proposed in the literature. For example Baldi and Long (2001), Dudoit, Yang, Speed and Callow (2002), Kerr, Martin and Churchill (2000) and Thomas, Olson, Tapscott and Zhao (2001) proposed parametric or partially nonparametric methods.

Here, we have considered an alternative that is totally nonparametric. Furthermore, the simulation studies show that, if the true state of nature is the normal mixture, our methods yield the expected results. However, as in most kernel estimation methods, the proposed approach is sensitive to distributional edge effects. We adapted the reflection method to study this problem and found a practical optimal solution to minimize the edge effects. Nevertheless, more investigations are necessary for controlling the additional data. It will be genious to develop a method which associates β to the initial number of data.

For further studies, we will use the so-called local polynomial method to estimate the densities, see Hyndman and Yao (1991). The log-spline based method may be also used. New insights about the tails of distribution can be gained by considering these nonparametric estimation approaches. Comparisons can also be made with kernel and normal mixture approaches.

Bibliography

Baldi, P. and Long, A. D. (2001). A Bayesian framework for the analysis of microarray expression data: regularized t-test and statistical inferences of gene changes. *Bioinformatics*, **17**, 509-519.

Bosq, D. and Lecoutre, J. P. (1987). *Théorie de l'estimation fonctionnelle.* Economica: Paris.

Brown, P. O. and Botstein, D. (1999). Exploring the New World of the genome with DNA microarrays. *Nature Genetics*, **21**, 33-37.

Chen, Y., Dougherty, E. R. and Bittner, M. (1999). Ratio-based decisions and the quantitative analysis of cDNA microarray images. *Biomedical Optics*, **2**, 364-374.

Cline, D. B. H. and Hart, J. D. (1991). Kernel estimation of densities with discontinuities or discontinuous derivatives. *Statistics*, **22**, 69-84.

Dempster, A. P., Laird, N. M. and Rubin, D. B. (1977). Maximum likelihood estimation from incomplete data, via the EM algorithm (with discussion). *Journal of the Royal Statistical Society, Series B*, **39**, 1-38.

Deheuvels, P. (1977). Estimation non paramétrique de la densité par histogrammes généralisés. *Revue de Statistique Appliquée*, **25**, 35-42.

Dudoit, S., Yang, Y. H., Speed, T. P. and Callow, M. J. (2002). Statistical methods for identifying differentially expressed genes in replicated cDNA microarray experiments. *Statistica Sinica*, **12**, 111-139.

Efron, B., Tibshirani, R., Goss, V. and Chu, G. (2000). Microarrays and their use in a comparative experiment. *Technical report: Stanford University.*

Efron, B., Storey, J. and Tibshirani, R. (2001). Microarrays, empirical Bayes methods, and false discovery rates. *Technical report:Univ. California, Berkeley.*

Golub, T. R. , Slonim, D. K., Tamayo, P., Huard, C., Gaasenbeek, M., Mesirov, J. P., Coller, H., Loh, M. L., Downing, J. R., Caligiuri, M. A., Bloomfield, C. D., and Lander, E. S. (1999). Molecular classification of cancer: class discovery and class prediction by gene expression monitoring. *Science*, **286**, 531-537.

Hall, P. and Wehrly, T.E. (1991). A geometrical method for removing edge effects from kernel-type nonparametric regression estimators. *J. Amer. Stat. Assoc.*, **86**, 665-672.

Hall, P. and Yao, Q. (1991). Nonparametric estimation and symetry tests for conditional density function. *Journal of Nonparametric Statistics*, **14**, 259-278.

Kerr, M. K., Martin, M. and Churchill, G.A. (2000). Analysis of variance for gene expression microarray data. *Journal of Computational Biology*, **7**, 819-837.

Lander, E. S. (1999). Array of hope. *Nature Genetics*, **21**, 3-4.

Lee, M. L. T., Kuo, F. C., Whitmore, G. A. and Sklar, J. (2000). Importance of microarray gene expression studies: Statistical methods and evidence from repetitive cDNA hybridizations. *Proceedings of the National Academy of Sciences of the United States of America*, **97**, 9834-9839.

Li, C. and Wong, W.H. (2001). Model-based analysis of oligonucleotide arrays: Expression index computation and outlier detection. *Proceedings of the National Academy of Sciences of the United States of America*, **98**, 31-36.

McLachlan, G. and Peel, D. (1999). The EMMIX Algorithm for the Fitting of Normal and t-Components. *Journal of Statistical Software*, **4** (http://www.jstatsoft.org/).

Newton, M. A., Kendziorski, C. M., Richmond, C. S., Blattner, F.R. and Tsui, K. W. (2001). On differential variability of expression ratios: Improving statistical inference about gene expression changes from microarray data. *Journal of Computational Biology*, **8**, 37-52.

Newton, M. A., Noueiry, A., Sarkar, D. and Ahlquist, P. (2004). Detecting differential gene expression with a semiparametric hierarchical mixture method. *Biostatistics*, **5**, 155-176.

Pan, W. (2002). A comparative review of statistical methods for discovering differentially expressed genes in replicated microarray experiments. *Bioinformatics*, **12**, 546-554.

Pan, W., Lin, J. and Le, C. T. (2004). A mixture model approach to detecting differentially expressed genes with microarray data. *Functional and Integrative Genomics*, (To appear).

Press, W. H., Teukolsky, C. M., Vetterling, W. T. and Flannery, B. P. (1992). *Numerical recipes in C, The Art of Scientific Computing.* 2nd ed. Cambridge: New York.

Quackenbush, J. (2001). Computational analysis of microarray data. *Nature Reviews - Genetics*, **2**, 418-427.

Schwarz, G. (1978). Estimating the dimension of a model. *Annals of Statistics*, **6**, 461-464.

Schuster, E. F. (1985). Incorporating support constraints into nonparametric estimation of densities. *Communications in Statistics, Theory and Methods*, **14**, 1123-1136.

Silverman, B. W. (1986). *Density estimation for statistics and data analysis*. Monographs on Statistics and Applied Probability. Chapman & Hall, London.

Thomas, J. G., Olson, J. M., Tapscott, S. J. and Zhao, L. P. (2001). An efficient and robust statistical modeling approach to discover differentially expressed genes using genomic expression profiles. *Genome Research*, **11**, 1227-1236.

Tusher, V.G., Tibshirani, R. and Chu, G. (2001). Significance analysis of microarrays applied to the ionizing radiation response. *Proceedings of the National Academy of Sciences of the United States of America*, **98**, 5116-5121.

4 Kernel Estimates of Hazard Functions for Biomedical Data Sets

Ivana Horová and Jiří Zelinka

4.1 Introduction

The purpose of this chapter is to present a method of kernel estimates in modelling survival data. Within the framework of kernel estimates we draw our attention to the choice of the bandwidth and propose a special iterative method for estimation of it. The chapter also provides a bibliographical recent survey. As regards the applications we focus on applications in cancer research.

In recent years considerable attention has been paid to methods for analyzing data on events observed over time and to the study of factors associated with occurence rates for these events. In summarizing survival data, there are two functions of central interest, namely, the survival and the hazard functions. The well-know product-limit estimation of the survival function was proposed by Kaplan and Meier (1958). A single sample of survival data may also be summarized through the hazard function, which shows the dependence of the instantaneous risk of death on time. We will use the model of random censorship where the data are censored from the right. This type of censorship is often met in many applications, especially in clinical research or in the life testing of complex technical systems (see e.g. Collet (1997), Hougaard (2001), Thernau and Grambsch (2001) and the references therein).

We focus on nonparametric estimates of the hazard function and their derivatives. Among nonparametric methods kernel estimates represent one of the most effective methods (see e.g. Härdle (1991), Wand and Jones (1995), Härdle, Müller, Sperlich and Werwatz (2004)).

These methods are simple enough which makes the numerical calculation easy and fast and the possibilities for mathematical analysis of properties of obtained estimates are very good, too.

Kernel estimates depend on a bandwidth and on a kernel. Since the choice of the bandwidth is a crucial problem in kernel estimates, we draw our attention to this problem and propose a special iterative procedure for finding an estimate of the optimal bandwidth.

As far as the biomedical application is concerned the attention will be paid not only to the estimates of hazard functions but also to the estimation of the second derivatives of these functions since the dynamics of the underlying curve is often of the great interest. For this reason the points where the most rapid changes of the hazard function occur will be detected.

4.2 Kernel Estimate of the Hazard Function and Its Derivatives

Let $T_1, T_2, \ldots, T_n$ be independent and identically distributed lifetimes with distribution function F. Let $C_1, C_2, \ldots, C_n$ be independent and identically distributed censoring times with distribution function G which are usually assumed to be independent from the lifetimes. In the random censorship model we observe pairs $(X_i, \delta_i), i = 1, 2, \ldots, n$, where $X_i = \min{(T_i, C_i)}$ and $\delta_i = I\{X_i = T_i\}$ indicates whether the observation is censored or not. It follows that the $\{X_i\}$ are independent and identically distributed with distribution function L satisfying $\bar{L}(x) = \bar{F}(x)\bar{G}(x)$ where $\bar{E} = 1 - E$ is the survival function for any distribution function E.

The survival function $\bar{F}$ is the probability that an individual survives for a time greater or equal to x. Kaplan and Meier (1958) proposed the product-limit estimate of $\bar{F}$:

$$\hat{\bar{F}}(x) = \prod_{\{j:X_{(j)}<x\}} \left(\frac{n-j}{n-j+1} \right)^{\delta_{(j)}} \tag{4.1}$$

where $X_{(j)}$ denotes the j-th order statistics of $X_1, X_2, \ldots, X_n$ and $\delta_{(j)}$ the corresponding indicator of the censoring status.

The hazard function λ is the probability that an individual dies at time x, conditional on he or she having survived to that time. If the life distribution F has a density f, for $\bar{F}(x) > 0$ the hazard function is defined by

$$\lambda(x) = \frac{f(x)}{\bar{F}(x)} \tag{4.2}$$

and the cumulative hazard function as

$$H(x) = -\log \bar{F}(x). \tag{4.3}$$

Nelson (1972) proposed to estimate the cumulative hazard function H by

$$H_n(x) = \sum_{X_{(i)} \leq x} \frac{\delta_{(i)}}{n-i+1} \tag{4.4}$$

Parametric methods of the estimate of the hazard function are investigated e.g. in Hurt (1992), Collet (1997), Hougaard (2001), Thernau and Grambsch (2001) and many others.

We will focus on nonparametric estimates, namely, on kernel estimates. These estimates were proposed and studied by many authors, see e.g. Watson and Leadbetter (1964), Ramlau-Hansen (1983), Tanner and Wong (1983), Tanner and Wong (1984), Yandell (1983), Mielniczuk (1986), Müller and Wang (1990a), Müller and Wang (1990b), Müller and Wang (1994), Uzunogullari and Wang (1992), Patil (1993a), Patil (1993b), Patil, Wells and Marron (1994), Nielsen and Linton (1995), Youndjé, Sarda and Vieu (1996), Jiang and Marron (2003).

Our approach is based on the model introduced by Tanner and Wong (1983), Müller and Wang (1990a) and Jiang and Marron (2003).

Let $[0, T], T > 0$, be such an interval for which $L(T) < 1$. First, let us make some assumptions:

1° $\lambda \in C^{k_0}[0, T], k_0 \geq 2$

2° Let ν, k be nonnegative integers satisfying $0 \leq \nu \leq k - 2, 2 \leq k \leq k_0$

3° Let K be a real valued function on $\mathbb{R}$ satisfying conditions

(i) support $(K) = [-1, 1], K(-1) = K(1) = 0$

(ii) $K \in Lip[-1, 1]$

(iii) $\int\limits_{-1}^{1} x^j K(x) dx \begin{cases} 0, 0 \leq j < k, j \neq \nu \\ (-1)^{\nu}\nu!, j = \nu \\ \beta_k \neq 0, j = k. \end{cases}$

Such a function is called a kernel of order k and the class of these kernels is denoted by $S_{\nu k}$

4° Let $\{h(n)\}$ be a non-random sequence of positive numbers satisfying

$$\lim_{n\to\infty} h(n) = 0, \lim_{n\to\infty} h(n)^{2\nu+1} n = \infty.$$

These numbers are called bandwidths or smoothing parameters. To keep the notation less cumbersome the dependence of h on n will be suppressed in our calculations.

The definition of the kernel given above is very suitable for our next considerations and moreover it will be very reasonable to assume that ν and k have the same parity. This fact enables us to choose an optimal kernel.

The kernel estimate of the νth derivative of the hazard function λ is the following convolution of the kernel K with the Nelson estimator H_n:

$$\hat{\lambda}_{h,K}^{(\nu)}(x) = \frac{1}{h^{\nu+1}} \int K\left(\frac{x-u}{h}\right) dH_n(u) = \tag{4.5}$$

$$= \frac{1}{h^{\nu+1}} \sum_{i=1}^{n} K\left(\frac{x-X_{(i)}}{h}\right) \frac{\delta_{(i)}}{n-i+1}, K \in S_{\nu k}.$$

In the paper by Müller and Wang (1990a) the properties of these estimate have been investigated under additional assumptions:

$$nh^{k+1}(\log n)^{-1} \to \infty, nh(\log n)^{-2} \to \infty \text{ as } n \to \infty.$$

Let us denote

$$V(K) = \int_{-1}^{1} K^2(x)dx, \beta_k = \int_{-1}^{1} x^k K(x)dx$$

and

$$D_k = \int_0^T \left\{\frac{\lambda^{(k)}(x)}{k!}\right\}^2 dx, \Lambda = \int_0^T \frac{\lambda(x)}{\bar{L}(x)}dx.$$

Then, the bias and the variance can be expressed as (Müller and Wang, 1990a):

$$Bias \ \hat{\lambda}_{h,K}^{(\nu)}(x) = h^{k-\nu}\lambda^{(k)}(x)\left\{\frac{(-1)^k\beta_k}{k!} + o(1)\right\}, 0 < x \le T \tag{4.6}$$

$$Var \ \hat{\lambda}_{h,K}^{(\nu)}(x) = \frac{1}{nh^{2\nu+1}}\left\{\frac{\lambda(x)V(K)}{\bar{L}(x)} + o(1)\right\}, 0 \le x \le T. \tag{4.7}$$

The use of (4.6) and (4.7) provides the form of the Mean Squared Error. The global quality of this estimate can be described by means of the Mean Integrated Squared Error ($MISE \ \hat{\lambda}_{h,K}^{(\nu)}$).

Now we focus on the leading term $\overline{MISE}(\hat{\lambda}_{h,K}^{(\nu)})$ of $MISE(\hat{\lambda}_{h,K}^{(\nu)})$. Evidently, $\overline{MISE}(\hat{\lambda}_{h,K}^{(\nu)})$ takes the form

$$\overline{MISE}(\hat{\lambda}_{h,K}^{(\nu)}) = h^{2(k-\nu)}\beta_k^2 D_k + \frac{V(K)\Lambda}{nh^{2\nu+1}}. \qquad (4.8)$$

Consider a special parameter

$$\gamma_{\nu,k}^{2k+1} = \frac{V(K)}{\beta_k^2}, K \in S_{\nu,k}. \qquad (4.9)$$

This parameter is called a canonical factor and was introduced by Marron and Nolan (1989), see also Härdle, Müller, Sperlich and Werwatz (2004).

Then, the asymptotically optimal bandwidth $h_{opt,\nu,k}$ minimizing $\overline{MISE}(\hat{\lambda}_{h,K}^{(\nu)})$ with respect to h is given by

$$h_{opt,\nu,k}^{2k+1} = \frac{\Lambda(2\nu+1)}{2n(k-\nu)D_k}\gamma_{\nu,k}^{2k+1}. \qquad (4.10)$$

Further, getting along in a similar way as in the paper by Horová, Vieu and Zelinka (2002) we arrive at the formula

$$\overline{MISE}\left(\hat{\lambda}_{h_{opt,\nu,k}K}^{(\nu)}\right) = \Lambda\, T(K)^{\frac{2}{2k+1}}\frac{(2k+1)\gamma_{\nu,K}^{2\nu+1}}{2n(k-\nu)h_{opt,\nu,k}^{2\nu+1}}, \qquad (4.11)$$

where

$$T(K) = \left|\int_{-1}^{1} x^k K(x)dx\right|^{2\nu+1}\left(\int_{-1}^{1} K^2(x)dx\right)^{k-\nu}, K \in S_{\nu,k}. \qquad (4.12)$$

This formula shows the effects of the kernel as well as the bandwidth on the estimate.

The formula (4.10) offers a very useful tool for calculation of the optimal bandwidth for derivatives of $\hat{\lambda}$.

Let ν, k be even integers. Then

$$h_{opt,\nu,k} = \left\{\frac{(2\nu+1)k}{k-\nu}\right\}^{\frac{1}{2k+1}}\frac{\gamma_{\nu,k}}{\gamma_{0,k}}h_{opt,0,k}. \qquad (4.13)$$

Further, for ν and k being odd integers this formula provides

$$h_{opt,\nu,k} = \left\{\frac{(2\nu+1)k}{3(k-\nu)}\right\}^{\frac{1}{2k+1}}\frac{\gamma_{\nu,k}}{\gamma_{1,k}}h_{opt,1,k}. \qquad (4.14)$$

Such a procedure is called a factor method (see e.g. Müller, Stadmüller and Schmitt (1987), Härdle, Müller, Sperlich and Werwatz (2004), Horová, Vieu and Zelinka (2002).

4.3   Choosing the Shape of the Kernel

The formula (4.11) suggests naturally to look for a kernel that minimizing the functional (4.12). This problem has been investigated in most of the existing literature (see e.g. Mammitzsch (1988), Granovsky and Müller (1991), Granovsky and Müller (1995), Horová, Vieu and Zelinka (2002).

Let us briefly describe this problem. Let $\mathcal{N}_{k-2} = \{g \in L^2, g$ has exactly $k - 2$ changes of sign on $\mathbb{R}\}$. Kernels $K \in \mathcal{N}_{k-2} \cap S_{\nu k}$ minimizing the functional $T(K)$ are called optimal kernels. These kernels are polynomials of degree k having $k - 2$ different roots inside the interval $[-1, 1]$. In order to emphasize the dependence on ν and k we denote these kernels by $K_{opt,\nu,k}$. Table 4.1, 4.2, 4.3 bring some of these optimal kernels as well as the corresponding factors $\gamma_{\nu,k}$. Below each table are the XploRe quantlets that allow for computing and viewing these optimal kernels.

Table 4.1: Optimal kernel of order $(0, k)$

k	$\gamma_{0,k}$	$K_{opt,0,k}$
2	1.7188	$-\frac{3}{4}(x^2 - 1)\boldsymbol{I}(|x| \leq 1)$
4	2.0165	$\frac{15}{32}(x^2 - 1)(7x^2 - 3)\boldsymbol{I}(|x| \leq 1)$
6	2.0834	$-\frac{105}{256}(x^2 - 1)(33x^4 - 30x^2 + 5)\boldsymbol{I}(|x| \leq 1)$

Q XCSoptker02.xpl

Q XCSoptker04.xpl

Q XCSoptker06.xpl

Table 4.2: Optimal kernel of order $(1, k)$

k	$\gamma_{1,k}$	$K_{opt,1,k}$
3	1.4204	$\frac{15}{4}x(x^2 - 1)\boldsymbol{I}(|x| \leq 1)$
5	1.7656	$-\frac{105}{32}x(x^2 - 1)(9x^2 - 5)\boldsymbol{I}(|x| \leq 1)$
7	1.8931	$\frac{315}{32}x(x^2 - 1)(143x^4 - 154x^2 + 35)\boldsymbol{I}(|x| \leq 1)$

Q XCSoptker13.xpl

Q XCSoptker15.xpl

Q XCSoptker17.xpl

Table 4.3: Optimal kernel of order $(2, k)$

k	$\gamma_{2,k}$	$K_{opt,2,k}$
4	1.3925	$-\frac{105}{16}(x^2 - 1)(5x^2 - 1)\boldsymbol{I}(|x| \leq 1)$
6	1.6964	$\frac{315}{64}(x^2 - 1)(77x^4 - 58x^2 + 5)\boldsymbol{I}(|x| \leq 1)$
8	1.8269	$-\frac{3465}{2048}(x^2 - 1)(1755x^6 - 2249x^4 + 721x^2 - 35)\boldsymbol{I}(|x| \leq 1)$

Q XCSoptker24.xpl

Q XCSoptker26.xpl

Q XCSoptker28.xpl

4.4 Choosing the Bandwidth

The problem of finding the optimal bandwidth belongs to the crucial problem of kernel estimates. This problem arises in the kernel estimates of regression functions, densities and as well as in kernel estimates of hazard functions.

Due to censoring modified cross-validation methods can be applied for the estimate the optimal bandwidth (see e.g. Marron and Padgett (1987), Uzunogullari and Wang (1992), Nielsen and Linton (1995)). In the paper by Tanner and Wong (1984) the modified likelihood method was proposed. Other methods for an estimate of the bandwidth can be also found e.g. in papers by Sarda and Vieu (1991), Patil (1993a), Patil (1993b), Patil, Wells and Marron (1994), Gonzales-Mantiega, Cao and Marron (1996).

Let $\hat{h}_{opt,0,k}$ be an estimate of $h_{opt,0,k}$. In view of the fact that we will only focus on the estimate $\hat{\lambda}^{(0)}$ and $\hat{\lambda}^{(2)}$ it is sufficient to estimate the optimal bandwidth $\hat{h}_{opt,0,k}$ since the formula (4.13) can be rewritten with $\hat{h}_{opt,0,k}$ and $\hat{h}_{opt,2,k}$ instead of $h_{opt,0,k}$ and $h_{opt,2,k}$. Here, we propose a special method for estimating $\hat{h}_{opt,0,k}$. Our approach is based on two facts.

Firstly, let us notice that the use of $h_{opt,0,k}$ given in (4.10) means that the leading term of variance $\overline{Var}(\hat{\lambda}_{h_{opt,0,k},K})$ and the leading term of the bias $\overline{Bias}(\hat{\lambda}_{h_{opt,0,k},K})$ satisfy

$$\overline{Var}\left(\hat{\lambda}_{h_{opt,0,k},K}\right) = 2k\left\{\overline{Bias}(\hat{\lambda}_{h_{opt,0,k},K})\right\}^2. \tag{4.15}$$

In the second place, we start from the suitable representation of MISE given in the papers by Müller and Wang (1990b), Müller and Wang (1994).

The aforementioned estimate of MISE is defined as

$$\widehat{MISE}\left(\hat{\lambda}_{h,K}\right) = \int_0^T \left\{\hat{v}(x,h) + \hat{b}^2(x,h)\right\} dx, \tag{4.16}$$

where $\hat{v}(x,h) = \widehat{Var}\left(\hat{\lambda}_{h,K}(x)\right)$ and $\hat{b}(x,h) = \widehat{Bias}\left(\hat{\lambda}_{h,K}(x)\right)$ are the estimates of variance and bias, respectively, and

$$\begin{cases} \hat{v}(x,h) = \frac{1}{nh} \int K^2(y) \frac{\hat{\lambda}_{h,K}(x-hy)}{\bar{L}_n(x-hy)} dy \\[2mm] \hat{b}(x,h) = \int \hat{\lambda}_{h,K}(x-hy)K(y)dy - \hat{\lambda}_{h,K}(x) \end{cases} \tag{4.17}$$

where $k \in S_{0\,k}$ and

$$\bar{L}_n(x) = 1 - \frac{1}{n+1}\sum_{i=1}^{n} I\{X_i \le x\} \tag{4.18}$$

is the modified empirical survival function.

The global bandwidth estimate

$$\hat{h}_{opt,0,k} = \arg\min_{h \in H_n} \widehat{MISE}\left(\hat{\lambda}_{h,K}\right)$$

satisfies $\hat{h}_{opt,0,k}/h_{opt,0,k} \to 1$ in probability, H_n denotes the set of acceptable bandwidths. This set will be dealing with below.

Taking the relations (4.15) and (4.17) into account we arrive at the formula for $\hat{h}_{opt,0,k}$:

$$
h = \frac{1}{2kn} \frac{\int_0^T \int K^2(y) \frac{\hat{\lambda}_{h,K}(x-hy)}{\hat{L}_n(x-hy)} dy dx}{\int_0^T \left\{ \int \hat{\lambda}_{h,K}(x-hy) K(y) dy - \hat{\lambda}_{h,K}(x) \right\}^2 dx} \tag{4.19}
$$

for sufficiently large n. Denoting the right hand side of this equation by ψ, the last equation can be rewritten as

$$
h = \psi(h).
$$

It means that asymptotically in terms of $\overline{MISE}$ we are looking for the fixed point $\hat{h}_{opt,0,k}$ of the function ψ. Consider one step iterative method. Starting with the initial approximation $\hat{h}^{(0)}_{opt,0,k}$ the sequence $\{\hat{h}^{(j)}_{opt,0,k}\}_{j=0}^\infty$ is generated by

$$
\hat{h}^{(j+1)}_{opt,0,k} = \psi\left(\hat{h}^{(j)}_{opt,0,k}\right), j = 0,1,2 \ldots
$$

Since it would be very difficult to verify whether the conditions for the convergence of this process are satisfied we propose to use the Steffensen's method. This method consists in the following steps:

$$
\begin{aligned}
t^{(j)} &= \psi(\hat{h}^{(j)}_{opt,0,k}) \\
z^{(j)} &= \psi(t^{(j)}) \\
\hat{h}^{(j+1)}_{opt,0,k} &= \hat{h}^{(j)}_{opt,0,k} - \\
&- \left(t^{(j)} - \hat{h}^{(j)}_{opt,0,k}\right)^2 / \left(z^{(j)} - 2t^{(j)} + \hat{h}^{(j)}_{opt,0,k}\right), j = 0,1,2,\ldots.
\end{aligned} \tag{4.20}
$$

In terms of one step iterative methods the Steffensen's method can be described by the iterative function

$$
\Psi(h) = \frac{h\psi\{\psi(h)\} - \psi^2(h)}{\psi\{\psi(h)\} - 2\psi(h) + h}
$$

i.e.,

$$
\hat{h}^{(j+1)}_{opt,0,k} = \Psi\left(\hat{h}^{(j)}_{opt,0,k}\right), \qquad j = 0,1,2,\ldots
$$

The Steffensen's method (Steffensen, 1933) is based on application $\triangle^2$ Aitken's methods for accelerating the convergence to a linearly convergent sequence obtained from fixed-point iteration (see Isaacson and Keller (1966), Stoer and Bulirsch (1980) in greater details).

It is clear that $\hat{h}_{opt,0,k}$ is the simple fixed point, i.e., $\psi'(\hat{h}_{opt,0,k}) \neq 1$. Then both iterative functions ψ and Ψ have the same fixed point and Ψ yields at least a second - order method for this point, i.e. a locally quadratically convergent method. The relative error can be taken as a criterion for obtaining the suitable approximation $\hat{h}_{opt,0,k}$:

$$\left| \frac{\hat{h}_{opt,0,k}^{(j+1)} - \hat{h}_{opt,0,k}^{(j)}}{\hat{h}_{opt,0,k}^{(j)}} \right| \leq \epsilon,$$

where $\epsilon > 0$ is a given tolerance, and we put $\hat{h}_{opt,0,k} = \hat{h}_{opt,0,k}^{(j+1)}$.

The evaluation of the right hand side in the equation (4.19) looks rather complicated, but these integrals can be easily evaluated by suitable discretization; here the composite trapeziodal rule is recommended.

Let us come back to the set H_n of acceptable bandwidths. The good choice of the initial approximation $\hat{h}_{opt,0,k}^{(0)} \in H_n$ is very important for the iterative process above.

We are going to show how a kernel density estimate could be useful for this aim.

Let us describe the motivation for our procedure. First, the Koziol-Green model is reminded (Koziol and Green, 1976). There is a natural question about the distribution of the time censor C. There are both theoretical and practical reasons to adopt the Koziol-Green model of random censorship under which it is assumed that there is a nonnegative constant ρ such that

$$\bar{F}(x)^\rho = \bar{G}(x),$$

$\rho = 0$ corresponds to the case without censoring.

Let l, f and g be densities of L, F and G, respectively. Then (Hurt, 1992):

$$l(x) = \frac{1}{p}\bar{F}(x)^\rho f(x), \tag{4.21}$$

$$p = \frac{1}{1+\rho}$$

Let

$$\hat{l}_{h,K}(x) = \frac{1}{nh}\sum_{i=1}^{n} K\left(\frac{x - X_i}{h}\right) \tag{4.22}$$

be the kernel estimate of the density l and keep now $\bar{F}(x)$ as a known quantity. Then, with respect to (4.21)

$$\tilde{f}_{h,K}(x) = \frac{p\hat{l}_{h,K}(x)}{\bar{F}^p(x)}$$

and $\tilde{f}_{h,K}(x)$ is an estimate of f.

Consider now an alternative estimate $\tilde{\lambda}_{h,K}$ of λ:

$$\tilde{\lambda}_{h,K}(x) = \frac{\tilde{f}_{h,K}(x)}{\bar{F}(x)}. \tag{4.23}$$

Hence

$$\tilde{\lambda}_{h,K}(x) = \frac{p\hat{l}_{h,K}(x)}{\bar{F}^{1/p}(x)}. \tag{4.24}$$

Now it is easy to verify that the optimal bandwidth for $\hat{l}_{h,K}$ is also the optimal bandwidth for $\tilde{\lambda}_{h,K}$. The properties of the estimate $\tilde{\lambda}_{h,K}$ can be investigated in a similar way as those in the paper by Uzunogullari and Wang (1992). Let $\hat{h}^*_{opt,0,k}$ be an optimal bandwidth for $\hat{l}_{h,K}$. Due to the aforementioned facts it is reasonable to take this value as a suitable initial approximation for the process (4.20).

The idea of the bandwidth choice for the kernel density estimate $\hat{l}_{h,K}$ is very similar to that presented for the hazard function but with the difference that here an upper bound for the set of acceptable bandwidth is known (see e.g. Terrell and Scott (1985), Terrell (1990), Horová and Zelinka (2004)). Getting along in a similar way as earlier we obtain the equation

$$h = \frac{1}{2nk} \frac{\int\int K^2(y)\hat{l}_{h,K}(x-hy)dydx}{\int\{\int \hat{l}_{h,K}(x-hy)K(y)dy - \hat{l}_{h,K}(x)\}^2dx}, K \in S_{0,k}$$

where $h = \hat{h}^*_{opt,0,k}$ is a fixed point.

We can take $\hat{h}^{*(0)}_{opt,0,k} = h_u$ where h_u is the upper bound defined as

$$h_u = \hat{\sigma}b_k n^{-1/2k+1} \tag{4.25}$$

where $\hat{\sigma}^2$ is an estimate of an unknown variance σ^2 of the data and

$$b_k = 2\sqrt{2k+5}\left\{\frac{(2k+1)(2k+5)(k+1)^2\Gamma^4(k+1)V(K)}{k\Gamma(2k+4)\Gamma(2k+3)\beta_k^2}\right\}^{\frac{1}{2k+1}}, \tag{4.26}$$

Γ is the gamma function.

The estimate of σ^2 can be done, e.g. by

$$\hat{\sigma}^2 = \frac{1}{n-1} \sum_{i=1}^{n} \left(X_i - \bar{X} \right)^2 . \tag{4.27}$$

Now the Steffensen's method is used in the same way as above. It seems that this process looks very complicated but our experience shows that this procedure is faster and more reliable than the cross - validation method.

The construction of the confidence intervals is described in the paper by Müller and Wang (1990a). The asymptotic $(1 - \alpha)$ confidence interval for $\lambda_{h,K}^{(\nu)}(x)$ is given by

$$\hat{\lambda}_{h,K}^{(\nu)}(x) \pm \left\{ \frac{\hat{\lambda}_{h,K}(x) V(K)}{(1 - L_n(x))n\hat{h}^{2\nu+1}} \right\}^{1/2} \Phi^{-1}(1 - \alpha/2) \tag{4.28}$$

where Φ is the normal cumulative distribution function and L_n is the modified empirical distribution function of L

$$L_n(x) = \frac{1}{n+1} \sum_{i=1}^{n} 1_{\{X_i \leq x\}}.$$

Remark. When we estimate near 0 or T then boundary effects can occur because the "effective support" $[x-h, x+h]$ of the kernel K is not contained in $[0, T]$. This can lead to negative estimates of hazard functions near endpoints. The same can happen if kernels of higher order are used in the interior. In such cases it may be reasonable to truncate $\hat{\lambda}_{h,K}$ below at 0, i.e. to consider $\hat{\lambda}_{h,K}(x) = max(\hat{\lambda}_{h,K}(x), 0)$. The similar considerations can be made for the confidence intervals. The boundary effects can be avoided by using kernels with asymmetric supports (Müller and Wang, 1990a), (Müller and Wang, 1994).

4.5   Description of the Procedure

In the biomedical application the points θ of the most rapid change, i.e., points of the extreme of the first derivative of λ, are also of a great interest. These points can be detected as zeros of the estimated second derivatives. Thus, we will only concentrate on the estimate of $\lambda^{(0)}$ and $\lambda^{(2)}$. We focus on such points $\hat{\theta}$, $\hat{\lambda}_{h,K}^{(2)}(\hat{\theta}) = 0$, where $\lambda_{h,K}^{(2)}$ changes its sign from - to + since only the local minima of $\hat{\lambda}_{h,K}^{(1)}$ are important. It can be shown that $\hat{\theta} \to \theta$ in probability (Müller and Wang, 1990a).

According to our experience the kernel $K \in S_{04}$

$$K_{opt,0,4}(x) = \frac{15}{32}(x^2 - 1)(7x^2 - 3)\boldsymbol{I}(|x| \leq 1), \gamma_{04} = 2.0165 \qquad (4.29)$$

is very convenient for the estimate of the hazard function. In this case the value of b_4 defined in (4.26) is equal to $b_4 = 3.3175$.

In connection with theoretical results the following kernel should be chosen for the estimate of $\lambda^{(2)}$:

$$K_{opt,2,4}(x) = \frac{105}{16}(1 - x^2)(5x^2 - 1)\boldsymbol{I}(|x| \leq 1), \gamma_{24} = 1.3925 \qquad (4.30)$$

Now, our procedure is briefly described. It consists in the following steps:

Step 1: Estimate the density l with (4.29) and find the estimated optimal bandwidth $\hat{h}^*_{opt,0,4}$ by Steffensen's method.

Step 2: Put $\hat{h}^*_{opt,0,4} = \hat{h}^{(0)}_{opt,0,4}$ and use this value as the initial approximation for iterative method (4.20) which yields the suitable estimate $\hat{h}_{opt,0,4}$.

Step 3: Construct the estimate $\hat{\lambda}^{(0)}_{h,K}$ with the kernel (4.29) and the bandwidth obtained in the step 2.

Step 4: Compute the optimal bandwidth for the estimate $\hat{\lambda}^{(2)}_{h,K}$ using the formula (4.13):
$\hat{h}_{opt,2,4} = (10)^{1/9}\frac{\gamma_{24}}{\gamma_{04}}\hat{h}_{opt,0,4} = 1.87031\hat{h}_{opt,0,4}$

Step 5: Get the kernel estimate of $\lambda^{(2)}$ with the kernel (4.30) and bandwidth selected in the step 4.

Step 6: Detect the zeros of $\lambda^{(2)}_{h,K}$ and construct the confidence intervals.

4.6   Application

Note that all our procedures have been programmed with XploRe and are accessible in the library `hazker`. The quantlet `XCSdensestim` is computing kernel density estimation while `XCSdensiterband` is computing the Steffensen's optimal bandwidth.

Q `XCSdensestim.xpl`

Q `XCSdensiterband.xpl`

The quantlet XCSHFestim computes the kernel estimate of the hazard function and its derivatives, while the quantlet XCSHFestimci gives in addition confidence bands.

Q XCSHFestim.xpl

Q XCSHFestimci.xpl

Finally, the Steffensen's optimal bandwidth for hazard estimation is computed with the quantlet XCSHFiterband.

Q XCSHFiterband.xpl

Now, we are going to apply the procedure described in the Section 4.5 to the data which were kindly provided by the Masaryk Memorial Cancer Institute in Brno (Soumarová *et al.*, 2002), (Horová *et al.*, 2004).

The first set of data (data file HFdata1) involves 236 patients with breast carcinoma. The study was carried out based on the records of women who had received the breast conservative surgical treatment and radiotherapy as well in the period 1983-1994. The patients with the breast carcinoma of the I. and II. clinical stage and with T1 and T2 tumors where only included to this study. Of 236 patients 47 died by the end of the study and 189 were thus censored. The study was finished in the year 2000.

The period of time from the time origin to the death of a patient is the survival time; the time of the remaining individuals is right censored – i.e. those who have been alive in the end of study in 2000.

In this study patients were not recruited at exactly the same time, but accrued over a period of months. The period of time that a patient spent in the study, measured from the date of surgery (month/year), is often referred to as patient's time (Collet, 1997). Figure 4.1 shows the individual patients' time for the complete data set of 236 patients.

First patients entered the study in 1983, the last patients in 1995 and the study was finished in 2000. Each of 236 vertical segments shows the time which individual patients spent in the study.

In Figure 4.2 the Kaplan-Meier estimate of the survival function $\bar{F}$ is presented. Figure 4.3 shows the estimate of the density l. In Figure 4.4 the shape of the function defined in (4.19) is presented. Figure 4.5 brings the estimate $\hat{\lambda}_{h,K}^{(0)}$ constructed by the proposed procedure including the confidence

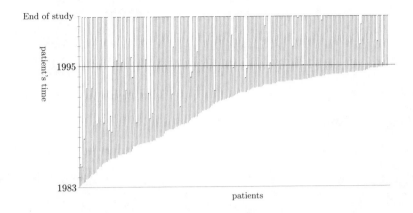

Figure 4.1: The patients' time for the complete data set of 236 patients

intervals and Figure 4.6 shows the estimate $\lambda^{(2)}_{h,K}$. Estimated points of the most rapid change $\hat{\theta}_1, \hat{\theta}_2$ are defined as zero of the estimated second derivatives with sign changes from $-$ to $+$. The main change obviously occurs for $\hat{\theta}_1 \doteq 51.39$ months whereas the second change at $\hat{\theta}_2 \doteq 128.87$ months. These figures indicated that patients run a high risk about 50 months after surgical treatment. Then it is followed by a low risk and higher risk occurs again in the 100th month approximately.

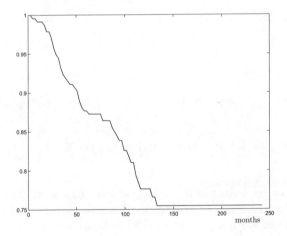

Figure 4.2: The Kaplan-Meier estimate of the survival function $\bar{F}$

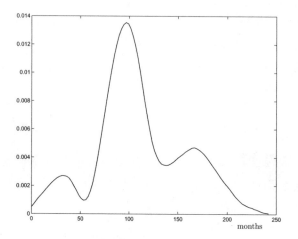

Figure 4.3: The estimate of the density l

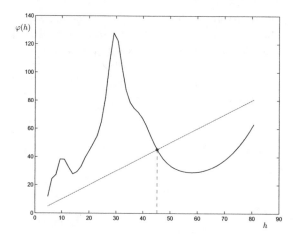

Figure 4.4: Iterative function and the fixed point

The influence of the bandwidth h to the shape of the estimate $\hat{\lambda}_{h,K}^{(0)}$ of the hazard function λ can be seen on Figure 4.7 where the family of estimates indexed by the bandwidth is presented. The estimate for $\hat{h}_{opt,0,4}$ is highlighted in the figure.

Table 4.6 brings the sequence of iterations generated by the method (4.20)

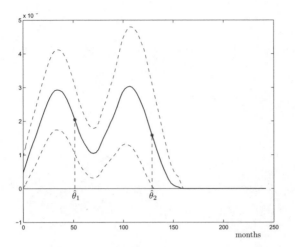

Figure 4.5: The estimate $\hat{\lambda}_{h,K}^{(0)}$ of the hazard function (solid line), the confidence intervals (dashed line)

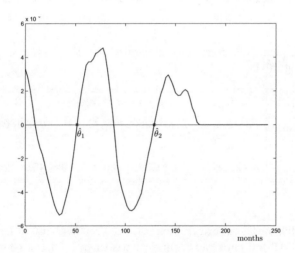

Figure 4.6: The estimate $\hat{\lambda}_{h,K}^{(2)}$

for tolerance $\epsilon = 1.0 \times 10^{-6}$.

The second study is concerning the retrospective study of 222 patients with uterine carcinoma (data file HFdata1). These patients were treated in the pe-

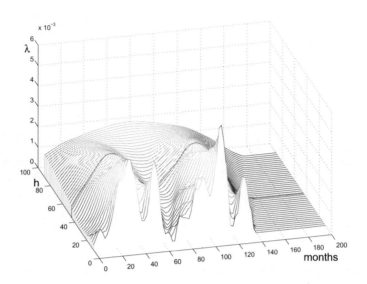

Figure 4.7: 3D view of the family of estimates

Table 4.4: Sequence of iterations generated by the iterative function in Figure 4.4

j	0	1	2	3
$\hat{h}^{(j)}_{opt,0,k}$	22.526490	51.517280	47.411171	45.548046
j	4	5	6	7
$\hat{h}^{(j)}_{opt,0,k}$	45.222855	45.205395	45.205249	45.205249

riod 1980 – 1998 at the Masaryk Memorial Cancer Institute in Brno (Horová *et al.*, 2004). All patients had a surgical treatment. Of the complete set of 222 patients 27 died of cancer causes. The patients of the first clinical stage were included to this study.

Figures 4.8, 4.9 and 4.10 present the Kaplan-Meier estimate of the survival function $\bar{F}$, the estimate $\hat{\lambda}^{(0)}_{h,K}$ of the hazard function including the confidence intervals and the estimate of $\lambda^{(2)}_{h,K}$ with points of the most rapid change $\hat{\theta}_1, \hat{\theta}_2$.

Iterations generated by the method (4.20) for this data set and tolerance

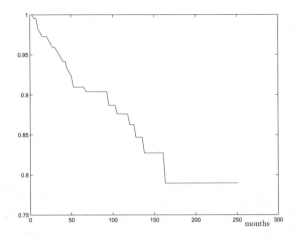

Figure 4.8: The Kaplan-Meier estimate of the survival function $\bar{F}$

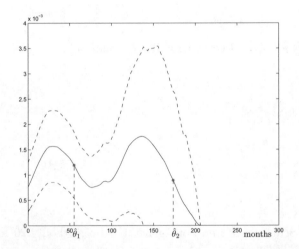

Figure 4.9: The estimate $\hat{\lambda}_{h,K}^{(0)}$ of the hazard function (solid line), the confidence intervals (dashed line)

$\epsilon = 1.0 \times 10^{-6}$ are presented by Table 4.6.

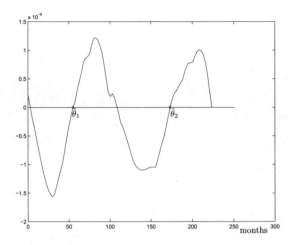

Figure 4.10: The estimate $\hat{\lambda}_{h,K}^{(2)}$

Table 4.5: Sequence of iterations generated by method 4.20 for the set of 222 patients

j	0	1	2	3	4
$\hat{h}_{opt,0,k}^{(j)}$	44.467283	69.586408	69.335494	69.330511	69.330523

Bibliography

Chaubey P. Y. and Sen K. P. (1996). On Smooth Estimation of Survival and Density Functions *Statistics & Decision*, **14**, 11-22.

Collet D. (1997). *Modelling Survival Data in Medical Research*. Chapman & Hall/CRC, Boca Raton, London, New York, Washington D.C.

Gonzales-Mantiega W., Cao R. and Marron J. S. (1996). Bootstrap Selection of the Smoothing Parameter in Nonparametric Hazard Rate Estimation. *J. Amer. Stat. Assoc.*, **91**, 435.

Granovsky B. L. and Müller H. G. (1991). Optimizing Kernel Methods. A unifying Variational Principle. *Int. Stat. Review*, **59**, 3, 378-388.

Granovsky B. L. and Müller H. G. (1995). Remarks of Optimal Kernel Functions. *Statistics & Decision*, **13**, 101-116.

Härdle W., Müller M., Sperlich S. and Werwatz A. (2004). *Nonparametric and Semiparametric Models*, Springer

Härdle W. (1991). Applied Nonparametric Regression, *Cambridge University Press*.

Horová H., Růžičková J., Ježková B., Horová I., Budíková M. and Dörr A. (2004). Adjuvant Radiotherapy in the Treatment of the Carcinoma of Uterus of the First Clinical Stage (in Czech, English summary), *to appear in Česká a slovenská gynekologie*.

Horová I., Vieu P. and Zelinka J. (2002). Optimal Choice of Nonparametric Estimates of a Density and of its Derivatives, *Statistics & Decision*, **20**, 355-378.

Horová I. and Zelinka J. (2004). A Contribution to the Bandwidth Choice for the Kernel Density Estimates, *submitted to Comput. Statistics*.

Horová I., Zelinka J. and Budíková M. (2004). Estimates of Hazard Functions for Carcinoma Data Sets, *accepted for publication in Environmetrics*.

Hougaard P. (2001). *Analysis of Multivariate Survival Data*, Springer-Verlag, New York, Berlin, Heidelberg.

Hurt J. (1992). Statistical Methods for Survival Data Analysis, *Proceedings ROBUST'92, Eds. J.Antoch & G.Dohnal*, 54-74.

Isaacson E. and Keller H. B. (1966). *Analysis of Numerical Methods.*, John Wiley& Sons, Inc., New York, London, Sydney.

Jiang J. and Marron J. S. (2003). SiZer for Censored Density and Hazard Estimation *prerpint*.

Kaplan E. I. and Meier P. V. (1958). Nonparametric Estimation from Incomplete Observations, *J. Amer. Stat. Assoc.*, **53**, 282, 457-481.

Koziol J. A. and Green S.B. (1976). Cramer-von Mises Statistics for Randomly Censored Data, *Biometrika*, **63**, 3, 465-474.

Mammitzsch V. (1988). A note on kernels of order ν, k, *Proceedings of the fourth Prague symposium on asymptotic statistics*, Charles University, Prague, 405-412.

Marron J. S. and Nolan D. (1989). Canonical Kernels for Density Estimation, *Statistics & Probability Letters*, **7**, 195-199.

Marron J. S. and Padgett W. J. (1987). Asymptotically Optimal Bandwidth Selection for Kernel Density Estimators from Randomly Right-Censored Samples, *Annals of Statistics*, **15**, 4, 1520-1535.

Mielniczuk J. (1986). Asymptotic Propertics of Kernel Estimators of a Density Function in Case of Censored Data, *The Annals of Statistics*, **14**, 2, 766-773.

Müller H. G., Stadmüller U. and Schmitt T. V. (1987). Bandwidth Choice and Confidence Intervals for Derivatives of Noisy Data, *Biometrika*, **74**, 4, 743-749.

Müller H. G. and Wang J. L. (1990). Nonparametric Analysis of Changes in Hazard Rates for Censored Survival Data: An alternative Change-Point Models, *Biometrika*, **77**, 2, 305-314.

Müller H. G. and Wang J. L. (1990). Nonparametric Locally Addaptive Hazard Smoothing, *Prob. Th. Rel. Fields*, **85**, 523-538.

Müller H. G. and Wang J. L. (1994). Hazard Rate Estimation under Random Censoring with Varying Kernels and Bandwidths, *Biometrics*, **50**, 61-76.

Nelson W. (1972). Theory and Applications of Hazard Plotting for Censored Data, *Technometrics*, **14**, 945-966.

Nielsen J. P. and Linton O. B. (1995). Kernel Estimation in a Nonparametric Marker Dependent Hazard model, *Annals of Statistics*, **23**, 5, 1735-1748.

Patil P. N. (1993). Bandwidth Choice for Nonparametric Hazard Rate Estimation, *Journal of Stat. Plann. and Inf.*, **35**, 15-30.

Patil P. N. (1993). On the Least Squares Cross-Validation Bandwidth in Hazard Rate Estimation, *The Annals of Statistics*, **21**, 1792-1810.

Patil P. N., Wells M. T. and Marron J. S. (1994). Some Heuristics of Kernel Based Estimators of Ratio Functions, *Nonparametrics Statistics*, **4**, 203-209.

Ramlau-Hansen (1983). Counting Processes Intensities by Means of Kernel Functions, *The Annals of Statistics*, **11**, 2, 453-466.

Sarda P. and Vieu P. (1991). Smoothing Parameter Selection in Hazard Estimation, *Statistics & Probability Letters*, **11**, 429-434.

Soumarová R., Horová H., Růžičková J., Čoupek P., Šlampa P., Šeneklová Z., Petráková K., Budíková M. and Horová I. (2002). Local and Distant Failure in Patients with Stage I and II Carcinoma of the Breast Treated with Breat-Conserving Surgery and Radiation Therapy (in Czech, English summary), *Radiační onkologie*, **2**, 1, 17-24.

Steffensen J. F. (1933). Remarks on Iteration, *Skand. Aktuarie Tidskr.*, **16**, 64-72.

Stoer J. and Bulirsch R. (1980). *Introduction to Numerical Analysis*, Springer-Verlag, New York, Heidelberg, Berlin.

Tanner M. A. and Wong W. H. (1983). The Estimation of the Hazard Function from Randomly Censored Data by the Kernel Method, *The Annals of Statistics*, **11**, 3, 989-993.

Tanner M. A. and Wong W. H. (1984). Data-Based Nonparametric Estimation of the Hazard Function with Applications to Model Diagnostis and Exploratory Analysis, *J. Amer. Stat. Assoc.*, **79**, 35, 174-182.

Terrell, G. R. (1990). The maximal smoothing principle in density estimation, *J. Amer. Stat. Assoc.*, **85**, 470-477.

Terrell, G. R. and Scott, D. E. (1985). Oversmoothed nonparametric density estimations, *J. Amer. Stat. Assoc.*, **80**, 209-214.

Thernau T. M. and Grambsch P.M. (2001). *Modelling Survival Data. Extending the Cox Model*, Springer-Verlag, New York, Berlin, Heidelberg.

Uzunogullari U. and Wang J. L. (1992). A comparision of Hazard Rate Estimators for Left Truncated and Right Censored Data, *Biometrika*, **79**, 2, 297-310.

Wand, I. P. and Jones, I. C. (1995). *Kernel smoothing*, Chapman & Hall.

Watson G. S. and Leadbetter M. R. (1964). Hazard Analysis I., *Biometrika*, **51**, 1/2, 175-184.

Yandell B. S. (1983). Nonparametric Inference for Rates with Censored Survival Data, *The Annals of Statistics*, **11**, 4, 1119-1135.

Youndjé E., Sarda P. and Vieu P. (1996). Optimal Smooth Hazard Estimates, *Test*, **5**, 2, 379-394.

5 Partially Linear Models

Wolfgang Härdle and Hua Liang

5.1 Introduction

Partially linear models (PLM) are regression models in which the response depends on some covariates linearly but on other covariates nonparametrically. PLMs generalize standard linear regression techniques and are special cases of additive models. This chapter covers the basic results and explains how PLMs are applied in the biometric practice. More specifically, we are mainly concerned with least squares estimators of the linear parameter while the nonparametric part is estimated by e.g. kernel regression, spline approximation, piecewise polynomial and local polynomial techniques. When the model is heteroscedastic, the variance functions are approximated by weighted least squares estimators. Numerous examples illustrate the implementation in practice.

PLMs are defined by

$$Y = X^\top \beta + g(T) + \varepsilon, \tag{5.1}$$

where X and T are d-dimensional and scalar regressors, β is a vector of unknown parameters, $g(\cdot)$ an unknown smooth function and ε an error term with mean zero conditional on X and T.

The PLM is a special form of the additive regression models Hastie and Tibshrani (1990); Stone (1985), which allows easier interpretation of the effect of each variables and may be preferable to a completely nonparametric regression since the well-known reason "curse of dimensionality". On the other hand, PLMs are more flexible than the standard linear models since they combine both parametric and nonparametric components.

Several methods have been proposed to estimate PLMs. Suppose there are n observations $\{X_i, T_i, Y_i\}_{i=1}^n$. Engle, Granger, Rice and Weiss (1986), Heckman (1986) and Rice (1986) used spline smoothing and defined estimators of β and g as the solution of

$$\arg\min_{\beta,g} \frac{1}{n}\sum_{i=1}^{n}\{Y_i - X_i^{\top}\beta - g(T_i)\}^2 + \lambda \int \{g''(u)\}^2 du. \qquad (5.2)$$

Speckman (1988) estimated the nonparametric component by $\mathcal{W}\gamma$, where $\mathcal{W}$ is a $(n \times q)$−matrix of full rank and γ is an additional parameter. A PLM may be rewritten in a matrix form

$$Y = X\beta + \mathcal{W}\gamma + \varepsilon. \qquad (5.3)$$

The estimator of β based on (5.3) is

$$\widehat{\beta}_S = \{X^{\top}(I - P_{\mathcal{W}})X\}^{-1}\{X^{\top}(I - P_{\mathcal{W}})Y\}, \qquad (5.4)$$

where $P_{\mathcal{W}} = \mathcal{W}(\mathcal{W}^{\top}\mathcal{W})^{-1}\mathcal{W}^{\top}$ is a projection matrix and I is a d−order identity matrix. Green, Jennison and Seheult (1985) proposed another class of estimates

$$\widehat{\beta}_{\mathrm{GJS}} = \{X^{\top}(I - \mathcal{W}_h)X)\}^{-1}\{X^{\top}(I - \mathcal{W}_h)Y)\}$$

by replacing $\mathcal{W}$ in (5.4) by another smoother operator $\mathcal{W}_h$. Chen (1988) proposed a piecewise polynomial to approximate nonparametric function and then derived the least squares estimator which is the same form as (5.4). Recently Härdle, Liang and Gao (2000) have systematically summarized the different approaches to PLM estimation.

No matter which regression method is used for the nonparametric part, the forms of the estimators of β may always be written as

$$\{X^{\top}(I - W)X\}^{-1}\{X^{\top}(I - W)Y\},$$

where W is a projection operation. The estimators are asymptotically normal under appropriate assumptions.

The next section will be concerned with several nonparametric fit methods for $g(t)$ because of their popularity, beauty and importance in nonparametric statistics. In Section 5.4, the Framingham heart study data are investigated for illustrating the theory and the proposed statistical techniques.

5.2 Estimation and Nonparametric Fits

As stated in the previous section, different ways to approximate the nonparametric part yield the corresponding estimators of β. The popular nonparametric methods includes kernel regression, local polynomial, piecewise polynomial and smoothing spline. Related works are referred to Wand and Jones (1995), Eubank (1988), and Fan and Gijbels (1996). Härdle (1990) gives an extensive discussion of various nonparametric statistical methods based on the kernel estimator. This section mainly mentions the estimation procedure for β when one adapts these nonparametric methods and explains how to use XploRe quantlets to calculate the estimates.

5.2.1 Kernel Regression

Let $K(\cdot)$ be a kernel function satisfying certain conditions and h_n be a bandwidth parameter. The weight function is defined as:

$$\omega_{ni}(t) = K\left(\frac{t - T_i}{h_n}\right) \Big/ \sum_{j=1}^{n} K\left(\frac{t - T_j}{h_n}\right).$$

Let $g_n(t, \beta) = \sum_{i=1}^{n} \omega_{ni}(t)(Y_i - X_i^\top \beta)$ for a given β. Substitute $g_n(T_i, \beta)$ into (5.1) and use least square criterion. Then the least squares estimator of β is obtained as

$$\widehat{\beta}_{\mathrm{KR}} = (\widetilde{\mathbf{X}}^\top \widetilde{\mathbf{X}})^{-1} \widetilde{\mathbf{X}}^\top \widetilde{\mathbf{Y}},$$

where $\widetilde{\mathbf{X}}^\top = (\widetilde{X}_1, \ldots, \widetilde{X}_n)$ with $\widetilde{X}_j = X_j - \sum_{i=1}^{n} \omega_{ni}(T_j)X_i$ and $\widetilde{\mathbf{Y}}^\top = (\widetilde{Y}_1, \ldots, \widetilde{Y}_n)$ with $\widetilde{Y}_j = Y_j - \sum_{i=1}^{n} \omega_{ni}(T_j)Y_i$. The nonparametric part $g(t)$ is estimated by:

$$\widehat{g}_n(t) = \sum_{i=1}^{n} \omega_{ni}(t)(Y_i - X_i^\top \widehat{\beta}_{\mathrm{KR}}).$$

When $\varepsilon_1, \ldots, \varepsilon_n$ are identically distributed, their common variance σ^2 may be estimated by $\widehat{\sigma}_n^2 = (\widetilde{\mathbf{Y}} - \widetilde{\mathbf{X}}\widehat{\beta}_{\mathrm{KR}})^\top (\widetilde{\mathbf{Y}} - \widetilde{\mathbf{X}}\widehat{\beta}_{\mathrm{KR}})$.

For detailed discussion on asymptotic theories of these estimators we refer to Härdle, Liang and Gao (2000) and Speckman (1988). A main result on the estimator $\widehat{\beta}_{\mathrm{KR}}$ is:

THEOREM 5.1 *Suppose (i)* $\sup_{0 \leq t \leq 1} E(\|X\|^3 | t) < \infty$ *and* $\Sigma = Cov\{X - E(X|T)\}$ *is a positive definite matrix. (ii)* $g(t)$ *and* $E(x_{ij}|t)$ *are Lipschitz continuous; and (iii) the bandwidth* $h \approx \lambda n^{-1/5}$ *for some* $0 < \lambda < \infty$*. Then*

$$\sqrt{n}(\widehat{\beta}_{\mathrm{KR}} - \beta) \overset{\mathcal{L}}{\longrightarrow} N(0, \sigma^2 \Sigma^{-1}).$$

In XploRe the quantlet `plmk` calculates the estimates $\widehat{\beta}_{\mathrm{KR}}$, $\widehat{\sigma}_n^2$ and $\widehat{g}_n(t)$. Its syntax is the following:

```
plmest=plmk(x,t,y,h)
```

                                                     Q plmk.xpl

Input parameters:
x: the linear regressors
t: represents the non-linear regressors
y: the response
h: determines the bandwidth

Output parameters:
plmest.hbeat: estimate the parameter of X
plmest.hsigma: estimate the variance of the error
plmest.hg: estimate the nonparametric part

5.2.2 Local Polynomial

The kernel regression (or local constant) can be improved by using local linear, more generally, local polynomial smoothers since they have appealing asymptotic bias and variance terms that are not adversely affected at the boundary, Fan and Gijbels (1996).

Suppose that the $(p+1)$-th derivative of $g(t)$ at the point t_0 exists. We then approximate the unknown regression function $g(t)$ locally by a polynomial of order p. A Taylor expansion gives, for t in a neighborhood of t_0,

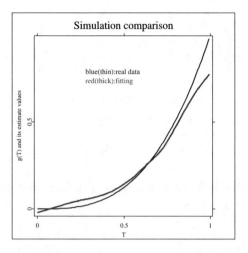

Figure 5.1: The simulation results for nonparametric function via quantlet plmk. Real data (thin) and the fitting (thick)

⊙ XCSplm01.xpl

$$g(t) \approx g(t_0) + g'(t_0)(t - t_0) + \frac{g^{(2)}(t_0)}{2!}(t - t_0)^2 + \cdots + \frac{g^{(p)}(t_0)}{p!}(t - t_0)^p$$

$$\overset{\text{def}}{=} \sum_{j=0}^{p} \alpha_j(t - t_0)^j. \tag{5.5}$$

To estimate β and $g(t)$, we first estimate α_j as the functions of β, denoted as $\alpha_j(\beta)$, by minimizing

$$\sum_{i=1}^{n} \left\{ Y_i - X_i^\top \beta - \sum_{j=0}^{p} \alpha_j(T_i - t_0)^j \right\}^2 K_h(T_i - t_0), \tag{5.6}$$

where h is a bandwidth controlling the size of the local neighborhood, and $K_h(\cdot) = K(\cdot/h)/h$ with K a kernel function. Minimize

$$\sum_{i=1}^{n} \left\{ Y_i - X_i^\top \beta - \sum_{j=0}^{p} \alpha_j(\beta)(T_i - t_0)^j \right\}^2 . \tag{5.7}$$

Denote the solution of (5.7) by β_n. Let $\alpha_j(\beta_n)$ be the estimate of α_j, and denote by $\widehat{\alpha}_{jn}$ $j = 0, \ldots, p$. It is clear from the Taylor expansion in (5.5) that $\nu! \widehat{\alpha}_{jn}$ is an estimator of $g^{(j)}(t_0)$ for $j = 0, \ldots, p$. To estimate the entire function $g^{(j)}(\cdot)$ we solve the above weighted least squares problem for all points t_0 in the domain of interest.

It is more convenient to work with matrix notation. Denote by $\mathbf{Z}$ the design matrix of T in problem (5.6). That is,

$$\mathbf{Z} = \begin{pmatrix} 1 & (T_1 - t_0) & \cdots & (T_1 - t_0)^p \\ \vdots & \vdots & \vdots & \vdots \\ 1 & (T_n - t_0) & \cdots & (T_n - t_0)^p \end{pmatrix} .$$

Set $\mathbf{Y} = (Y_1, \cdots, Y_n)^\top$ and $\alpha(\beta) = (\alpha_0(\beta), \cdots, \alpha_p(\beta))^\top$. Let $\mathbf{W}$ be the $n \times n$ diagonal matrix of weights: $\mathbf{W} = \operatorname{diag}\{K_h(T_i - t_0)\}$. The weighted least squares problems (5.6) and (5.7) can be rewritten as

$$\min_{\beta} (\mathbf{Y} - \mathbf{X}\beta - \mathbf{Z}\alpha)^\top \mathbf{W} (\mathbf{Y} - \mathbf{X}\beta - \mathbf{Z}\alpha),$$

$$\min_{\alpha} \{\mathbf{Y} - \mathbf{X}\beta - \mathbf{Z}\alpha(\beta)\}^\top \{\mathbf{Y} - \mathbf{X}\beta - \mathbf{Z}\alpha(\beta)\},$$

with $\alpha(\beta) = (\alpha_0(\beta), \ldots, \alpha_p(\beta))^\top$. The solution vectors are provided by weighted least squares and are given by

$$\widehat{\beta}_{\mathrm{LP}} = [\mathbf{X}^\top \{\mathbf{I} - \mathbf{Z}(\mathbf{Z}^\top \mathbf{W}\mathbf{Z})^{-1} \mathbf{Z}^\top \mathbf{W}\} \mathbf{X}]^{-1} \mathbf{X}^\top \{\mathbf{I} - \mathbf{Z}(\mathbf{Z}^\top \mathbf{W}\mathbf{Z})^{-1} \mathbf{Z}^\top \mathbf{W}\} \mathbf{Y}$$

$$\widehat{\alpha} = (\mathbf{Z}^\top \mathbf{W}\mathbf{Z})^{-1} \mathbf{Z}^\top \mathbf{W} (\mathbf{Y} - \mathbf{X}\widehat{\beta}_{\mathrm{LP}})$$

Theoretically the asymptotic normality is still valid under the conditions similarly to those of Theorem 5.1. More detailed theoretical discussions are referred to Hamilton and Truong (1997).

The quantlet `plmp` is assigned to handle the calculation of $\widehat{\beta}_{\mathrm{LP}}$ and $\widehat{\alpha}$. Its syntax is similar to that of the quantlet `plmk`:

```
plmest=plmp(x,t,y,h,{p})
```

where x, t, y, h are the same as in the quantlet `plmk`. p is the local polynomial order. The default value is $p = 1$, meaning the local linear estimator.

As a consequence, the estimate of the parameter equals

$$(1.2019, 1.2986, 1.3968)$$

and the estimates of the nonparametric function is shown in Figure 5.2. There exist obvious differences between these results from the quantlet `plmk` and `plmp`. More specifically, the results for parametric and nonparametric estimation from the quantlet `plmp` are preferable to those from the quantlet `plmk`.

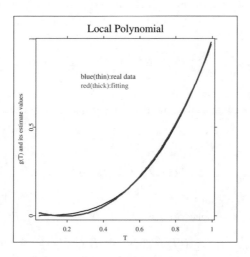

Figure 5.2: The simulation results for nonparametric function via quantlet `plmp`. Real data (thin) and the fitting (thick).

Q XCSplm02.xpl

5.2.3 Piecewise Polynomial

We assume g is Hölder continuous smooth of order $p = (m + r)$, that is, let r and m denote nonnegative real constants $0 < r \leq 1$, m is nonnegative integer such that

$$|g^{(m)}(t') - g^{(m)}(t)| < M|t' - t|^r, \text{ for } t, t' \in [0, 1].$$

Piecewise polynomial approximation for the function $g(\cdot)$ on $[0, 1]$ is defined as follows. Given a positive M_n, divide $[0, 1]$ in M_n intervals with equal length $1/M_n$. The estimator has the form of a piecewise polynomial of degree m based on the M_n intervals, where the $(m + 1)M_n$ coefficients are chosen by the method of least squares on the basis of the data. The basic principle is concisely stated as follows.

Let $I_{n\nu}(t)$ be the indicator function of the ν-th interval, and d_ν be the midpoint of the ν-th interval, so that $I_{n\nu}(t) = 1$ or 0 according to $t \in [(\nu - 1)/M_n, \nu/M_n)$ for $\nu = 1, \ldots, M_n$ and $[1 - 1/M_n, 1]$ or not. $P_{n\nu}(t)$ be the m-order Taylor expansion of $g(t)$ at the point d_ν. Denote

$$P_{n\nu}(t) = \sum_{j=0}^{m} a_{ju} t^j \text{ for } t \text{ in the } \nu\text{-th interval.}$$

Consider the piecewise polynomial approximation of g of degree m given by

$$g_n^*(t) = \sum_{\nu=1}^{M_n} I_\nu(t) P_{n\nu}(t).$$

Suppose we have n observed data $(X_1, T_1, Y_1), \ldots, (X_n, T_n, Y_n)$. Denote

$$\mathbf{Z} = \begin{pmatrix} I_{n1}(T_1) & \cdots & I_{n1}(T_1)T_1^m & \cdots & I_{nM_n}(T_1) & \cdots & I_{nM_n}(T_1)T_1^m \\ \vdots & \vdots & \vdots & \vdots & \vdots & \vdots & \vdots \\ I_{n1}(T_n) & \cdots & I_{n1}(T_n)T_n^m & \cdots & I_{nM_n}(T_n) & \cdots & I_{nM_n}(T_n)T_n^m \end{pmatrix}$$

and

$$\eta_{\mathbf{g}} = (a_{01}, \ldots, a_{m1}, a_{02}, \ldots, a_{m2}, \ldots, a_{0M_n}, \ldots, a_{mM_n})^\top.$$

Then

$$\begin{pmatrix} g_n^*(T_1) \\ \vdots \\ g_n^*(T_n) \end{pmatrix} = \begin{pmatrix} \sum_{u=1}^{M_n} I_{nu}(T_1) P_{n\nu}(T_1) \\ \vdots \\ \sum_{u=1}^{M_n} I_{nu}(T_n) P_{n\nu}(T_n) \end{pmatrix} = \mathbf{Z}\eta_{\mathbf{g}}.$$

Hence we need to find β and η_g to minimize

$$(\mathbf{Y} - \mathbf{X}\beta - \mathbf{Z}\eta_{\mathbf{g}})^\top (\mathbf{Y} - \mathbf{X}\beta - \mathbf{Z}\eta_{\mathbf{g}}).$$

Suppose that the solution of minimization problem exists. The estimators of β and η_g are

$$\widehat{\beta}_{\mathrm{PP}} = \{\mathbf{X}^\top (\mathbf{I} - \mathbf{P})\mathbf{X}\}^{-1}\mathbf{X}^\top (\mathbf{I} - \mathbf{P})\mathbf{Y}$$

and $\eta_{ng} = \mathbf{A}(\mathbf{Y} - \mathbf{X}\widehat{\beta}_{\mathrm{PP}})$, where $\mathbf{A} = (\mathbf{Z}^\top\mathbf{Z})^{-1}\mathbf{Z}^\top$ and $\mathbf{P} = \mathbf{Z}\mathbf{A}$. The estimate of $g(t)$ may be described

$$g_n(t) = z(\mathbf{Z}^\top\mathbf{Z})^{-1}\mathbf{Z}^\top(\mathbf{Y} - \mathbf{X}\widehat{\beta}_{\mathrm{PP}})$$

for a suitable z.

THEOREM 5.2 *There exist positive definite matrices Σ_{00} and Σ_{01} such that both $Cov(X|t) - \Sigma_{00}$ and $\Sigma_{01} - Cov(X|t)$ are nonnegative definite for all $t \in [0, 1]$. Suppose that $\lim_{n\to\infty} n^{-\lambda}M_n = 0$ for some $\lambda \in (0, 1)$ and $\lim_{n\to\infty} \sqrt{n}M_n^{-p} = 0$. Then $\sqrt{n}(\widehat{\beta}_{\mathrm{PP}} - \beta) \overset{\mathcal{L}}{\longrightarrow} N(0, \sigma^2\Sigma^{-1})$.*

The quantlet `plmp` evaluates the estimates $\widehat{\beta}_{\mathrm{PP}}$ and $g_n(t)$ stated above. Its syntax is similar to those of the two previous quantlets:

```
plmest=plmp(x,t,y,m,mn)
```

where `m` and `mn` represent m and M_n, respectively. We now use the quantlet `plmp` to investigate the example considered in the quantlet `plmk`. We assume $m = 2$ and $M_n = 5$ and compute the related estimates via the quantlet `plmp`. The implementation works as follows.

Q XCSplm03.xpl

The result for parameter β is `plmest.hbeta`$= (1.2, 1.2999, 1.3988)^\top$. Alternatively the estimates for nonparametric part are also given.

5.2.4   Least Square Spline

This subsection introduces least squares splines. We only state its algorithm rather than the theory, which can be found in Eubank (1988) for an overall discussion.

Suppose that g has $m-1$ absolutely continuous derivatives and m-th derivative that is square integrable and satisfies $\int_0^1 \{g^{(m)}(t)\}^2 dt < C$ for a specified $C > 0$. Via a Taylor expansion, the PLM can be rewritten as

$$Y = X^\top \beta + \sum_{j=1}^{m} \alpha_j T^{j-1} + Rem(T) + \varepsilon,$$

where $Rem(s) = (m-1)!^{-1} \int_0^1 \{g^{(m)}(t)(t-s)_+^{m-1}\}^2 dt$. By using a quadrature rule, $Rem(s)$ can be approximated by a sum of the form $\sum_{j=1}^{k} d_j (t-t_j)_+^{m-1}$ for some set of coefficients $d_1, \ldots, d_k$ and points $0 < t_1, \ldots, < t_k < 1$. Take a basis $V_1(t) = 1$, $V_2(t) = t$, $\ldots$, $V_m(t) = t^{m-1}$, $V_{m+1}(t) = (t-t_1)^{m-1}$, $\ldots$, $V_{m+k}(t) = (t-t_k)^{m-1}$ and set

$$\eta = (\alpha_1, \ldots, \alpha_m, d_1, \ldots, d_k) \stackrel{\text{def}}{=} (\eta_1, \ldots, \eta_{m+k})^\top$$

The least squares spline estimator is to minimize

$$\underset{\beta, \eta}{\arg\min} \frac{1}{n} \sum_{i=1}^{n} \left\{ Y_i - X_i^\top \beta - \sum_{j=1}^{m+k} \eta_j V_j(T_i) \right\}^2 .$$

Conveniently with matrix notation, denote $\mathbf{Z} = (Z_{ij})$ with $Z_{ij} = \{V_j(T_i)\}$ for $i = 1, \ldots, n$ and $j = 1, \ldots, m+k$ and $\mathbf{X} = (X_1, \ldots, X_n)^\top$. The least squares spline estimator is equivalent to the solution of the minimizing problem

$$(\mathbf{Y} - \mathbf{X}\beta - \mathbf{Z}\eta)^\top (\mathbf{Y} - \mathbf{X}\beta - \mathbf{Z}\eta).$$

If the problem has an unique solution, its form is the same as $(\widehat{\beta}_{\text{PP}}, \eta_{ng})$ in the subsection about piecewise polynomial. Otherwise, we may use a ridge estimator idea to modify the estimator. plmls is concerned with implementation of the above algorithm in XploRe.

```
plmest=plmls(x,t,y,m,knots)
```

Q XCSplm04.xpl

Input parameters:
x: $n \times d$ matrix of the linear design points
t: $n \times 1$ vector of the non-linear design points
y: $n \times 1$ vector of the response variables
m: the order of spline
knots: $k \times 1$ vector of knot sequence knots

Output parameters:
plmest.hbeat: $d \times 1$ vector of the estimate of the parameter
plmest.hg: the estimate of the nonparametric part

5.3 Heteroscedastic Cases

When the variance function given covariates (X, T) is non-constant, the estimators of β proposed in former section is inefficient. The strategy of overcoming this drawback is to use weighted least squares estimation. Three cases will be briefly discussed. Let $\{(Y_i, X_i, T_i), i = 1, \ldots, n\}$ denote a sequence of random samples from

$$Y_i = X_i^\top \beta + g(T_i) + \sigma_i \xi_i, i = 1, \ldots, n, \qquad (5.8)$$

where X_i, T_i are the same as those in model (5.1). ξ_i are i.i.d. with mean 0 and variance 1, and σ_i^2 are some functions, whose concrete forms will be discussed later.

In general, the least squares estimator $\widehat{\beta}_{\mathrm{LS}}$ is modified to a weighted least squares estimator

$$\beta_W = \left(\sum_{i=1}^n \gamma_i \widetilde{X}_i \widetilde{X}_i^\top \right)^{-1} \left(\sum_{i=1}^n \gamma_i \widetilde{X}_i \widetilde{Y}_i \right) \qquad (5.9)$$

for some weight γ_i, $i = 1, \ldots, n$. In our model (5.8) we take $\gamma_i = 1/\sigma_i^2$. In principle the weights γ_i (or σ_i^2) are unknown and must be estimated. Let

$\{\widehat{\gamma}_i, i = 1, \ldots, n\}$ be a sequence of estimators of γ. One may define an estimator of β by substituting γ_i in (5.9) by $\widehat{\gamma}_i$. Let

$$\widehat{\beta}_{\text{WLS}} = \left(\sum_{i=1}^{n} \widehat{\gamma}_i \widetilde{X}_i \widetilde{X}_i^\top \right)^{-1} \left(\sum_{i=1}^{n} \widehat{\gamma}_i \widetilde{X}_i \widetilde{Y}_i \right)$$

be the estimator of β.

Under suitable conditions, the estimator $\widehat{\beta}_{\text{WLS}}$ is asymptotically equivalent to that supposed the function σ_i^2 to be known. Therefore $\widehat{\beta}_{\text{WLS}}$ is more efficient than the estimators given in the previous section. The following subsections present three variance functions and construct their estimators. Three non-parametric heteroscedastic structures will be studied. In the remainder of this section, $H(\cdot)$ is always assumed to be unknown Lipschitz continuous.

5.3.1   Variance Is a Function of Exogenous Variables

Suppose $\sigma_i^2 = H(W_i)$, where $\{W_i; i = 1, \ldots, n\}$ are design points, which are assumed to be independent of ξ_i and (X_i, T_i) and defined on $[0, 1]$ in the case where $\{W_i; i = 1, \ldots, n\}$ are random design points. Let $\widehat{\beta}_{\text{LS}}$ and $\widehat{g}_n(\cdot)$ be initial estimators of β and $g(\cdot)$, for example, given by kernel regression in Section 5.2.1. Define

$$\widehat{H}_n(w) = \sum_{j=1}^{n} \widetilde{W}_{nj}(w)\{Y_j - X_j^\top \widehat{\beta}_{\text{LS}} - \widehat{g}_n(T_i)\}^2$$

as the estimator of $H(w)$, where $\{\widetilde{W}_{nj}(t); i = 1, \ldots, n\}$ is a sequence of weight functions satisfying appropriate assumptions. Then let $\widehat{\sigma}_{ni}^2 = H_n(W_i)$.

Quantlet `plmhetexog` performs the weighted least squares estimate of the parameter. In the procedure of estimating the variance function, the estimate given by `plmk` is taken as the primary one.

Q `XCSplm05.xpl`

5.3.2 Variance Is an Unknown Function of T

Suppose that the variance σ_i^2 is a function of the design points T_i, i.e., $\sigma_i^2 = H(T_i)$, with $H(\cdot)$ an unknown Lipschitz continuous function. Similarly to subsection 5.3.1, we define the estimator of $H(\cdot)$ as

$$\widehat{H}_n(t) = \sum_{j=1}^{n} \widetilde{W}_{nj}(t)\{Y_j - X_j^\top \widehat{\beta}_{\mathrm{LS}} - \widehat{g}_n(T_i)\}^2.$$

Quantlet `plmhett` calculates the weighted least squares estimate of the parameter in this case. In the procedure of estimating the variance function, the estimate given by `plmk` is taken as the primary one.

    plmest=plmhett(x,t,y,h,h1)

Q XCSplm06.xpl

5.3.3 Variance Is a Function of the Mean

We consider the model (5.8) with $\sigma_i^2 = H\{X_i^\top \beta + g(T_i)\}$, which means that the variance is an unknown function of the mean response.

Since $H(\cdot)$ is assumed to be completely unknown, the standard method is to get information about $H(\cdot)$ by replication, i.e., we consider the following "improved" partially linear heteroscedastic model

$$Y_{ij} = X_i^\top \beta + g(T_i) + \sigma_i \xi_{ij}, \quad j = 1, \ldots, m_i; \quad i = 1, \ldots, n,$$

where Y_{ij} is the response of the j-th replicate at the design point (X_i, T_i), ξ_{ij} are i.i.d. with mean 0 and variance 1, β, $g(\cdot)$ and (X_i, T_i) are the same as before.

We compute the predicted value $X_i^\top \widehat{\beta}_{\mathrm{LS}} + \widehat{g}_n(T_i)$ by fitting the least squares estimator $\widehat{\beta}_{\mathrm{LS}}$ and nonparametric estimator $\widehat{g}_n(T_i)$ to the data and the residuals $Y_{ij} - \{X_i^\top \widehat{\beta}_{\mathrm{LS}} + \widehat{g}_n(T_i)\}$, and estimate σ_i^2 by

$$\widehat{\sigma}_i^2 = \frac{1}{m_i} \sum_{j=1}^{m_i} [Y_{ij} - \{X_i^\top \widehat{\beta}_{\mathrm{LS}} + \widehat{g}_n(T_i)\}]^2,$$

where each m_i is unbounded.

Quantlet `plmhetmean` executes the above algorithm in XploRe. For calculation simplicity, we use the same replicate in practice. The estimate given by `plmk` is taken as the primary one.

```
plmest=plmhetmean(mn,x,t,y,h)
```

Q XCSplm07.xpl

5.4 Real Data Examples

In this section we analyze the well known Framingham data set and illustrate the calculation results when using the quantlets introduced in Section 5.2.

EXAMPLE 5.1 *We use the data from the* Framingham Heart Study *which consists of a series of exams taken two years apart, to illustrate one of the applications of PLM in biometrics. There are 1615 men, aged between 31 to 65, in this data set. The outcome Y represents systolic blood pressure (SBP). Covariates employed in this example are patient's age (T) and the serum cholesterol level (X). Empirical study indicates that SBP linearly depends upon the serum cholesterol level but nonlinearly on age. For this reason, we apply PLM to investigate the function relationship between Y and (T, X).*

Specifically, we estimate β and $g(\cdot)$ in the model

$$Y_i = X_i\beta + g(T_i) + \varepsilon_i, \quad i = 1, \cdots, 1615.$$

For nonparametric fitting, we use a Nadaraya-Watson weight function with quartic kernel

$$(15/16)(1 - u^2)^2 \boldsymbol{I}(|u| \leq 1)$$

and choose the bandwidth using cross-validation.

The estimated value of the linear parameter equals to 10.617, and the estimate of $g(T)$ is given in Figure 5.3. The figure shows that with the age increasing, SBP increases but looks like a straight line. The older the age, the higher the SBP is.

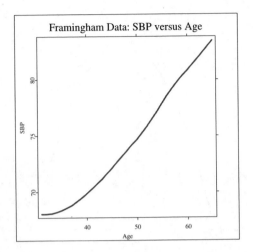

Figure 5.3: Relationship SBP and serum cholesterol level in Framingham Heart Study.

Q XCSplm08.xpl

EXAMPLE 5.2 *This is an example of using PLM to analyze the* NHANES *Cancer data. This data set is a cohort study originally consisting of 8596 women, who were interviewed about their nutrition habits and when later examined for evidence of cancer. We restrict attention to a sub-cohort of 3145 women aged 25 − 50 who have no missing data the variables of interest. The outcome Y is saturated fat, while the predictors include age, body mass index (BMI), protein and vitamin A and B intaken. Again it is believable that Y depends as in (5.2) nonlinearly on age but linear upon other dummy variables.*

In this example we give an illustration of the `plmls` for the real data. We select $m = 3$ and the knots at $(35, 46)$. As a consequence, the estimates of linear parameters are $(-0.162, 0.317, -0.00002, -0.0047)$, and the nonparametric estimated are shown in Figure 5.4. The curve of the nonparametric part in this data set is completely different from that of the above example and looks like arch-shape. The pattern reaches to maximum point at about age 35.

We also run other quantlets for these two data sets. We found that the estimates of nonparametric parts from different quantlets have similar shapes,

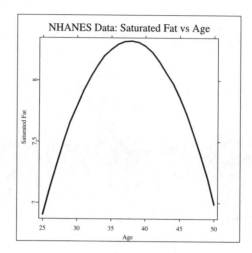

Figure 5.4: NHANES regression of saturated fat on age.

Q XCSnhanes.xpl

although differences in the magnitude of the estimates from different estimation methods are visible.

Bibliography

de Boor, C. (1978). *A Practical Guide to Splines.* New York:Springer-Verlag.

Chen, H.(1988). Convergence rates for parametric components in a partly linear model. *Annals of Statistics,* **16**, 136-146.

Engle, R. F., Granger, C. W. J., Rice, J. and Weiss, A. (1986). Semiparametric estimates of the relation between weather and electricity sales. *J. Amer. Stat. Assoc.,* **81**, 310-320.

Eubank, R. L. (1988). *Spline Smoothing and Nonparametric Regression.* New York: Marcel Dekker.

Fan, J. and Gijbels, I. (1996). *Local Polynomial Modelling and Its Applications.* Vol. 66 of *Monographs on Statistics and Applied Probability,* Chapman and Hall, New York.

Green, P., Jennison, C. and Seheult, A. (1985). Analysis of field experiments by least squares smoothing. *Journal of the Royal Statistical Society, Series B*, **47**, 299-315.

Härdle, W. (1990). *Applied Nonparametric Regression*. Cambridge University Press, New York.

Härdle, W., Liang, H. and Gao, J. T. (2000). *Partially Linear Models*. Springer-Physica-Verlag, Heidelberg.

Hastie, T. J. and Tibshirani, R. J. (1990). *Generalized Additive Models*. Vol. 43 of *Monographs on Statistics and Applied Probability*, Chapman and Hall, London.

Hamilton, S. A. and Truong, Y. K. (1997). Local linear estimation in partly linear models. *Journal of Multivariate Analysis*, **60**, 1-19.

Heckman, N.E. (1986). Spline smoothing in partly linear models. *Journal of the Royal Statistical Society, Series B*, **48**, 244-248.

Rice, J.(1986). Convergence rates for partially splined models. *Statistics & Probability Letters*, **4**, 203-208.

Robinson, P.M.(1988). Root-n-consistent semiparametric regression. *Econometrica*, **56**, 931-954.

Speckman, P. (1988). Kernel smoothing in partial linear models. *Journal of the Royal Statistical Society, Series B*, **50**, 413-436.

Stone, J. C. (1985). Additive regression and other nonparametric models. *Annals of Statistics*, **13**, 689-705.

Wand, M.P. and Jones, M. C.(1995). *Kernel Smoothing*. Vol. 60 of *Monographs on Statistics and Applied Probability*, Chapman and Hall, London.

6 Analysis of Contingency Tables

Masahiro Kuroda

6.1 Introduction

This chapter presents analysis of log-linear models for contingency tables. In analysis of contingency tables, we are interested in associations and interactions among the categorical variables or interpretations of the parameters describing the model structure. Then our goal is to find a best model such that the model structure is simple and the model has few parameters.

The log-linear models which is used in analysis of contingency tables are a generalized linear model for counted data and can easily describe the variety of associations and interactions among the variables. To search a best model, we assess the effects on interaction terms in log-linear models by goodness of fit tests. The methodology for analysis of contingency tables is described in many books, for example, Bishop et al. (1975), Everitt (1977) and Agresti (2002).

This chapter is organized as follows: Section 11.2 introduces log-linear models and generalized linear models. Moreover we provide the procedures to find the best model by using goodness of fit tests for independence and comparing two log-linear models. Section 11.3 presents the XploRe functions to make inferences for log-linear models. Contingency table analysis using XploRe are illustrated in Section 11.4.

6.2 Log-linear Models

Let $Y = (Y_1, Y_2, \ldots, Y_D)$ be categorical variables. Then a rectangular $(N \times D)$ data matrix consisting of N observations on Y can be rearranged as a D-way contingency table with cells defined by joint levels of the variables. Let $n_{ij\ldots t}$ denote the frequency for a cell $Y = (i, j, \ldots, t)$ and $n = \{n_{ij\ldots t}\}$. Suppose that

Y has a multinomial distribution with an unknown parameter $\theta = \{\theta_{ij...t}\}$, where $\theta_{ij...t} \geq 0$ and $\sum \theta_{ij...t} = 1$. The log-linear model is expressed in the form

$$\log \theta = X\lambda, \tag{6.1}$$

where X is a $D \times r$ design matrix and λ is an $r \times 1$ parameter vector. When Y has a Poisson distribution, the log-linear model is re-written by

$$\log m = X\lambda, \tag{6.2}$$

where $m = \{m_{ij...t} = N\theta_{ij...t}\}$ is the vector of expected frequencies.

6.2.1   Log-linear Models for Two-way Contingency Tables

Consider an $I \times J$ contingency table. The log-linear model is represented by

$$\log \theta_{ij} = \lambda_0 + \lambda_i^1 + \lambda_j^2 + \lambda_{ij}^{12}, \tag{6.3}$$

for all i and j, under the constraints of the λ terms to sum to zero over any subscript such as

$$\sum_{i=1}^{I} \lambda_i^1 = 0, \quad \sum_{j=1}^{J} \lambda_j^2 = 0, \quad \sum_{i=1}^{I} \lambda_{ij}^{12} = \sum_{j=1}^{J} \lambda_{ij}^{12} = 0. \tag{6.4}$$

The log-linear model given by (6.3) is called the *saturated model* or the *full model* for the statistical dependency between Y_1 and Y_2.

By analogy with analysis of variance models, we define the overall mean by

$$\lambda_0 = \frac{1}{IJ} \sum_{i=1}^{I} \sum_{j=1}^{J} \log \theta_{ij},$$

the main effects of Y_1 and Y_2 by

$$\lambda_i^1 = \frac{1}{J} \sum_{j=1}^{J} \log \theta_{ij} - \lambda_0,$$

$$\lambda_j^2 = \frac{1}{I} \sum_{i=1}^{I} \log \theta_{ij} - \lambda_0,$$

and the two-factor effect between Y_1 and Y_2 by

$$\lambda_{ij}^{12} = \log \theta_{ij} - (\lambda_i^1 + \lambda_j^2) - \lambda_0.$$

Then the main and two-factor effects are determined by the odds and odds ratios, and can be written by

$$\lambda_i^1 = \frac{1}{IJ} \sum_{i'=1}^{I} \sum_{j=1}^{J} \log \frac{\theta_{ij}}{\theta_{i'j}},$$

$$\lambda_j^2 = \frac{1}{IJ} \sum_{i=1}^{I} \sum_{j'=1}^{J} \log \frac{\theta_{ij}}{\theta_{ij'}}$$

and

$$\lambda_{ij}^{12} = \frac{1}{IJ} \sum_{i'=1}^{I} \sum_{j'=1}^{J} \log \frac{\theta_{ij}\theta_{i'j'}}{\theta_{i'j}\theta_{ij'}}.$$

For the *independence model* that Y_1 is statistically independent of Y_2, the cell probability θ_{ij} can be factorized into the product of marginal probabilities θ_{i+} and θ_{+j}, that is,

$$\theta_{ij} = \theta_{i+}\theta_{+j},$$

where $\theta_{i+} = \sum_{j=1}^{J} \theta_{ij}$ and $\theta_{+j} = \sum_{i=1}^{I} \theta_{ij}$. Then the two-factor effect is

$$\lambda_{ij}^{12} = \frac{1}{IJ} \sum_{i'=1}^{I} \sum_{j'=1}^{J} \log \frac{\theta_{i+}\theta_{+j}\theta_{i'+}\theta_{+j'}}{\theta_{i'+}\theta_{+j}\theta_{i+}\theta_{+j'}} = 0,$$

so that the log-linear model for the independence model is expressed by

$$\log \theta_{ij} = \lambda_0 + \lambda_i^1 + \lambda_j^2,$$

for all i and j.

6.2.2 Log-linear Models for Three-way Contingency Tables

For an $I \times J \times K$ contingency table, the saturated log-linear model for the contingency table is

$$\log \theta_{ijk} = \lambda_0 + \lambda_i^1 + \lambda_j^2 + \lambda_k^3 + \lambda_{ij}^{12} + \lambda_{ik}^{13} + \lambda_{jk}^{23} + \lambda_{ijk}^{123},$$

for all i, j and k. The λ terms satisfy the constraints:

$$\sum_{i=1}^{I} \lambda_i^1 = \sum_{j=1}^{J} \lambda_j^2 = \sum_{k=1}^{K} \lambda_k^3 = 0,$$

$$\sum_{i=1}^{I} \lambda_{ij}^{12} = \sum_{j=1}^{J} \lambda_{ij}^{12} = \cdots = \sum_{k=1}^{K} \lambda_{jk}^{23} = 0,$$

$$\sum_{i=1}^{I} \lambda_{ijk}^{123} = \sum_{j=1}^{J} \lambda_{ijk}^{123} = \sum_{k=1}^{K} \lambda_{ijk}^{123} = 0.$$

We define the λ terms as follows: The overall mean is given by

$$\lambda_0 = \frac{1}{IJK} \sum_{i=1}^{I} \sum_{j=1}^{J} \sum_{k=1}^{K} \log \theta_{ijk}.$$

The main effects of Y_1, Y_2 and Y_3 are

$$\lambda_i^1 = \frac{1}{JK} \sum_{j=1}^{J} \sum_{k=1}^{K} \log \theta_{ijk} - \lambda_0,$$

$$\lambda_j^2 = \frac{1}{IK} \sum_{i=1}^{I} \sum_{k=1}^{K} \log \theta_{ijk} - \lambda_0,$$

$$\lambda_k^3 = \frac{1}{IJ} \sum_{i=1}^{I} \sum_{j=1}^{J} \log \theta_{ijk} - \lambda_0.$$

Each interaction effect is given by

$$\lambda_{ij}^{12} = \frac{1}{K} \sum_{k=1}^{K} \log \theta_{ijk} - (\lambda_i^1 + \lambda_j^2) - \lambda_0,$$

$$\lambda_{ik}^{13} = \frac{1}{J} \sum_{j=1}^{J} \log \theta_{ijk} - (\lambda_i^1 + \lambda_k^3) - \lambda_0,$$

$$\lambda_{jk}^{23} = \frac{1}{I} \sum_{i=1}^{I} \log \theta_{ijk} - (\lambda_j^2 + \lambda_k^3) - \lambda_0$$

and

$$\lambda_{ijk}^{123} = \log \theta_{ijk} - (\lambda_{ij}^{12} + \lambda_{ik}^{13} + \lambda_{jk}^{23}) - (\lambda_i^1 + \lambda_j^2 + \lambda_k^3) - \lambda_0.$$

Like log-linear models for two-ways contingency tables, the λ terms in the log-linear models for three-way contingency tables directly relate to the odds and odds ratios.

Here we introduce an important class of independence models that are called *hierarchical log-linear models*. In the hierarchical models, if high-order λ terms with certain variables are contained in the model, all lower-order λ terms with these same variables are included. For instance, when a log-linear model contains $\{\lambda_{ij}^{12}\}$, the log-linear model also contains $\{\lambda_i^1\}$ and $\{\lambda_j^2\}$. Table 6.1 is the list of the hierarchical log-linear models for three-way contingency tables. Interpretations of parameters in the log-linear models refer then to the highest-order terms.

In log-linear models for conditional independence models, the two-factor effects correspond to *partial associations*. For instance, the log-linear model $[Y_1Y_2][Y_2Y_3]$ permits two-factor terms for associations between Y_1 and Y_2, and Y_2 and Y_3, but does not contain a two-factor term for an association between Y_1 and Y_3. Then the log-linear model $[Y_1Y_2][Y_2Y_3]$ specifies conditional independence between Y_1 and Y_3 given Y_2. In the log-linear model $[Y_1Y_2][Y_1Y_3][Y_2Y_3]$ called the *no three-factor interaction model*, there exists conditional dependence for all three pairs. Then the no three-factor interaction model has equal conditional odds ratios between any two variables at each level of the third variable. For example, the conditional odds ratio of Y_1 to Y_2 in the k-th level of Y_3 does not depend on k, and is given by

$$\log \frac{m_{ijk}m_{IJk}}{m_{iJk}m_{Ijk}} = \lambda_{ij}^{12} + \lambda_{IJ}^{12} - \lambda_{iJ}^{12} - \lambda_{Ij}^{12},$$

for $i = 1, \ldots, I-1$, $j = 1, \ldots, J-1$ and all k.

With multi-way contingency tables, the independence models are more complicated than the models for three-way contingency tables. The log-linear models can also describe several models for multi-way contingency tables easily. The basic principles of log-linear models for three-way contingency tables can be extended readily to multi-way contingency tables.

6.2.3 Generalized Linear Models

The log-linear model is a special case of generalized linear models (McCullagh and Nelder, 1989). For cell frequencies in contingency tables, the generalized linear models assume a Poisson distribution as the link function. Thus the log-linear models are given by equation (6.2).

Table 6.1: Independence models for three-way contingency tables

Symbol	Log-linear model
Mutual independence	
$[Y_1][Y_2][Y_3]$	$\log\theta_{ijk} = \lambda_0 + \lambda_i^1 + \lambda_j^2 + \lambda_k^3$
Joint independence from two-factors	
$[Y_1][Y_2Y_3]$	$\log\theta_{ijk} = \lambda_0 + \lambda_i^1 + \lambda_j^2 + \lambda_k^3 + \lambda_{jk}^{23}$
$[Y_1Y_2][Y_3]$	$\log\theta_{ijk} = \lambda_0 + \lambda_i^1 + \lambda_j^2 + \lambda_k^3 + \lambda_{ij}^{12}$
$[Y_1Y_3][Y_2]$	$\log\theta_{ijk} = \lambda_0 + \lambda_i^1 + \lambda_j^2 + \lambda_k^3 + \lambda_{ik}^{13}$
Conditional independence	
$[Y_1Y_2][Y_1Y_3]$	$\log\theta_{ijk} = \lambda_0 + \lambda_i^1 + \lambda_j^2 + \lambda_k^3 + \lambda_{ij}^{12} + \lambda_{ik}^{13}$
$[Y_1Y_3][Y_2Y_3]$	$\log\theta_{ijk} = \lambda_0 + \lambda_i^1 + \lambda_j^2 + \lambda_k^3 + \lambda_{ik}^{13} + \lambda_{jk}^{23}$
$[Y_1Y_2][Y_2Y_3]$	$\log\theta_{ijk} = \lambda_0 + \lambda_i^1 + \lambda_j^2 + \lambda_k^3 + \lambda_{ij}^{12} + \lambda_{jk}^{23}$
No three-factor interaction	
$[Y_1Y_2][Y_1Y_3][Y_2Y_3]$	$\log\theta_{ijk} = \lambda_0 + \lambda_i^1 + \lambda_j^2 + \lambda_k^3 + \lambda_{ij}^{12} + \lambda_{ik}^{13} + \lambda_{jk}^{23}$

Consider a 2×3 contingency table. From the constraints

$$\sum_{i=1}^{2}\lambda_i^1 = 0, \qquad \sum_{j=1}^{3}\lambda_j^2 = 0, \qquad \sum_{i=1}^{2}\lambda_{ij}^{12} = \sum_{j=1}^{3}\lambda_{ij}^{12} = 0, \tag{6.5}$$

the parameter vector is identified by

$$\lambda = \left(\lambda_0, \lambda_1^1, \lambda_1^2, \lambda_2^2, \lambda_{11}^{12}, \lambda_{12}^{12}\right)^{\top}.$$

Thus the log-linear (6.2) can be written as

$$\begin{pmatrix} \log m_{11} \\ \log m_{12} \\ \log m_{13} \\ \log m_{21} \\ \log m_{22} \\ \log m_{23} \end{pmatrix} = \begin{pmatrix} 1 & 1 & 1 & 0 & 1 & 0 \\ 1 & 1 & 0 & 1 & 0 & 1 \\ 1 & 1 & -1 & -1 & -1 & -1 \\ 1 & -1 & 1 & 0 & -1 & 0 \\ 1 & -1 & 0 & 1 & 0 & -1 \\ 1 & -1 & -1 & -1 & -1 & -1 \end{pmatrix} \begin{pmatrix} \lambda_0 \\ \lambda_1^1 \\ \lambda_1^2 \\ \lambda_2^2 \\ \lambda_{11}^{12} \\ \lambda_{12}^{12} \end{pmatrix}.$$

When the maximum likelihood estimates (MLEs) of λ can not be found directly, iterative algorithms such as the Newton-Raphson and Fisher-scoring algorithms or the iterative proportional fitting procedure are applied. To compute the MLEs $\hat{\lambda}$ in log-linear models, XploRe uses the Newton-Raphson and Fisher-scoring algorithms.

6.2.4   Fitting to Log-linear Models

Chi-squared Goodness of Fit Tests

To test a log-linear model against the saturated model, we estimate the expected frequencies of the log-linear model and evaluate the adequacy by the Pearson chi-squared statistic. When the MLEs $\hat{\lambda}$ in a log-linear model are obtained, the expected frequencies are estimated from

$$\hat{m} = \exp(X\hat{\lambda}).$$

To assess a log-linear model fitting to the data by comparing n to $\hat{m}$, the Pearson chi-squared statistic

$$\chi^2 = \sum_{i,j,\dots,t} \frac{(n_{ij\dots t} - \hat{m}_{ij\dots t})^2}{\sqrt{\hat{m}_{ij\dots t}}}$$

is computed. As another measure of goodness of fit, the likelihood ratio test statistic is used. This test statistic is computed from

$$G^2 = 2 \sum_{i,j,\dots,t} n_{ij\dots t} \log \frac{n_{ij\dots t}}{\hat{m}_{ij\dots t}}.$$

If the sample size is sufficiently large, χ^2 and G^2 have an asymptotic chi-squared distribution with degrees of freedom (df) equal to the difference of the number of free parameters in the saturated model and a log-linear model. Then the chi-squared goodness of fit test can be conducted by the value of χ^2 or G^2.

Moreover the likelihood ratio test statistic G^2 can be used to compare two log-linear models M_1 and M_2. Then M_2 is nested in M_1, such that every nonzero λ terms in M_2 is contained in M_1. For example, the log-linear model $[Y_1 Y_2][Y_3]$ is the nested model in the log-linear model $[Y_1 Y_2][Y_2 Y_3]$ and these models are expressed by

$$\begin{aligned} M_1: &\quad \log \theta_{ijk} = \lambda_0 + \lambda_i^1 + \lambda_j^2 + \lambda_k^3 + \lambda_{ij}^{12} + \lambda_{jk}^{23}, \\ M_2: &\quad \log \theta_{ijk} = \lambda_0 + \lambda_i^1 + \lambda_j^2 + \lambda_k^3 + \lambda_{ij}^{12}. \end{aligned}$$

Thus M_2 is simpler than M_1 and M_1 must hold when M_2 holds. Assuming that M_1 holds, we test whether M_2 fits the data as well as M_1. To compare two models, the following test statistic is used:

$$\triangle G^2 = G_2^2 - G_1^2, \tag{6.6}$$

where G_1^2 and G_2^2 are the likelihood ratio test statistics for M_1 and M_2. Then $\triangle G^2$ also has an asymptotic chi-squared distribution with *df* equal to $(df \text{ for } M_1) - (df \text{ for } M_2)$.

When the value of $\triangle G^2$ is in a critical region, we conclude that M_2 provides a better description of the data. Furthermore $\triangle G^2$ is computed to compare a nested model in M_2 with M_2. If the value of $\triangle G^2$ is outside a critical region, we re-compare another nested model in M_1 with M_1. Repeating goodness of fit tests to compare nested models, we find a best model.

Other criteria to compare nested models, the Akaike information criteria (AIC) and the Bayesian information criteria (BIC) are well known.

Model Residuals

The goodness of fit statistic gives the summary of how well a log-linear model fits to the data. We examine lack of fit by comparing observed data to the fitted data individually.

For cell (i, j) in a two-way contingency table, the Pearson standardized residual is defined by

$$e_{ij} = \frac{n_{ij} - \hat{m}_{ij}}{\sqrt{\hat{m}_{ij}}}.$$

The Pearson residual is also related to the Pearson chi-squared test statistics by

$$\chi^2 = \sum_{i,j} e_{ij}^2.$$

When a log-linear model holds, the residuals $\{e_{ij}\}$ have an approximate normal distribution with mean 0. Then, by checking whether the Pearson residuals are larger than about ± 2 that is standard normal percentage points, we detect the presence of the data that are influential on the fit of a log-linear model.

6.3   Inference for Log-linear Models Using XploRe

To make inferences for log-linear models, we use the functions in the `glm` library. The library is available by

    library("glm")

6.3.1   Estimation of the Parameter Vector λ

The parameter vector λ can be estimated by using the `glmest` function

    glmest("polog", x, n)

where `polog` is a Poisson distribution with logarithm link function, `x` is the design matrix and `n` is the cell frequencies for contingency tables. Executing

    lambda = glmest("polog", x, n)

the estimates of λ are assigned to the variable `lambda`. Then `lambda` contains the following output:

`b` : the estimated parameter vector λ

`bv` : the estimated covariance of `b`

`stat` : several statistics

The expected frequencies `m` are also computed from

    m = exp(x*lambda.b)

Moreover the `glmest` function and other functions in `glm` library can be also specified several options by defining `opt` with `glmopt`. For the optional parameters, refer to Härdle et al. (1999) or Help function in XploRe.

6.3.2   Computing Statistics for the Log-linear Models

A number of statistical characteristics can be computed using the `glmstat` function. Then statistical characteristics can be obtained from

```
stat = glmstat("polog", x, m, lambda.b, lambda.bv)
```

and are stored in the output `stat`:

`df` : degrees of freedom

`deviance` : the deviance of the estimated model

`pearson` : the Pearson statistic

`loglik` : the log-likelihood of the estimated model, using the estimated dispersion parameter

`aic, bic` : Akaike's AIC and Schwarz' BIC criterion, respectively

`r2, adr2` : the (pseudo) coefficient of determination and its adjusted version, respectively

`it` : the number of iterations needed

`ret` : the return code

`nr` : the number of replicated observation in `x`, if they were searched for.

6.3.3   Model Comparison and Selection

The computation of the likelihood ratio test statistic for comparing nested models can be performed by the `glmlrtest` function:

```
{lr, pvalue} = glmlrtest(loglik2, df2, loglik1, df1)
```

where `loglik1` and `loglik2` are the log-likelihoods for the log-linear models M_1 and M_2. Note that M_2 must be the nested model in M_1. These values are obtained from the `glmstat` function. The augments `df1` and `df2` are *df*s for each model. Executing the above call, the test statistic `lr` and the p-value `pvalue` are yielded.

Moreover, to select the best model automatically, XploRe has the `glmselect`, `glmforward` and `glmbackward` functions. The `glmselect` function performs a complete search model selection, the `glmforward` and `glmbackward` functions do the forward and backward search model selections, respectively. The syntax of these functions is the same as `glmest`. Note that best models found by these functions are not always hierarchical log-linear models. Then we repeat to compute the likelihood ratio statistics for comparing the nested models and finally find the best model. When the parameters λ_0, $\{\lambda_i^A\}$ and $\{\lambda_j^B\}$ are contained in all models, the optional parameter fix that specifies them is described as follows:

```
opt = glmopt("fix", 1|2|3)
```

To search the best model by using the backward search model selection, we type

```
select = glmbackward("polog", x, m, opt)
```

Then the output list select consists of five components:

best : the five best models

bestcrit : a list containing bestcrit.aic and bestcrit.bic, the Akaike and Schwarz criteria for the five best models

bestord : the best models of each order

beatordcrit : like bestcrit, but for the best model for each order

bestfit : containing bestfit.b, bestfit.bv and bestfit.stat, the estimation results for the best model

6.4 Numerical Analysis of Contingency Tables

6.4.1 Testing Independence

Chi-squared Test

The data in Table 11.1 are a cross-sectional study of malignant melanoma taken from Roberts et al. (1981) and treated in Dobson (2001). For the two-way table, we are interested in whether there exists a association between Tumor type and Site.

Let $m = \{m_{ij}\}$ be the expected frequencies for the contingency table. The log-linear model that Tumor type is independent of Site is expressed by

$$\log m_{ij} = \lambda_0 + \lambda_i^{Type} + \lambda_j^{Site}, \tag{6.7}$$

for all i and j. From the constraints

$$\lambda_H^{Type} + \lambda_S^{Type} + \lambda_N^{Type} + \lambda_I^{Type} = \lambda_{HN}^{Site} + \lambda_T^{Site} + \lambda_E^{Site} = 0,$$

Table 6.2: Contingency table with tumor type and site

Tumor Type (i)	Site (j)	Cell frequency
Hutchinson's melanotic freckle (H)	Head & neck (HN)	22
	Trunk (T)	2
	Extremities (E)	10
Superficial spreading melanoma (S)	Head & neck (HN)	16
	Trunk (T)	54
	Extremities (E)	115
Nodular (N)	Head & neck (HN)	19
	Trunk (T)	33
	Extremities (E)	73
Indeterminate (I)	Head & neck (HN)	11
	Trunk (T)	17
	Extremities (E)	28

Table 6.3: Expected frequencies for the independence model

Tumor Type	Site	Cell frequency
Hutchinson's melanotic freckle	Head & neck	5.78
	Trunk	9.01
	Extremities	19.21
Superficial spreading melanoma	Head & neck	31.45
	Trunk	49.03
	Extremities	104.52
Nodular	Head & neck	21.25
	Trunk	33.13
	Extremities	70.62
Indeterminate	Head & neck	9.52
	Trunk	14.84
	Extremities	31.64

the parameter vector λ for the independence model is identified by

$$\lambda = [\lambda_0, \lambda_H^{Type}, \lambda_S^{Type}, \lambda_N^{Type}, \lambda_{HN}^{Site}, \lambda_T^{Site}].$$

To find the expected frequencies, we estimate the MLEs $\hat{\lambda}$ using the following statements:

```
library("glm")
n=#(22,2,10,16,54,115,19,33,73,11,17,28)
x=read("design.dat")
lambda = glmest("polog", x, n)
```

where `design.dat` is specified by

```
1 -1 -1 -1 -1 -1
1 -1 -1 -1  1  0
1 -1 -1 -1  0  1
1  1  0  0 -1 -1
1  1  0  0  1  0
1  1  0  0  0  1
1  0  1  0 -1 -1
1  0  1  0  1  0
1  0  1  0  0  1
1  0  0  1 -1 -1
1  0  0  1  1  0
1  0  0  1  0  1
```

The expected frequencies shown in Table 11.2 can be obtained by

```
m = exp(x*lambda.b)
```

and are compared to the data in Table 11.1 by using χ^2. The value of χ^2 is computed from

```
lambda.stat
```

or

```
stat = glmstat("polog", x, m, lambda.b, lambda.bv)
stat.pearson
```

Then χ^2 of 65.8 is very significant compared to the chi-square distribution with 6 *df* and indicates that the independence model does not fit to the data. We can conclude that there exists the association between Tumor type and Site.

Note that the function `crosstable` provides the chi-squared statistic for testing independence for two-way contingency tables.

Model Residuals

Table 6.4: Pearson residuals for the independence model

Tumor Type	Site	Residual
Hutchinson's melanotic freckle	Head & neck	6.75
	Trunk	2.34
	Extremities	-2.10
Superficial spreading melanoma	Head & neck	-2.76
	Trunk	0.71
	Extremities	1.03
Nodular	Head & neck	-0.49
	Trunk	-0.02
	Extremities	0.28
Indeterminate	Head & neck	0.48
	Trunk	0.56
	Extremities	-0.65

Table 6.4 shows the Pearson standardized residuals for the fit of the independence model. The values are easily computed from

```
e = (n-m)/sqrt(m)
```

We can see that the residual for Hutchinson's melanotic freckle and Head & neck reflects the overall poor fit, because the value of $6.75^2 = 45.56$ is related to $\chi^2 = 65.8$.

6.4.2   Model Comparison

Chi-squared Test

The data in Table 11.3 summarize to a survey the Wright State University school of Medicine and the United Health Services in Dayton, Ohio. The analysis for the contingency table is given in Agresti (2002). For the three-way table, we search the best model by using the likelihood ratio tests.

Table 6.5: Alcohol, cigarette and marijuana use for high school seniors

Alcohol use (A)	Cigarette use (C)	Marijuana use (M)	Cell frequency
Yes	Yes	Yes	911
		No	538
	No	Yes	44
		No	456
No	Yes	Yes	3
		No	43
	No	Yes	2
		No	279

Table 6.6 shows the expected frequencies for log-linear models of no three-factor interaction and conditional independence models. The expected frequencies for each model are computed by using `glmest`.

The expected frequencies for the log-linear model $[AC][AM][CM]$ are found using the following statements:

```
library("glm")
n=#(911, 538, 44, 456, 3, 43, 2, 279)
x=read("design.dat")
lambda = glmest("polog", x, n)
m = exp(x*lambda.b)
```

Then, under the constraints with the λ terms, the parameter vector λ is identified by

$$\lambda = [\lambda_0, \lambda_{Yes}^A, \lambda_{Yes}^C, \lambda_{Yes}^M, \lambda_{Yes,Yes}^{AC}, \lambda_{Yes,Yes}^{AM}, \lambda_{Yes,Yes}^{CM}]^T,$$

and the design matrix x is specified by

Table 6.6: Expected frequencies for log-linear models applied to Table 11.3

			Log-linear model			
A	C	M	$[AC][AM]$	$[AM][CM]$	$[AC][CM]$	$[AC][AM][CM]$
Yes	Yes	Yes	710.00	909.24	885.88	910.38
		No	175.64	438.84	133.84	538.62
	No	Yes	131.05	45.76	123.91	44.62
		No	2005.80	555.16	470.55	455.38
No	Yes	Yes	5.50	4.76	28.12	3.62
		No	24.23	142.16	75.22	42.38
	No	Yes	1.02	0.24	3.93	1.38
		No	276.70	179.84	264.45	279.62

```
1  1  1  1  1  1  1
1  1  1 -1  1 -1 -1
1  1 -1  1 -1  1 -1
1  1 -1 -1 -1 -1  1
1 -1  1  1 -1 -1  1
1 -1  1 -1 -1  1 -1
1 -1 -1  1  1 -1 -1
1 -1 -1 -1  1  1  1
```

To compute the expected frequencies of the nested models in the log-linear model $[AC][AM][CM]$, we delete the columns of x corresponding to λ setting to zero in these models and then execute the above statements. For example, deleting the seventh column of x, we can obtain the expected frequencies of the log-linear model $[AC][AM]$. The command

```
x[,1|2|3|4|5|6]
```

produces the design matrix for the log-linear model $[AC][AM]$.

Table 6.7 shows results of the likelihood ratio and Pearson chi-squared tests for log-linear models. The statements to compute the values of G^2 for the saturated model M_1 and a log-linear model M_2 are

```
stat1 = glmstat("polog", x1, n, lambda1.b, lambda1.bv)
df1 = rows(lambda1.b)
stat2 = glmstat("polog", x2, n, lambda2.b, lambda2.bv)
```

```
df2 = rows(lambda2.b)
{lr,pvalue}=glmlrtest(stat2.loglik, df2, stat1.loglik, df1)
lr
pvalue
```

where the design matrix x1 for the saturated model is specified by

```
1  1  1  1  1  1  1  1
1  1  1 -1  1 -1 -1 -1
1  1 -1  1 -1  1 -1 -1
1  1 -1 -1 -1 -1  1  1
1 -1  1  1 -1 -1  1 -1
1 -1  1 -1 -1  1 -1  1
1 -1 -1  1  1 -1 -1  1
1 -1 -1 -1  1  1  1 -1
```

The value of χ^2 is also computed from

```
lambda = glmest("polog",x,n)
lambda.stat
```

Then the values of G^2 and χ^2 or p-value indicate that the model $[AC][AM][CM]$ fits well to the data.

Table 6.7: Goodness of fit tests for log-linear models

Log-linear model	G^2	χ^2	Degrees of freedom	p-value
$[AC][AM][CM]$	0.4	0.4	1	0.53
$[AC][AM]$	497.4	443.8	2	0.00
$[AM][CM]$	187.8	177.6	2	0.00
$[AC][CM]$	92.0	80.8	2	0.00

Model Residuals

To examine lack of fit to the data, we analyze the residuals for each log-linear model. Table 6.8 shows the Pearson standardized residuals for the log-linear models. All residuals for the log-linear model $[AC][AM][CM]$ are very small and demonstrate that the model well fits to the data. On the other hand, the residuals for conditional independence models indicate poorly fit to the data. In particular, the extremely large residuals of -34.604 for the model $[AC][AM]$ and of 34.935 for the model $[AC][CM]$ cause the lack of fit to the data.

Table 6.8: The Pearson standardized residuals for log-linear models

| | | | \multicolumn{4}{c}{Log-linear model} |
A	C	M	$[AC][AM]$	$[AM][CM]$	$[AC][CM]$	$[AC][AM][CM]$
Yes	Yes	Yes	7.543	0.058	0.844	0.020
		No	27.342	4.734	34.935	-0.027
	No	Yes	-7.604	-0.260	-7.179	-0.092
		No	-34.604	-4.209	-0.671	0.029
No	Yes	Yes	-1.077	-0.807	-4.737	-0.324
		No	3.813	-8.317	-3.715	0.095
	No	Yes	0.969	3.596	-0.975	0.524
		No	0.138	7.394	0.895	-0.037

Test for Partial Associations

Moreover, it is possible to compare nested log-linear models by testing partial associations. We test to compare the model $[AC][AM]$ with the model $[AC][AM][CM]$. Then the test examines whether there exists a partial association between Alcohol use and Cigarette use, that is,

$$\lambda_{11}^{CM} = \lambda_{12}^{CM} = \lambda_{21}^{CM} = \lambda_{22}^{CM} = 0.$$

Each log-linear model is expressed by

$$M_1: \quad \log m_{ijk} = \lambda_0 + \lambda_i^A + \lambda_j^C + \lambda_k^M + \lambda_{ij}^{AC} + \lambda_{ik}^{AM} + \lambda_{jk}^{CM},$$
$$M_2: \quad \log m_{ijk} = \lambda_0 + \lambda_i^A + \lambda_j^C + \lambda_k^M + \lambda_{ik}^{AC} + \lambda_{jk}^{AM}.$$

From Table 6.7,

$$\triangle G^2 = 497.4 - 0.4 = 497.0$$

and $df = 2 - 1 = 1$, so that $\triangle G^2$ provides strong evidence of a partial association between Cigarette use and Marijuana use. We can also test for partial associations by comparing the models $[AM][CM]$ and $[AC][CM]$ with the model $[AC][AM][CM]$.

Search for the Best Model

Next we illustrate the best model search using the `glmbackward` function. Using

```
opt = glmopt("fix", 1|2|3|4)
```

we specify to contain λ_0, $\{\lambda_i^A\}$, $\{\lambda_j^C\}$ and $\{\lambda_k^M\}$ in the model. To choose a best model, we execute

```
select=glmbackward("polog", x, n, opt)
select.best
```

where x is the design matrix for the saturated model. Then `select.best` displays the five best models for the data:

```
Contents of best
[1,]        1          1          1          1          1
[2,]        2          2          2          2          2
[3,]        3          3          3          3          3
[4,]        4          4          4          4          4
[5,]        5          5          0          5          5
[6,]        6          6          6          6          0
[7,]        7          7          7          0          7
[8,]        0          8          8          8          8
```

In the above output, each row corresponds to the parameter vector λ in the saturated log-linear model as follows:

row	λ term
1	λ_0
2	$\{\lambda_{Yes}^A\}$
3	$\{\lambda_{Yes}^C\}$
4	$\{\lambda_{Yes}^M\}$
5	$\{\lambda_{Yes,Yes}^{AC}\}$
6	$\{\lambda_{Yes,Yes}^{AM}\}$
7	$\{\lambda_{Yes,Yes}^{CM}\}$
8	$\{\lambda_{Yes,Yes,Yes}^{ACM}\}$

Those components that are not contained in a log-linear model are indicated by zero. The first column shows the no three-interaction model, since the row 8 is zero. The second column represents the saturated model. The last three columns are not the hierarchical models. Therefore the model $[AC][AM][CM]$ is also selected as the best model. The output `select.bestfit` includes all estimation results with the best model.

Bibliography

Agresti, A. (2002). *Categorical Data Analysis* 2nd edition, John Wiley & Sons, New York.

Bishop, Y.M., Fienberg, S. and Holland, P. (1975). *Discrete Multivariate Analysis*, M.I.T. Press, Cambridge, MA.

Dobson, A.J. (2001). *An Introduction to Generalized Linear Models* 2nd edition, Chapman & Hall, London.

Everitt, B.S. (1977). *The analysis of Contingency Tables*, Chapman & Hall, London.

Härdle, W., Klinke, S. and Müller, M. (1999). *XploRe—Learning Guide*, Springer-Verlag, Berlin.

McCullagh, P. and Nelder, J.A. (1989). *Generalized Linear Models* 2nd edition, Chapman & Hall, London.

Roberts, G., Martyn, A.L., Dobson, A.J. and McCarthy, W.H. (1981). Tumour thickness and histological type in malignant melanoma in New South Wales, Australia, 1970-76, *Pathology* **13**: 763-770.

7 Identifying Coexpressed Genes

Qihua Wang

Some gene expression data contain outliers and noise because of experiment error. In clustering, outliers and noise can result in false positives and false negatives. This motivates us to develop a weighting method to adjust the expression data such that the outlier and noise effect decrease, and hence result in a reduction in false positives and false negatives in clustering.

In this paper, we describe the weighting adjustment method and apply it to a yeast cell cycle data set. Based on the adjusted yeast cell cycle expression data, the hierarchical clustering method with a correlation coefficient measure performs better than that based on standardized expression data. The clustering method based on the adjusted data can group some functionally related genes together and yields higher quality clusters.

7.1 Introduction

In order to explore complicated biological systems, microarray expression experiments have been used to generate large amounts of gene expression data (Schena *et al.* (1995), DeRisi *et al.* (1997), Wen *et al.* (1998), Cho *et al.* (1998)). An important type of those experiments is to monitor each gene multiple times under some conditions (Spellman *et al.* (1998), Cho *et al.* (1998), Chu *et al.* (1998)). Those of this type have allowed for the identification of functionally related genes due to common expression patterns (Brown *et al.* (2000), Eisen *et al.* (1998), Wen *et al.* (1998), Roberts *et al.* (2000)). Because of the large number of genes and the complexity of biological networks, clustering is a useful exploring technique for analysis of gene expression data. Different clustering methods including the hierarchical clustering algorithm (Eisen *et al.* (1998), Wen *et al.* (1998)), the CAST algorithm (Ben-Dor *et al.*, 2000) and self-organizing maps (Tamayo *et al.*, 1999) have been employed to analyze expression data.

Given the same data set, different clustering algorithms can potentially generate very different clusters. A biologist with a gene expression data set is faced with the problem of choosing an appropriate clustering algorithm or developing a more appropriate clustering algorithm for his or her data set. Cho *et al.* (1998) recently published a 17-point time course data set measuring the expression level of each of 6601 genes for the yeast Saccharomyces Cerevisiae obtained from using an Affymetrix hybridization array. Cells in a yeast culture were synchronized, and cultured samples were taken at 10-minutes intervals until 17 observations were obtained. Heyer, Kruglyak and Yooseph (1999) presented a systematic analysis procedure to identify, group, and analyze coexpressed genes based on this 17-point time course data.

An important problem for clustering is to select a suitable pairwise measure of coexpression. Possible measures include the Euclidean distance, correlation and rank correlation. Euclidean distances and pattern correlation have a clear biological meaning: Euclidean distances are used when the interest is in looking for identical patterns, whereas correlation measures are used in the case of the trends of the patterns.

In the clustering, most measures scored curves with similar expression patterns well, but often gave high scores to dissimilar curves or low scores to similar ones. We will refer to a pair that is dissimilar, but receives a high score from the similarity measure as a false positive (Heyer, Kruglyak and Yooseph, 1999), and a pair that is similar, but receives a low score as a false negative. As pointed out by Heyer, Kruglyak and Yooseph (1999) that the correlation coefficient performed better than the other measures, but resulted in many false positives. It is noted that the reason for false positive to occur is outlier effect. Hence, Heyer, Kruglyak and Yooseph (1999) proposed a new measure called jackknife correlation. For a data set with t observations, the jackknife correlation J_{ij} is defined as $J_{ij} = \min\{\rho_{ij}^{(1)}, \rho_{ij}^{(2)}, \cdots, \rho_{ij}^{(t)}, \rho_{ij}\}$, where ρ_{ij} denotes the correlation of the gene pair i, j and $\rho_{ij}^{(l)}$ denotes the correlation of the pair i, j computed with the lth observation deleted. An advantage of this method is that it results in a reduction in false positives. However, this method might be radical and lead to false negatives since it takes the least value of these correlation coefficients as the measure of the similarity. On the other hand, the method may lose much valuable information since it works by deleting data. Also, the jackknife correlation is only robust to a single outlier. For n outliers, a more general definition of jackknife correlation is needed. For this case, however, this method is computationally intensive for even small values of n and can result in the loss of much valuable information since it deletes n data points.

If the expression level of a gene at each time point is viewed as a coordinate, then the standardized expression level of each gene at all t time points describes a point in the t dimensional space, and the Euclidean distance between any two points in this space can be computed. Euclidean distances are more affected by small variations in the patterns and produce less interpretable clusters of sequences. As pointed by Heyer, Kruglyak and Yooseph (1999) the two points for which the distance is minimized are precisely the points that have the highest correlation. However, the opposite is not true. That is, a pair of genes that are dissimilar and have large Euclidean distance may have high correlation because of outlier effect and hence receive a high score from the similarity measure of correlation coefficient.

This shows that the Euclidean distance measure with standardized data performs better than the correlation coefficient measure in the sense of resulting in less false positive. However, the Euclidean distance measure still result in many false negatives due to the effect of outliers. If the expression levels of two genes are close to each other but one of the time points, and one of the two genes has a high peak or valley at the remaining time point, then the Euclidean distance may be large and hence the pair which closes to each other except for the outlier may be considered as dissimilarity.

It seems difficult to avoid outlier effect by selecting similarity measure. A possible method to reduce the outlier effect is to adjust the expression data.

Wang (2002) proposes a weighting adjustment method and applies it to the 17 time-point time course data such that a similarity measure assigns higher score to coexpressed gene pairs and lower scores to gene pairs with unrelated expression patterns, and hence results in not only a reduction of false positives but also a reduction of false negatives in clustering. Here, we present the work.

7.2   Methodology and Implementation

We consider the Saccharomyces cerevisiae data set by Cho *et al.* (1998). This data set measures the expression level of each of the 6601 genes of Saccharomyces cerevisiae at 17 time points, sampled every ten minutes during roughly two complete cell cycles. Before giving and applying our method to the data set, we first filter away the genes that were either expressed at very low levels or did not vary significantly across the time points (Heyer, Kruglyak and Yooseph, 1999). The reason to do so is that the fluctuations were more likely noise than signal if the expression levels were below a detection threshold or that the gene that showed so little variation over time may be inactive or not involved in regulation. We remove the genes whose expression values across all the time points are less than 250 and those whose maximum expression levels are not larger than 1.1 times of their average expression levels. After filtering, 3281 genes remained in the data set.

7.2.1   Weighting Adjustment

Many of the false positives and false negatives occurred due to the effect of outliers by standard clustering methods. A possible method to reduce the effect of outliers is to adjust the raw data by a certain method. It is noted that the expression level of a gene at any time point is closely related to the expression levels of the gene at the time points in the nearest neighbor of this point. It is likely that the closer the two time points, the higher the relationship between the two expression levels at the two time points.

This leads us to use a weighting method to adjust the expression values so that not only the effect of outliers decreases but also data analysis is less sensitive to small perturbation in the data. The data have been standardized by subtracting the mean and dividing by the standard deviation. Let $x_{i,j}$ be the standardized expression level of the ith gene at the j time point for $i = 1, 2, \ldots, 3281$ and $j = 1, 2, \ldots, 17$. We get the following adjusted expression level

$$x'_{i,j} = \begin{cases} \frac{1}{2}x_{i,j} + \frac{1}{3}x_{i,j+1} + \frac{1}{6}x_{i,j+2}, & \text{if } j = 1 \\ \frac{1}{5}x_{i,j-1} + \frac{1}{2}x_{i,j} + \frac{1}{5}x_{i,j+1} + \frac{1}{10}x_{i,j+2}, & \text{if } j = 2 \\ \frac{1}{12}x_{i,j-2} + \frac{1}{6}x_{i,j-1} + \frac{1}{2}x_{i,j} + \frac{1}{6}x_{i,j+1} + \frac{1}{12}x_{i,j+2}, & \text{if } 3 \leq j \leq 15 \\ \frac{1}{10}x_{i,j-2} + \frac{1}{5}x_{i,j-1} + \frac{1}{2}x_{i,j} + \frac{1}{5}x_{i,j+1}, & \text{if } j = 16 \\ \frac{1}{2}x_{i,j} + \frac{1}{3}x_{i,j-1} + \frac{1}{6}x_{i,j-2}. & \text{if } j = 17 \end{cases}$$

It is easily seen that the adjusted expression level of a gene at the jth time point is the weighting average of the expression levels of the gene at the time points in the nearest neighbor of the j time point for $j = 1, 2, \ldots, 17$.

Actually, the adjusted expression level of the jth time point is given by assigning weight $1/2$ to jth time point and total weight $1/2$ to other points. The symmetric points about the jth time point such as $j + 1$ and $j - 1$ are assigned the equal weights for $j = 3, 2, \ldots, 15$.

The weights which are assigned to time points k with $|k - j| > 2$ are zero and to time point $j + 2$ or $j - 2$ is $1/2$ time of that for the time point $j + 1$ or $j - 1$. One intuitive method for seeing how the weighting method behaves is to plot the expression data and the adjusted ones for some gene pairs.

From Figure 7.1 to Figure 7.4, it seems that the curves of the functionally related gene pairs with coexpression become more similar to each other after adjustment. From Figures 7.5 and 7.6, the unrelated gene pair which is

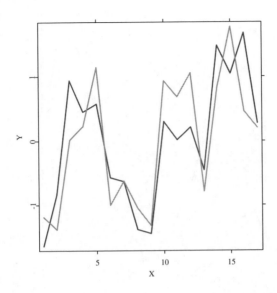

Figure 7.1: Standardized expression level curves for YDR224c/HTB1 and YDR225w/HTA1_i. The gene pair has a correlation coefficient of 0.8094 based on the standardized data.

XCSclust01.xpl

not coexpressed seems to become further away from each other. Another more exact method is to compare the correlation coefficients of gene pairs or Euclidean distances of them based on the expression data with those based on the adjusted ones. It is interesting to find that the correlation coefficients of the most of highly correlated gene pairs become larger and those of lowly correlated gene pairs become smaller after the expression values are adjusted. This can be seen from Table 7.1 and Figure 7.7.

From Figure 7.7, it is easy to see that the correlation coefficients of the most gene pairs whose correlation coefficients are larger than 0.6 before adjustment become larger after adjustment, and those whose correlation coefficients are less than 0.2 before adjustment become less after adjustment. That is, this method gives higher score to similar gene pairs and lower score to dissimilar ones. This may be due to the fact that the weighting adjustment method can lead to a reduction of effect of outliers and noise in expression data.

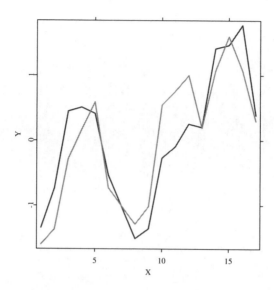

Figure 7.2: Adjusted expression level curves for YDR224c/HTB1 and
YDR225w/HTA1_i. The gene pair has a correlation coefficient
of 0.8805 based on the adjusted data.

Q XCSclust02.xpl

From Figure 7.7 and Table 7.1, we also see that some of the highly correlated pairs are given lower correlation coefficient score after the expression data are adjusted. The reason may be that outliers or data noise lead to the high correlation between these gene pairs, or that, randomly, some of them display very similar pattern before adjustment.

After weighting adjustment for the expression values, the correlation coefficients for these pairs will decrease since the adjustment method leads to a reduction of effect of outliers, data noisy and randomization. Also, it is observed that some lowly correlated gene pairs are given much higher correlation coefficient score after the expression data are adjusted. The reason may be that only one of a gene pair contains outliers at the same time points or one of the two genes has high peaks and another gene have high valleys at the same time points, and these outliers lead to the low correlation between the gene pair. After adjustment, effect of outliers decreases and hence the

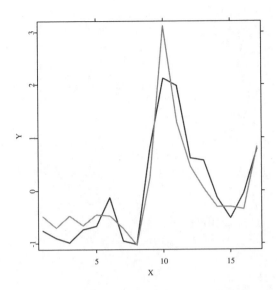

Figure 7.3: Standardized expression level curves for YDL179w/PCL9 and YLR079w/SIC1. The gene pair has a correlation coefficient of 0.9106 based on the standardized data.

Q XCSclust03.xpl

correlation coefficient for the gene pair will increase. This, for example, can be seen from Figures 7.8 and 7.9, which contain plots of the expression level curves for gene pair YAR002w and YBL102w/SFT2 based on standardized expression data and adjusted ones, respectively. From Figure 7.8, we see that YBL102w/SFT2 and YAR002w seem to be overly expressed at two different time points of 90 minutes and 150 minutes, respectively. At the time point of 90 minutes, only YBL102w/SFT2 has a high peak. At the time point of 150 minutes, YAR002w has a high peak and YBL102w/SFT2 has a low valley.

If one removes the expression values of the two genes at the two time points, the correlation coefficient of the two genes increase to 0.6036 from 0.3150. This shows that the two special expression values lead to a low correlation between the two genes. From Figure 7.9, it is easily seen that the weighting adjustment method leads to a reduction of effect of the expression values at the two time points so that the correlation coefficient of the two genes

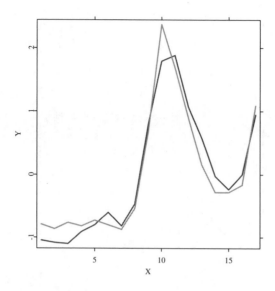

Figure 7.4: Standardized expression level curves for YDL179w/PCL9 and
         YLR079w/SIC1. The gene pair has a correlation coefficient of
         0.9675 based on the adjusted data.

Q XCSclust04.xpl

increase to 0.8113.

By the above important features, we can expect that this adjustment method
will lead to a reduction of both the false positives and false negatives when
Pearson correlation coefficient clustering algorithm is used.

7.2.2 Clustering

We clustered the gene expression time series according to the Pearson correlation coefficient since it not only conforms well to the intuitive biological
notion and performs better than other measures, but also the correlation coefficient measure has the important features in Section 7.2.1 for the adjusted
expression data.

The clustering method that we use is the popular hierarchical method. This

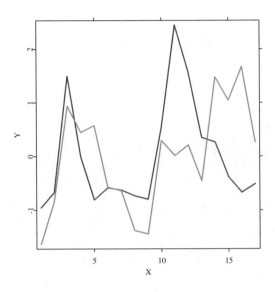

Figure 7.5: Standardized expression level curves for YDL227c/HO and
YDR224c/HTB1. The gene pair has a correlation coefficient of
0.3172 based on the standardized data based on the standardized
expression data.

Q XCSclust05.xpl

method computes a dendrogram that assembles all the genes into a single
tree. Starting with N clusters containing a single gene each, at each step
in the iteration the two closest clusters are merged into a larger cluster by
calculating an upper-diagonal similarity matrix by the metric described above
and scanning the matrix to identify the highest value. Similarity measure
between clusters is defined as that between their average expression pattern.
After $N - 1$ steps, all the genes are merged together into an hierarchical tree.

Once the tree is constructed, the data can be partitioned into any number of
clusters by cutting the tree at the appropriate level. For large data sets, however, it is not easy to choose an appropriate location for cutting the tree. We
will not address this problem here since our purpose in this paper is to show
how our weighting adjustment method improves the classification results. To
evaluate how 'good' our clustering is, let us identify some applications.

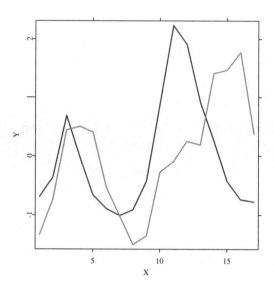

Figure 7.6: Standardized expression level curves for YDL227c/HO and
           YDR224c/HTB1. The gene pair has a correlation coefficient of
           0.1401 based on the adjusted expression data.

Q XCSclust06.xpl

YDR224c/HTB1 and YDR225w/HTA1 are late G1 and G2 regularly genes
which have the same biological function (DNA replication, (Cho *et al.*,
1998)). A natural question is: Can the two genes be grouped together based
on the adjusted expression levels? To answer this question, let us find the
clusters including the two genes.

In our hierarchical tree, it can be found the smallest cluster including
YDR224c/HTB1 contains two genes, YDR224c/HTB1 and YDR225w/HTA1.
It is interesting to note that the two genes are just known functionally related
by Cho *et al.* (1998).

The above result implies that this cluster is also the smallest one which
includes the two genes. This shows that our method can group the two
functionally related genes together.

Another intuitive method to evaluate objectively the quality of the clustering

Table 7.1: Correlation coefficients for some gene pairs based on the standarized and adjusted expression data

Gene	Pairs	BA	AA
YKL130c/SHEI	YNL053w/MSG5	0.8047	0.8474
YDL179w/PCL9	YLR079w/SICI	0.9106	0.9676
YJL157c/FAR1	YKL185w/ASH1	0.9293	0.9535
YJR092w/BUD4	YLR353w/BUD8	0.6904	0.9684
YIL009w/FAA3	YLL040c/VPS13	0.7519	0.8798
YJL196c/EL01	YJR148w/TWT2	0.6815	0.7433
YBL023c/MCM2	YBR202w/CDC47	0.7891	0.8383
YHR005c/GPA1	YJL157c/FAR1	0.8185	0.8320
YOR373w/NUD	YJL157c/FAR	-0.1256	-0.2090
YOR373w/NVD1	YAL040c/c	-0.1133	-0.2222
YDR225w/HTA1i	YLL022c	0.3493	0.0673
YJR018w	YJR068w/RFe2	0.9046	0.8968
YJR068/RFC2	YJR132w/NMD5	0.8700	0.7121

BA: Before Adjustment, AA: After Adjustment

for the particular application is to plot the expression data for the genes in the clustering and determine whether the plots look similar and how the plots look similar. Figure 7.1 plots the expression level curves for the two genes. By Figure 7.1, their expression patterns are indeed similar to each other.

It is known there are 19 late G1 regulatory genes and two of them are just YDR224c/HTB1 and YDR225w/HTA1 (Cho *et al.*, 1998). In our clustering tree, the cluster including the two genes whose gene number is the closest to 19 contains 17 genes, 4 of them are known to be late G1 regulary and functionally related with DNA replication. It is known that some unrelated genes also may have similar expression patterns. Hence, the remaining 13 genes are not necessarily functionally related with the 4 genes even though they are coexpressed. However, the 13 genes provide excellent candidates for further study.

We also try to find the smallest cluster including the 19 genes in late G1 group. Unfortunately, this cluster contains 2930 genes and hence is not of high quality since it contains many lowly related genes. This reason may be that some gene pairs in the late G1 group are lowly related. For example, the correlation coefficient of the gene pair, YDR225w/HTA1 and YPR175w/DPB2, in the late G1 group is 0.0471.

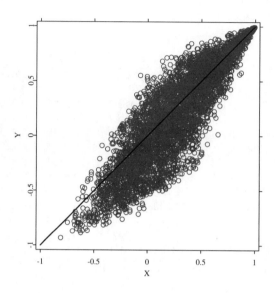

Figure 7.7: Correlation coefficients of 10,000 gene pairs. ρ and ζ are the correlation coefficients based on the standardized expression data and the adjusted expression data, respectively. 869 gene pairs have correlation coefficients which are larger than 0.6. The correlation coefficients of 556 pairs of them become larger after adjustment. 2303 gene pairs have correlation coefficients which are less than 0.2. The correlation coefficients of 1520 pairs of them become less after adjustment.

Q XCSclust07.xpl

Another problem we should answer is whether the adjustment method improves the classification result compare to the corresponding hierarchical method based on standardized expression data. Let us consider the above example again and see how the clustering method based on standard expression data behaves. From the hierarchical tree based on the standardized data without adjustment, the smallest cluster including YDR224c/HTB1 is {YDR224c/HTB1, YDR134C/_f}. However, YDR134C/_f is not known to be functionally related with YDR224c/HTB1 though it provides a possible candidate. Figure 7.10 plots the expression level curves of the two genes.

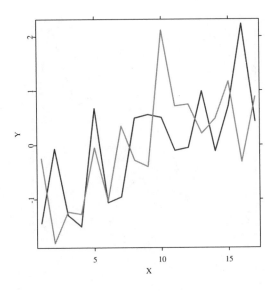

Figure 7.8: Standardized expression level curves for YAR002w and YBL102w/SFT2. The gene pair has a correlation coefficient of 0.3750 based on the standardized expression data.

XCSclust08.xpl

In the clustering tree based on the standardized expression data without adjustment, the cluster including all the 3281 genes is the only one including both YDR224c/HTB1 and YDR225w/HTA1. This shows that this method cannot group the two functionally related genes together.

Both YDR224c/HTB1 and YDR225w/HTA1 are also in the late G1 group mentioned above, which contains 19 genes. Hence, the cluster including the 3281 genes are also the only one including the 19 genes. This shows that this clustering method with standardized expression data yields much lower quality clusters and also cannot group the 19 genes together.

Let us consider another example. YJR092W/BUD4 and YLR353W/BUD8 are M regulatory genes which are functionally related to directional growth (Cho *et al.*, 1998). In our clustering tree, the smallest cluster including the two genes contains four genes. The other two genes are YNL066W and

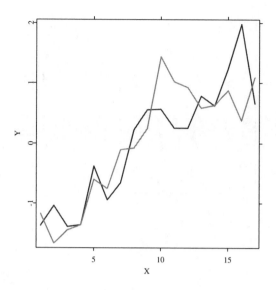

Figure 7.9: Standardized expression level curves for YAR002w and
            YBL102w/SFT2. The gene pair has a correlation coefficient of
            0.8113 based on the adjusted expression data.

Q XCSclust09.xpl

YOR025W/HST3. Figure 7.11 plots the standardized expression level curves
of the four genes.

From Figure 7.11, all the expression level curves are similar to each other
except YNL066W. It is easy to see that YOR025W/HST3 is coexpressed with
YJR092W/HUD4 and YLR353W/BUD8. Hence, YOR025W/HST3 provides
an excellent candidate for further study whether it is functionally related with
YJR092W/HUD4 and YLR353W/BUD8.

Let us apply the clustering method with standardized data without adjustment to the above example. The smallest cluster including YJR092W/BUD4
and YLR353W/BUD8 contains 11 genes.

YJL157c/FAR1 is an early G1 regulary gene which is functionally related
with mating pathway. In our hierarchical tree, the smallest cluster including this gene contains two genes, YJL157c/FAR1 and YGR183C/QCR9_ex1.

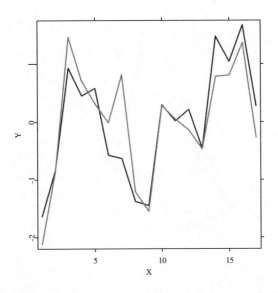

Figure 7.10: Standardized expression level curves for YDR224c/HTB1 and
YDR134c/_f in the clustering tree based on the standardized
expression data.

🔍 XCSclust10.xpl

From Figure 7.12, we can see that YGR183C/QCR9_ex1 is coexpressed with
YJL157c/FAR1 though it is not known to be early G1 regularly gene which
is functionally related with YJL157c/FAR1. The second smallest cluster contains 5 genes in addition to YJL157c/FAR1. One of them is YKL185w/ASH1,
which is known to be functionally related with YJL157c/FAR1. Actually, this
cluster is also the smallest one including the two functionally related genes.

For the clustering method with standardized expression data, the smallest
cluster including YJL157c/FAR1 contains 6 genes. The second smallest cluster contains 7 genes. No genes in the two clusters are known to be functionally related. The smallest cluster including the two functionally related
genes, YJL157c/FAR1 and YKL185w/ASH1, contains 96 genes.

It is known that YIL140w/SRO4 is the only one which is known to be S regulatory and to be related with directional growth. Are there any functionally

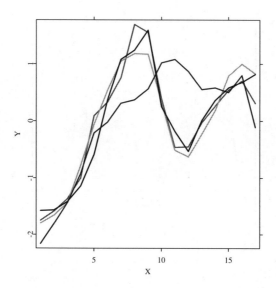

Figure 7.11: Standardized expression level curves for the genes in the smallest
            cluster including YJR092w/HUD4 and YLR353w/HUD8 in the
            clustering tree based on the adjusted data. The remaining two
            genes are YNL066w and YOR025w/HST3.

Q XCSclust11.xpl

related genes with it? Which genes are coexpressed with it? In our clustering
tree, the first smallest cluster including this gene is
{YIL140w/SRO4, YPL163c/SVS1}. The second smallest cluster contains another gene, YOR373w/NUD1, in addition to the above two genes. From the
standardized data without adjustment, different clusters are obtained. The
smallest cluster including YIL140w/SRO4 is {YIL140w/SRO4, YLR326w}.
The second smallest cluster contains YNL243w/SLA2 and YPR052c/NHP6A
in addition to the two genes in the smallest cluster. Figures 7.13 and 7.14 plot
the expression level curves for the genes in the two second smallest clusters,
respectively.

From Figures 7.13 and 7.14, we see that the expression level curves for the
genes in the cluster by our method are more closer to each other. This also
can be seen by their correlation coefficients. In our cluster, other genes are

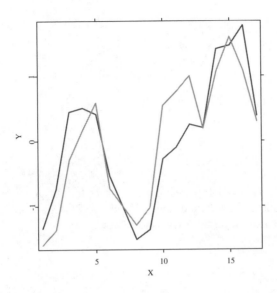

Figure 7.12: Standardized expression level curves for the genes in the smallest cluster including YJL157c/FAR1 in the clustering tree based on the adjusted data.

Q XCSclust12.xpl

more highly related with YIL140w/SRO4. This shows that our clusters have higher quality for this special example. From Figure 7.14, the cluster based on the standardized expression data is of much more lowly quality since it contains some lowly related genes.

From the above examples, we see that the clustering method based on the adjusted expression data behave better than that based on the standardized expression data without adjustment. Our method can group coexpression genes and some functionally related genes together. However, We have not found that any known functionally related genes can be in the same clusters with high quality in the clustering tree based on the standard expression data. Figure 7.13 shows that two functionally related gene pairs, YJR092w/BUD4 and YLR353w/BUD8, are in a cluster with 11 genes. However, this cluster is clearly not of high quality since it contains some lowly related genes with YJR092w/BUD4 and YLR353w/BUD8.

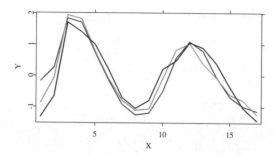

Figure 7.13: Standardized expression level curves for the genes in the second
              smallest cluster including YIL140w/SRO4 in the clustering tree
              based on adjusted expression data.

Q XCSclust13.xpl

It should be pointed out some functionally related genes cannot also group
together based on the adjusted data. This reason may be that some functionally related genes are not coexpressed. Also, genes in the same high quality
cluster are not necessarily functionally related since some functionally unrelated genes have similar expression patterns. Because there is a connection
between coexpression and functional relation, the clusters are an exploratory
tool that meant to identify candidate functionally related genes for further
study though they do not reveal the final answer whether these genes in the
same clusters are functionally related.

7.3   Concluding Remarks

Our purpose to use the weighting method to adjust the expression data is
to decrease the the effect of the outliers and noise. It is reasonable to assign
a weight of 1/2 to the point that one hopes to adjust and a total weight of
1/2 to other points which are located in its nearest neighbor. This method
of assigning weights used in this paper can effectively result in a reduction of
effect of outliers and noise and does not change the normal expression levels
too much. Also, the weighting method is robust for the slight change of the

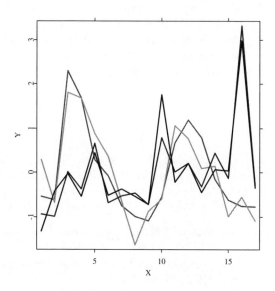

Figure 7.14: Standardized expression level curves for the genes in the second
            smallest cluster including YIL140w/SRO4 in the clustering tree
            based on the standardized expression data.

Q XCSclust14.xpl

weights. If one assigns a much larger weight than $1/2$ to the point which
is adjusted, effect of outlier or noise may not decrease effectively. If one
assigns a much less weight than $1/2$ to the point, the adjusted expression level
may not provide correct information and hence the weighting method may
result in wrong clustering results since such a method changes the expression
levels too much. It should be pointed out that the weighting adjustment
method can be applied to any analysis procedures for any gene expression
data to decrease the effect of outlier and noise though we apply it only to a
hierarchical clustering for the yeast cell cycle data in this paper.

Heyer, Kruglyak and Yooseph (1999) proposed a jackknife correlation measure to resolve false positive. As pointed out before, this method may
be radical and may lead to false negatives. An improved method which
can avoid the false negatives may be to use another jackknife correlation
$\rho_{ij,JK} = \frac{1}{n}\sum_{k=1}^{n}(n\rho_{ij} - (n-1)\rho_{ij}^{(k)})$ based on the adjusted data, where ρ_{ij}

and $\rho_{ij}^{(k)}$ are as defined in Introduction. On the other hand, the clustering method with the jackknife correlation measure $\rho_{ij,JK}$ based on the standardized expression data without adjustment may be conservative and cannot avoid the occurring of false positives very well. Based on the adjusted data, however, the jackknife correlation measure may avoid the false positives and false negatives very well. We will investigate the measure in future work.

Bibliography

Ben-Dor, A., Bruhn, L., Friedman, N., Nachman, I., Schummer, M. and Yakhini, Z. (2000). Tissue classification with gene expression profiles. In *Proceedings of the 4th Annual International Conference on Computational Molecular Biology (RECOMB)* Universal Academy Press, Tokyo.

Brown,M.P.S., Grundy, W.N., Lin,D., Cristianini,N., Sugnet, C.W., Furey,T.S., Jr, M.A. and Haussler, D. (2000). Knowledge-based analysis of microarray gene expression data by using support vector machines. *Proc. Natl Acad. Sci. USA*, **96**, 9112-9217.

Cho,R.J., Cambell,M.J., Winzeler,E.A., Steinmetz,E.A., Conway,A., Wodicka,L., Wolfsberg, T.J., Gabrielian, A.E., Landsman,D., Lockhart,D.J. and Davis, R.W. (1998). A genome-wide transcriptional analysis of the mitotic cell cycle. *Mol. Cell.*, **2**, 65-73.

Chu,S., J.DeRisi, M. eisen, J. Mulholland, D. Botstein, P. Brown, and I. Herskowize (1998). The transcriptional program of sporulation in budding yeast. *Science* **282**, 699-705.

DeRisi,J.L., Iyer,V.R.and Brown, P. O. (1997)Exploring the metabolic and genetic control of gene expression on a genomic scale. *Science*, **278**, 680-686.

Eisen,M.B., Spellman, P.T., Brown,P.O. and Botstein,D. (1998). Cluster analysis and display of genome-wide expression patterns. *Proc. Natl Acad.Sci USA*, **95**, 14863-14868.

Heyer, L.J., Kruglyak,S. and Yooseph,S. (1999). Exploring expression data: Identification and Analysis of coexpressed genes. *Genome Research*, **9**, 1106-1115.

Roberts,C., Nelson, B., Marton, M., Stoughton,R., Meyer, M., Bennett, H., He, Y., Dai, H., Walker,W., Hughes, T., Tyers, M., Boone,C. Friend, S. (2000). Signaling and circuitry of mutiple maps pathways revealed by a matrix of global gene expression profiles. *Science*, **287**, 873-880.

Schena,M., Shalon,D., Davis,R.W. andBrown,P.O.(1995)Quantitative monitoring of gene expression patterns with a DNA microarray. *Science*, **210**, 467-470.

Spellman, P.T., Sherlock, G., Zhang, M.Q., Iyer,V.R., Anders, K., Eisen, M.B., Brown,P.O., Botstein, D. and Futcher,B. (1998)Comprehensive identification of cell cycle-regulated genes of the yeast *Saccharomyces cerevisiae* by microarray hybridization. *Mol. Biol. Cell*, **9**, 3273-3297.

Tamayo, P., Slonim,D., Mesirov,J., Zhu,Q., Kitareewan,S., Dmitrovsky,E., Lander,E. and Golub,T. (1999)Interpreting patterns of gene expression with sely-organizing maps. *Proc. Natl. Acad. Sci. USA*, **96**, 2907-2912.

Wang, Q. H. (2002). Identifying Coexpressed Genes with Adjusted Time Course Macroarray Data using Weighting Method. Unpublished manuscript.

Wen,X., Fuhrman, S., Michaels, G. S., Carr, D. B., Smith, S., Barker, J. L. and Somogyi, R. (1998). Large-scale temporal gene expression mapping of central nervous system development. *Proc. Natl Acad. Sci. USA*, **95**, 334-339.

8 Bootstrap Methods for Testing Interactions in GAMs

Javier Roca-Pardiñas, Carmen Cadarso-Suárez
and Wenceslao González-Manteiga

8.1 Introduction

In many biomedical studies, parametric regression models are widely used to evaluate the effects of continuous exposures on a dependent variable. However, the relative lack of flexibility of parametric models has, in recent years, led to the development of nonparametric regression techniques based on the broad family of generalized additive models (GAMs; Hastie and Tibshirani, 1990). These techniques do not impose a parametric form on the effects of continuous predictors; instead, they assume only that these effects are reasonably smooth. In this work we focus our attention on logistic GAMs.

Let Y be the binary (0/1) response and $\mathbf{X} = (X_1, \ldots, X_p)^\top$ the p-vector of associated continuous covariates. Denoting by $p(\mathbf{X}) = p(Y = 1|\mathbf{X})$, the logistic GAM expresses $p(\mathbf{X})$ as

$$\log\left[p(\mathbf{X})/\left\{1 - p(\mathbf{X})\right\}\right] = \eta_{\mathbf{X}} = \alpha + f_1(X_1) + \ldots + f_p(X_p), \qquad (8.1)$$

where systematic component $\eta_{\mathbf{X}}$, is defined by the constant α, and the sets of unknown partial functions $\{f_j\}_{j=1}^p$ associated with each continuous covariate X_j.

Algorithms aspects of additive modeling by backfitting are discussed in Hastie and Tibshirani (1990). Alternative procedures based on marginal integration have also been suggested by Tjøstheim and Auestad (1994) and Linton and Nielsen (1995).

A disadvantage of (8.1) is that this model completely ignores the fact that the functional form of a covariate effect often varies according to the values tacken by one or more of the remaining covariates. A possible generalization of model (8.1) is the second-order continuous interactions GAM, resulting in the following curve-by-curve interactions model:

$$\log\left[p(\mathbf{X})/\left\{1 - p(\mathbf{X})\right\}\right] = \eta_{\mathbf{X}} = \alpha + \sum_{j=1}^{p} f_j\left(X_j\right) + \sum_{1 \leq j < k \leq p} f_{jk}\left(X_j, X_k\right), \quad (8.2)$$

where $\{f_{jk}\}$ $(1 \leq j < k \leq p)$ is now a set of unknown partial bidimensional functions.

Several methods for estimating (8.2) have already been proposed in the literature. Hastie and Tibshirani (1990) discussed algorithms for backfitting with cubic smoothing splines. More recently, Sperlich *et al.* (2002) used marginal integration for estimating additive models with interactions. Alternative procedures were suggested by Ruppert, Wand and Carroll (2003) using penalized splines.

Another generalization of "pure" GAM in (8.1) is the GAM with factor-by-curve interactions. In this type of model, the relationship between Y and each of the continuous covariates X_j can vary among the subsets defined by the levels of a categorical covariate Z with M levels $\{1, \ldots, M\}$. The possibility of incorporating this type of interaction in GAMs and using the local scoring algorithm for its estimation was already discussed by Hastie and Tibshirani (1990). Recently, Coull *et al* (2001) presented an algorithm based on penalized splines which would allow these types of interactions to be incorporated into GAMs.

The factor-by-curve logistic GAM takes the form:

$$\begin{aligned}\log\left[p(Z, \mathbf{X})/\left\{1 - p(Z, \mathbf{X})\right\}\right] &= \eta_{Z,\mathbf{X}} \\ &= \alpha + \sum_{j=1}^{p}\left\{f_j\left(X_j\right) + f_{Zj}\left(Z, X_j\right)\right\},\end{aligned} \quad (8.3)$$

where the interaction terms, $\{f_{Zj}\}$, are given by

$$f_{Zj}\left(Z, X_j\right) = \sum_{l=1}^{M} I\{Z = l\}g_j^l(X_j), \quad (8.4)$$

being g_j^l $(l = 1, \ldots, M)$ unidimensional functions depending on X_j.

Apart from estimation, it would be most interesting to have statistical tests available that were capable of detecting which effects depend on another covariate. For continuous interactions Hastie and Tibshirani (1990) proposed using the likelihood ratio test; Sperlich *et al.* (2002) presented interactions tests for additive models; and, insofar as factor-by-curve interactions are concerned, Coull *et al.* (2001) presented tests based on penalized spline estimators. Yet, until now, these types of interactions have not been emphasized in the literature.

The layout of this chapter is as follows. Logistic GAMs with interactions and the local scoring estimation algorithm based on local linear kernel smoothers are presented in Section 11.2. The testing problem is introduced in Section 11.3. In this section, different interaction tests are proposed, with bootstrap approximations being used to implement the tests. To check our test procedures, a simulation example is provided in Section 11.4 along with power results. In Section 8.5 we apply our methodology to real data. Section 8.5.1 describes an application to assess the relationship between neuronal activity data and decision making. In Section 8.5.2 we apply the proposed methodology to data drawn from a registry-based prospective cohort study to identify risk factors for post-operative infections. Finally, we conclude with a discussion section.

8.2   Logistic GAM with Interactions

Continuing with the notation introduced in Section 11.1, let Y be the binary $(0/1)$ response, $\mathbf{X} = (X_1, \ldots, X_p)^\top$ a vector of p continuous covariates and Z a categorical covariate with M levels $\{1, \ldots, M\}$. Denoting by $p(Z, \mathbf{X}) = p(Y = 1 | Z, \mathbf{X})$, in this work we consider the model

$$\log\left[p(Z, \mathbf{X}) / \{1 - p(Z, \mathbf{X})\}\right] = \eta_{Z, \mathbf{X}} = \alpha + \sum_{j=1}^{p} \{f_j(X_j) + \\ + f_{Zj}(Z, X_j)\} + \sum_{1 \leq j < k \leq p} f_{jk}(X_j, X_k), \qquad (8.5)$$

where α is a constant, f_j represent the main effects of the continuous covariates, f_{Zj} are the factor-by-curve interactions terms, and f_{jk} are the continuous-by-continuous interactions terms. Note that (8.5) is a generalization of models given in (8.1), (8.2) and (8.3). In order to guarantee the identification of (8.5) we assume zero mean for the main effect f_j, and zero mean marginal means for the interaction terms f_{Zj} and f_{jk}.

8.2.1 Estimation: the Local Scoring Algorithm

We have adapted the local scoring algorithm (Hastie and Tibshirani, 1990) with backfitting (Opsomer, 2000) for the purposes of estimating the GAM with interactions in (8.5). We present a new algorithm which, on the basis of a random independent sample $\{(Z_i, \mathbf{X}_i, Y_i)\}_{i=1}^n$ of $(Z, \mathbf{X}, Y)$, allows for the $f_j(X_{ij})$, $f_{Zj}(Z_i, X_{ij})$ and $p(Z_i, \mathbf{X}_i)$ estimates to be obtained. The steps of this algorithm are as follows:

Initialize. Compute the initial estimates, $\hat{\alpha} = \log\{\bar{Y}/(1-\bar{Y})\}$, $\hat{f}_j^0 = 0$, $\hat{f}_{Zj}^0 = 0 (1 \leq j < p)$, $\hat{f}_{jk}^0 = 0$ $(1 \leq j < k \leq p)$ and $\hat{p}_i^0 = \hat{p}^0(Z_i, \mathbf{X}_i) = \bar{Y}$ $(i = 1, \ldots, n)$ with $\bar{Y} = n^{-1}\sum_{i=1}^n Y_i$.

Step 1. Form the adjusted dependent variables $\tilde{\mathbf{Y}} = \left(\tilde{Y}_1, \ldots, \tilde{Y}_n\right)$ and the weights $\hat{\mathbf{W}} = \left(\hat{W}_1, \ldots, \hat{W}_n\right)$, so that $\tilde{Y}_i = \hat{\eta}_i^0 + (Y_i - \hat{p}_i^0)/\{\hat{p}_i^0(1 - \hat{p}_i^0)\}$ and $\hat{W}_i^{-1} = \hat{p}_i^0(1 - \hat{p}_i^0)$, where

$$\hat{\eta}_i^0 = \hat{\alpha} + \sum_{j=1}^p \left\{\hat{f}_j^0(X_{ij}) + \hat{f}_{Zj}^0(Z_i, X_{ij})\right\} + \sum_{1 \leq j < k \leq p} \hat{f}_{jk}^0(X_j, X_k)$$

Step 2. Fit an additive model (with factor-by-curve interactions) to $\tilde{Y}$ using backfitting, and compute the updates $\hat{f}_j$ and f_{Zj}, as follows:

Step 2.1. Cycle $j = 1, \ldots, p$, calculating the partial residuals

$$R_i^j = \tilde{Y}_i - n^{-1}\sum_{i=1}^n \tilde{Y}_i - \sum_{l<j}\left\{\hat{f}_l(X_{il}) + \hat{f}_{Zl}(Z_i, X_{il})\right\} -$$
$$- \sum_{l>j}\left\{\hat{f}_l^0(X_{il}) + \hat{f}_{Zl}^0(Z_i, X_{il})\right\} - \sum_{1 \leq l < m \leq p}\hat{f}_{lm}^0(X_{il}, X_{im}),$$

and for $i = 1, \ldots, n$, compute the local linear polynomial estimator updates (see (8.7) for details),

$$\hat{f}_j(X_{ij}) = \hat{\psi}\left(X_{ij}, \left\{\left(X_{sj}, R_s^j, \hat{W}_s\right)\right\}_{s=1}^n, h_j\right),$$

and then $\hat{f}_{Zj}(Z_i, X_{ij}) = \sum_{k=1}^M \hat{g}_j^k(X_{ik}) \mathbf{I}\{\{Z_i = k\}\}$, so that

$$\hat{g}_j^k(x) = \hat{\psi}\left(x, \left\{\left(X_i, R_i^{Zj}, \hat{W}_i^k\right)\right\}_{s=1}^n, h_j^k\right),$$

with $R_i^{Zj} = R_i^j - \hat{f}_j(X_{ij})$, $\hat{W}_i^k = \hat{W}_i I_{\{Z_i = k\}}$, h_j being the bandwidths associated with estimation of f_j, and $h_j^1, \ldots, h_j^M$ the bandwidths associated with estimation of f_{Zj} for each of the factors $Z = 1, \ldots, M$.

Step 2.2. Cycle $(j,k)_{1 \le j < k \le p}$ and calculate residuals

$$R_i^{jk} = \tilde{Y}_i - \bar{\tilde{Y}} - \sum_{j=1}^{p} \left\{ \hat{f}_j (X_{ij}) + \hat{f}_{Zj} (Z_i X_{ij}) \right\} - $$
$$- \sum_{(l,m)<(j,k)} \hat{f}_{lm} (X_{il}, X_{im}) - \sum_{(l,m)>(j,k)} \hat{f}_{lm}^0 (X_{il}, X_{im}),$$

$((l,m) < (j,k)$ if $l < j$, or $l = j$ and $m < k$) and compute compute the bidimensional local linear polynomial estimator updates (Ruppert and Wand, 1994, see (8.7) for details)

$$\hat{f}_{jk} (X_{ij}, X_{ik}) = \hat{\psi}_{2D} \left((X_{ij}, X_{ik}), \left\{ \left((X_{sj}, X_{sk}), R_s^{jk}, \hat{W}_s \right) \right\}_{s=1}^{n}, h_j \right),$$

being a bidimensional density function and $\mathbf{H}_{jk}$ a symmetric, positive definite 2×2 matrix (the bandwidth or smoothing parameter matrix).

Step 2.3. This process is repeated, with $\hat{f}_j^0$ being replaced by $\hat{f}_j$, $\hat{f}_{Zj}^0$ by $\hat{f}_{Zj}$, and $\hat{f}_{jk}^0$ by $\hat{f}_{jk}$, until $\sum_{i=1}^{n} \left(\hat{\eta}_i - \hat{\eta}_i^0 \right)^2 / \sum_{i=1}^{n} \left(\hat{\eta}_i^0 \right)^2 \le \varepsilon_{bf}$, where $\hat{\eta}_i = \hat{\alpha} + \sum_{j=1}^{p} \left\{ \hat{f}_j (X_{ij}) - \hat{f}_{Zj} (Z_i, X_{ij}) \right\} + \sum_{1 \le j < k \le p} \hat{f}_{jk} (X_j, X_k)$ and ε_{bf} is a small threshold.

Step 3. Repeat **Steps 1-2**, with $\hat{p}_i^0$ being replaced by $\hat{p}_i = \hat{p}(Z_i, \mathbf{X}_i) = \left(1 + \exp(\hat{\eta}_i)^{-1} \right)^{-1}$ for $i = 1, \ldots, n$, until $|D(\hat{\mathbf{p}}^0, \mathbf{Y}) - D(\hat{\mathbf{p}}, \mathbf{Y}) / D(\hat{\mathbf{p}}^0, \mathbf{Y})| \le \varepsilon$, where ε is a small threshold and

$$D(\hat{\mathbf{p}}, \mathbf{Y}) = -2 \sum_{i=1}^{n} \left\{ Y_i \log(\hat{p}_i) + (1 - Y_i) \log(1 - \hat{p}_i) \right\}.$$

Automatic Selection of the Smoothing Parameters

It is well known that the probability estimates $\hat{p}(Z_i, \mathbf{X}_i)$, depend heavily on the bandwidths $h_j; h_j^1, \ldots, h_j^M$ $(j = 1, \ldots, p)$, used in the estimation of the unidimensional partial functions $f_j; f_j^1, \ldots, f_j^M$, and on the 2×2 matrices of bandwidths $\mathbf{H}_{jk}$ $(1 \le j < k \le p)$, used in the estimation of the bidimensional partial functions f_{jk}. As a practical solution to this problem, we have used the cross-validation technique to choose (at each iteration of the algorithm) the windows $\{h_j; h_j^1, \ldots, h_j^M\}$ and $\{\mathbf{H}_{jk}\}$, used in the estimates $\hat{f}_j$, $\hat{f}_{Zj}$, and $\hat{f}_{jk}$. This mechanism is explained in detail in (8.7) below.

Cross-validation implies a high computational cost, in as much as it is necessary to repeat the estimation operations several times in order to select the optimal bandwidths. To speed up this process we used one- and two-dimensional binning-type acceleration techniques (see Wand (1994), Wand and Jones (1995), Fan and Marron (1994) and Härdle and Scott (1992)).

8.3   Bootstrap-based Testing for Interactions

In this section, bootstrap resampling techniques are used to test for interaction terms in the GAM specified in (8.5). We are interested in both the curve-by-curve and factor-by-curve interaction tests.

In the curve-by-curve tests, for any given fixed pair (j, k) the null hypothesis is

$$H^0 : \log \left[\left\{ p\left(Z, \mathbf{X}\right)^{-1} - 1 \right\}^{-1} \right] = \eta_{Z,\mathbf{x}} - f_{jk}\left(X_j, X_k\right), \qquad (8.6)$$

vs the general hypothesis

$$H : \log \left[\left\{ p\left(Z, \mathbf{X}\right)^{-1} - 1 \right\}^{-1} \right] = \eta_{Z,\mathbf{x}}.$$

Therefore the null hypothesis, $H^0 : f_{jk} = 0$, assumes that there is no interaction between the effect of the continuous covariates X_j and X_k.

In the factor-by-curve interaction tests, for a given continuous covariate, X_j, the interest is to contrast if the effect of this covariate depends on the modalities of the factor Z. In this case, the null hypothesis is given by

$$H^0 : \log \left[\left\{ p\left(Z, \mathbf{X}\right)^{-1} - 1 \right\}^{-1} \right] = \eta_{Z,\mathbf{x}} - f_{Zj}\left(Z, X_j\right). \qquad (8.7)$$

For testing purposes, we propose two test statistics, the first based on the likelihood ratio test and the second on a direct method based on the estimate of the interaction terms.

8.3.1 Likelihood Ratio-based Test

The likelihood ratio test is based on the statistic $\hat{R}$, defined as

$$\hat{R} = \sum_{i=1}^{n} \left[d\left\{ \hat{p}^0\left(Z_i, \mathbf{X}_i\right), Y_i \right\} - d\left\{ \hat{p}\left(Z_i, \mathbf{X}_i\right), Y_i \right\} \right], \qquad (8.8)$$

where $\hat{p}^0\left(Z_i, \mathbf{X}_i\right)$ denotes the estimations of $p\left(Z_i, \mathbf{X}_i\right)$ obtained under the null hypothesis $\mathbf{H}^0$, and deviance $d\left(p, y\right)$ is defined as

$$d\left(p, y\right) = -2\left\{ y \log\left(p\right) + \left(1 - y\right) \log\left(1 - p\right) \right\}.$$

Based on the test statistic $\hat{R}$, the test rule for checking $\mathbf{H}^0$, with asymptotic significance level $1 - \alpha$, is that the null hypothesis is rejected if $\hat{R} \geq \hat{R}^\alpha$, where R^p is the percentile $1 - p$ of the distribution (under the null hypothesis) of $\hat{R}$.

8.3.2 Direct Test

The direct test is based on the statistic $\hat{S} = \sum_{i=1}^{n} \left(\hat{f}_i^*\right)^2$ with:

$$\hat{f}_i^* = \hat{f}_{jk}\left(X_{ij}, X_{ik}\right)$$

(respectively $\hat{f}_i^* = \hat{f}_{jk}\left(Z_i, X_{ik}\right)$). The test rule based on the $\hat{S}$ is exactly the same as the one used for the $\hat{R}$ statistic, namely, the null hypothesis is rejected if $\hat{S} > \hat{S}^\alpha$, where $\hat{S}^\alpha$ is the percentile $1 - \alpha$ of the distribution (under the null hypothesis) of $\hat{S}$.

8.3.3 Bootstrap Approximation

Since our estimations are based on the local scoring algorithm (with backfitting), the theory for ascertaining the asymptotic distribution of $\hat{R}$ (and that of $\hat{S}$) is very difficult, which in turn renders it very difficult to calculate the critical values $\hat{R}^\alpha$ (and $\hat{S}^\alpha$ respectively). Binary bootstrap was thus used to calculate the critical values. Accordingly, the testing procedure consists of the following steps:

Step 1. Estimate the regression model (8.5) under the null hypothesis $\mathbf{H}^0$, and obtain the bootstrap pilot estimates $\tilde{p}^0\left(Z_i, \mathbf{X}_i\right)$, $i = 1, \ldots, n$.

For $b = 1, \ldots, B$

Table 8.1: Percentage of rejection under $\mathbf{H}_{12}^0$

Sample size	Test	Significance				
		1.0	5.0	10.0	15.0	20.0
250	T_1	0.2	2.2	6.1	9.6	14.4
	T_2	0.1	2.8	6.5	10.7	16.2
400	T_1	0.2	2.7	5.7	9.3	13.9
	T_2	1.0	4.7	9.5	16.5	21.6
1000	T_1	1.0	5.1	9.6	13.7	18.7
	T_2	1.0	3.9	8.4	12.7	17.2

Step 2. Generate a sample $\left\{\left(Z_i, \mathbf{X}_i, Y_i^{*b}\right)\right\}_{i=1}^n$, with $Y_i^{*b} \sim B\left(\tilde{p}^0\left(Z_i, \mathbf{X}_i\right)\right)$.

Step 3. Calculate the bootstrap test statistics $\hat{R}^{*b}$ and $\hat{S}^{*b}$ using the sample $\left\{\left(Z_i, \mathbf{X}_i, Y_i^{*b}\right)\right\}_{i=1}^n$ in the same way as the original $\hat{R}$ and $\hat{S}$ were calculated.

In **Step 1**, the use of slightly oversmoothing bandwidths is recommended (see Roca-Pardiñas, 2003; Kauermann and Opsomer, 2003). In particular, for the studies displayed throughout this work the length of the pilot bandwidhts is the double of that used in the estimation.

The test rule based on $\hat{R}$ consists of rejecting the null hypothesis if $\hat{R} > \hat{R}^{*(1-\alpha)}$, where $\hat{R}^{*(p)}$ is the empirical p-percentile of the values $\hat{R}^{*b}$ ($b = 1, \ldots, B$), obtained in **Step 3**. Likewise, if $\hat{S}$ is used, the null hypothesis is rejected if $\hat{S} > \hat{S}^{*(1-\alpha)}$, where $\hat{S}^{*(p)}$ is the empirical p-percentile of $\hat{S}^{*b}$ ($b = 1, \ldots, B$).

Hereafter, the test based on $\hat{T}$ will be denoted by **T1**, and the test based on $\hat{S}$ by **T2**.

8.4   Simulation Study

In this section, we report on a simulation study designed to assess the validity of the bootstrap-based interaction tests. Given the covariate vector $\mathbf{X} = (X_1, X_2, X_3)^t$, the binary outcome variable Y was generated on the basis of $Y \sim B\{p(\mathbf{X})\}$ where

$$p(\mathbf{X}) = \frac{\exp\{f_1(X_1) + f_2(X_2) + f_3(X_3) + f_{12}(X_1, X_2)\}}{1 + \exp\{f_1(X_1) + f_2(X_2) + f_3(X_3) + f_{12}(X_1, X_2)\}}. \tag{8.9}$$

Here, the covariates X_1, X_2 and X_3 were chosen as independent random variables uniformly distributed as $U[-2,2]$. One thousand independent samples $\{(X_i, Y_i)\}_{i=1}^n$ were generated from the model (8.9), under: $f_1(u) = \sin(180u)$, $f_2(u) = u^2$ and $f_{12}(u,v) = auv$, where a is a constant. Note that the value $a = 0$ corresponds to the hypothesis of no interaction ($f_{12} = 0$), and that the more constant a shifts from zero, the greater the degree of interaction in the model (8.9).

As regards the issue of testing, we considered the null hypothesis $\mathbf{H}_{12}^0 : f_{12} = 0$ (or equivalently $a = 0$), using the two different tests -**T1** and **T2**- explained in Section 11.3 above. To ascertain the results shown in Table 8.1 and Figure 8.1 we performed 1000 bootstrap replications of the three test statistics reviewed. Table 8.1 represents type 1 error for the two tests at different significance levels and different sample sizes, with the probability of rejection being determined by performing 1000 replications.

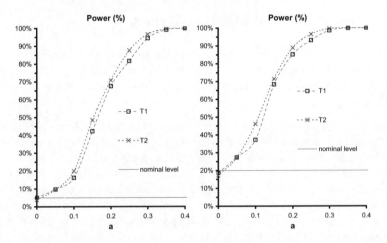

Figure 8.1: Power function at 5% and 20% significance levels for sample size $n = 1000$

As can be seen from Table 8.1, the two tests registered very satisfactory results overall, with a type 1 error very close to the nominal in evidence for $a = 0$. For small sample sizes (n=250, n=400), while **T2** proved to be the test that registered a type 1 error closest to the nominal, the two tests considered -**T1** and **T2**- rejected the null hypothesis less often than expected. For large sample sizes ($n = 1000$), **T1** showed a type 1 error practically equal to the nominal, whereas test **T2** tended to reject $\mathbf{H}_{12}^0$ less often than expected.

Power as a function of a is shown for different levels and sample size $n = 1000$

in Figure 8.1. All two tests registered satisfactory power curves, with the probability of rejection rising in response to any increase in the value of the constant a.

8.5 Application to Real Data Sets

In this section we apply the proposed methodology to two different real data sets. The first example comes from the physiological field, and the aim of this study is to assess the possible association between the temporal evolution of the neuronal firing rate and decision making. In the second example, the interest is focused on the potential influence of several continuous covariates on the risk of post-operative infection.

8.5.1 Neural Basis of Decision Making

A main goal in our case study, is to examine possible differences in single-neuron firing rate when the monkey decides whether a test bar (*test* stimulus) is oriented to the left or to the right of another bar shown previously (*reference* stimulus).

The data analyzed here come from studies of the extra-cellular single unit activity in the prefrontal cortex of behaving monkeys. Monkeys were trained to discriminate line orientations. A stimulus consisted of a stationary line segment subtending 3° of visual angle. Test lines, were presented clockwise or counter-clockwise to the reference. A trial was initiated with the presentation of the fixation target. Then, two stimuli (called *reference* and *test*), each of 500 ms of duration were presented in temporal sequence, with a fixed inter-stimulus interval (ISI: 1100 ms). At the end of the second stimulus, the subject released the key and pressed one of the two switches (left or right), indicating whether the orientation of the second stimulus was clockwise or counter-clockwise to the first stimulus.

To get enough data and to account for the cell response variability, the neuron was recorded over a number of $N = 80$ trials. For each of the $j = 1, \ldots, N$ trials, we have considered the orientation of the *test* stimuli ($Orien^j$): $Orien^j = 0$, if *test* stimulus is to the right of the *reference* stimulus, and $Orien^j = 1$, if *test* stimulus is to the left.

In this experiment, the outcome of interest is the neuronal activity. At each instant $t \in [t_{\min}, t_{\max}] = [-500, 4500]$, and trial $j = 1, \ldots, N$, this outcome may be then represented by a temporal binary sequence, Y_t^j, where

$Y_t^j = 1$ if there is a spike in $[t, t+1$ ms.) and 0 otherwise. Accordingly, for those blocks of N trials, the data set consists of the following information: $\left\{ t, Orien^j, Y_t^j \right\}$.

We use the GAM modeling to examine the temporal association between electrical activity of a single neuron and decision making. With this aim we consider the following logistic GAM:

$$p\left(Orien, t\right) = \left(1 + \exp\left[\alpha + f(t) + g\left\{Orien, t\right\}\right]^{-1}\right)^{-1} \qquad (8.10)$$

where $p\left(Orien, t\right) = p\left(Y_t = 1 | Orien, t\right)$, α is a fixed parameter, f a time function, and g the orientation-by-time interaction term given by

$$g\left(Orien, t\right) = g_0\left(t\right) \boldsymbol{I}\left\{Orien = 0\right\} + g_1\left(t\right) \boldsymbol{I}\left\{Orien = 1\right\},$$

being g_0 and g_1 two one-dimensional functions of time.

To assess the temporal association between firing probability (or equivalently, the firing rate) and decisions based on the orientation (1=left; 0=right) of the *test* stimulus, we propose the use of odds-ratios curve (OR) (Figueiras *et al.*, 2001). In accordance with model 8.10, we define $OR\left(t\right)$ at each instant t, as

$$OR(t) = \frac{p(1,t)/\left\{1 - p(1,t)\right\}}{p(0,t)/\left\{1 - p(0,t)\right\}} = \exp\left\{g_1(t) - g_0(t)\right\}, \qquad (8.11)$$

taking the 'right' orientation (i.e., $Orien = 0$) as the reference category. We then fit logistic GAM (8.10) to analyze the difference in firing rate, and its temporal evolution, when the monkey decides. The resulting fit is presented in Figure (8.2) (left column). As can be seen in thisigure, for decisions taken to the left, the firing rate is higher than that corresponding to decisions taken to the right. For both decisions, the increase of firing rate begins during the presentation of the test stimulus, and reaches its maximum close to the reaction time (RT), just before the beginning of the arm movement towards the buttons.

To determine the epoch(s) in which the discharge in both situations is different, i.e., when the cell firing rate discriminates between both decisions, we compute the temporal OR curve given in (8.11), taking the 'right' orientation as the reference. In the right plot of Figure (8.2), we present the resulting OR curve, along with the corresponding pointwise 95% bootstrap confidence bands. It is seen that the magnitude of the OR relating orientation to neural

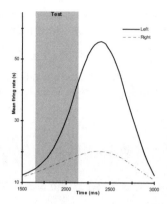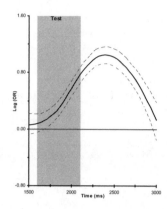

Figure 8.2: Left plot: Estimated firing rates grouped by orientation (left, right). Right plot: log OR curve for the association between firing rate and orientation together with the corresponding pointwise 95% confidence bands. Reference orientation: "Right". Grey boxes indicate the timing of the test stimulus

response becomes significantly greater than one, 77 ms after the beginning of the presentation of the test stimulus, reaches its maximum around the reaction time and then decreases, losing significance at 2959 ms, when the monkey finishes its arm movement. Therefore, a significant strength of association between firing rate and decisions –which might be interpreted as the *discrimination capability* of the neuron-, is maintained for 1282 ms. Applying the interaction tests, **T1** and **T2** (outlined in Section 11.3 above) yielded p-values lower than 0.01, thereby rendering the interaction term $g\,(Orien, t)$ statistically significant.

For the construction of the confidence intervals, displayed in Figure (8.2), we have used again the bootstrap technique. Given a point t, the steps for construction of the confidence interval for the true $OR\,(t)$ are as follows:

Step 1. Estimate the model (8.10) and obtain the pilot estimates $\tilde{p}_t^j = \tilde{p}\left(Y_t = 1 | Orien^j, t\right)$ for $(t = t_{\min}, \ldots, t_{\max}; \; j = 1, \ldots, N)$

and then the pilot estimate $\widetilde{OR}\,(t)$.

Step 2. For $b = 1, \ldots, B$ generate the sample $\left\{t, Orien^j, Y_t^{*b,j}\right\}$ with $Y_t^{*b,j} \sim \mathrm{B}\left(\tilde{p}_t^j\right)$ and obtain bootstrap estimates $\widehat{OR}^{*b}\,(t)$.

Once this process has been completed, the 95% limits of the confidence interval for the true $OR(t)$ are given by

$$\left(\widehat{OR}(t) - \widehat{OR}^{(0.975)}(t),\ \widehat{OR}(t) - \widehat{OR}^{(0.025)}(t)\right),$$

where $\widehat{OR}(t)$ is the estimate obtained with the original sample and $\widehat{OR}^{(p)}(t)$ represents the p-percentile of the differences $\widetilde{OR}^{*b}(t) - \widetilde{OR}(t)$ $(b = 1,\ldots,B)$.

8.5.2   Risk of Post-operative Infection

In this section we apply the proposed methodology to data drawn from a registry-based prospective cohort study of 2318 patients who underwent surgery at the University Hospital of Santiago de Compostela (NW Spain). Patients were characterized as follows: pre-operatively, in respect of a series of variables, including GLU=plasma glucose concentration (in mg/dl) and LYM=lymphocytes (expressed as relative counts (%) of the white blood cell count); and post-operatively, in respect of whether they suffered (POI=1) or did not suffer post-operative infection (POI=0).

The main goal of this analysis was to investigate the possible (main) effects of LYM and GLU on risk of POI, and also the potential modifying effect of GLU on the LYM-POI relationship. We first analyzed the main effects of LYM and GLU on risk of POI, adjusted for potential confounders, such as SEX (coded as 1=male; 0=female) and AGE, by fitting a logistic GAM as follows:

$$p(POI = 1|LYM, GLU, AGE, SEX) = \left\{1 + \exp\left(\eta^{\bullet}\right)^{-1}\right\}^{-1}, \qquad (8.12)$$

with

$$\eta^{\bullet} = \alpha + f_{LYM}(LYM) + f_{GLU}(GLU) + f_{AGE}(AGE) + \beta_{SEX} \times SEX.$$

According with (8.12) we define the OR curve for $GLUC$ and LYM as

$$OR_{GLU}^{95}(x) = \exp\left(f_{GLU}(x) - f_{GLU}(95)\right),$$

and

$$OR_{LYM}^{30\%}(x) = \exp\left(f_{LYM}(x) - f_{LYM}(30)\right)$$

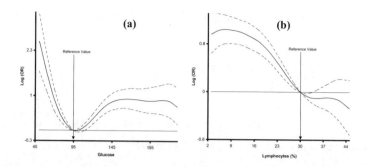

Figure 8.3: Estimated log OR curves and 95% pointwise confidence bands for the effect of pre-operative levels of (a) plasma glucose concentration and (b) lymphocytes (in percent), on the risk of post-operative infection

As reference values for the purposes of OR calculation, we took the midpoints of the ranges considered clinically "normal" (95mg/dl for GLU and 30% for LYM). Estimated OR curves with corresponding 95% pointwise confidence bands are depicted in Figure (8.3). Figure (8.3)(a) confirms the plausible results previously obtained by Figueiras and Cadarso-Suárez (2001), i.e., a "spoon-shaped" OR_{GLU}^{95} curve, as well as the existence of significant association between plasma glucose levels, both low and high, and increased risk of POI. As can be seen from Figure (8.3)(b), the estimated $OR_{LYM}^{30\%}$ curve appears to be non-linear, indicating that POI risk decreases with increasing LYM up to a value of around 30% and remains almost constant thereafter.

We next investigated the possibility that risk associated with lymphocytes (%) might vary with plasma glucose concentration levels. We then added the corresponding interaction term $f_{LYM,GLU}$, and fitted the "interaction" logistic GAM given in (8.12) with

$$\eta^{\bullet} = \alpha + f_{LYM}\left(LYM\right) + f_{GLU}\left(GLU\right) + f_{LYM,GLU}\left(LYM, GLU\right)$$
$$+ f_{AGE}\left(AGE\right) + \beta_{SEX} \times SEX,$$

Applying the interaction tests, **T1** and **T2** yielded p-values lower than 0.01, thereby rendering the interaction term $f_{LYM,GLU}$ statistically significant. According with the new model the bidimensional OR curve for LYM and GLU is defined as

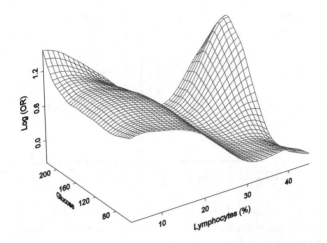

Figure 8.4: Estimated log $OR^{30\%}_{LYM,GLU}$ surface showing the nonparametric effect of percentage of lymphocytes (LYM) on the risk of post-operative infection, varying smoothly according to the values taken by plasma glucose concentration (GLU)

$$\log OR^{30\%}_{LYM,GLU}(x,y) = f_{LYM}(x) + f_{LYM,GLU}(x,y)$$
$$- f_{LYM}(30) - f_{LYM,GLU}(30,y),$$

A plot of the resulting estimate for the $OR^{30\%}_{LYM,GLU}$ surface from fitted model is depicted in Figure (8.4).

Nevertheless, to ascertain more clearly how the functional form of the LYM effect on POI varied with GLU values, we decided to plot cross-sections of the estimated surface separately. Two cross-sections for plasma glucose values (GLU=70, and 200) with their corresponding 95% pointwise confidence bands, are shown in Figure (8.5).

Examination of these and other sections showed that for plasma glucose values below a figure of approximately 150mg/dl, the estimated influence of lymphocytes (%) on risk of POI was qualitatively the same as when no (LYM,GLU)-interaction was included in the model. For higher plasma glucose values, however, risk of POI increased, not only as lymphocyte percentages fell below, but also as they rose above the reference value (30%); interestingly, the $OR^{30\%}_{LYM}$ curve was by now broadly U-shaped, with significant increasing risk attaching to both LYM<25% and LYM>35%, corresponding

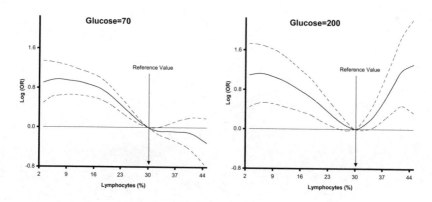

Figure 8.5: Cross-sections of the estimated surface of Figure (8.4) at two values of plasma glucose concentration, with the corresponding 95% pointwise confidence bands

to *LYM* values outside the normal clinical range.

8.6   Discussion

In this chapter local scoring (with backfitting) based on local linear kernel smoothers were used to estimate GAM with interactions. The main goal was to propose statistical tests for checking the presence of second-order interactions. As backfitting theory is very difficult, bootstrap procedure was used in the implementation of such tests.

The results obtained with the tests depend heavily on the smoothing parameter used in local scoring. Various proposals for an optimal selection have been suggested for GAMs, based on the minimization of some error criteria, such as Generalized Cross-Validation (GCV) or Akaike's Information Criterion (AIC) (Hastie and Tibshirani, 1990), yet the difficulty of asymptotic theory in a backfitting context means that nowadays optimal selection tends to be an opening problem. As a practical solution, we used cross-validation for the automatic choice of bandwidths in the estimation of the link and the partial functions.

As is well known, cross-validation implies a high computational cost. In our particular case, this cost was increased even further, given that the unidimensional uni and bidimensional partial functions had to be estimated in each cycle of the estimation algorithm. Moreover, in the use of the bootstrap procedure, these operations must be repeated a great number of (e.g., 1000) times. For these computational reasons, one-dimensional and bi-dimensional binning-type acceleration techniques were used to speed up the estimation process. Binning acelaration made it possible for the tests to be concluded in a reduced period of time, even when we have many data. For instance, in the post-operative infection data, presented in Section 8.5.2, with sample size of $n=2318$ the boostrap test based on 1000 bootstrap repetitions, was concluded in under 1.5 minutes (using a 1000 MHz Pentium III, 128MB RAM).

The performance of the proposed tests was verified in a simulation study, and by applying them to two biomedical problems: First, we applied our methods to neural data obtained while monkeys performed in discrimination tasks. Our testing methods reveal differences in neural firing rates associated with assessments of outcomes during decision making. Second, application of the methodology to data on potential risk factors for post-operative infection showed that for patients with high plasma glucose levels increased risk is associated not only with low percentages of lymphocytes, as is to be expected, but also with high percentages.

In this work, we focused on binary response, though all the procedures outlined are easily generalizable to the exponential family. Indeed, we conducted studies for Poisson response (results not reported here) and obtained similar results to those presented in this work for binary response. Moreover, our methodology, can be easily generalized to the case where the bivariate interaction terms associated with two continuous covariates (two-order continuous interactions) vary across levels of a categorical covariate.

8.7 Appendix

Unidimensional Weighted Local Linear Kernel Estimators

Given a sample $\{X_i, Y_i\}_{i=1}^n$ and a set of weights, $\{W_i\}_{i=1}^n$, the weighted local linear kernel estimator $\hat{\psi}(x) = \hat{\psi}(x, \{X_i, Y_i, W_i\}_{i=1}^n, h)$ at a localization x is defined as:

$$\hat{\psi}(x) = (1,0) \begin{pmatrix} s^0(x) & s^1(x) \\ s^1(x) & s^2(x) \end{pmatrix}^{-1} \begin{pmatrix} u^0(x) \\ u^1(x) \end{pmatrix},$$

where $s^r(x) = \sum_{i=1}^n (W_i \cdot L^r(x, X_i))$ and $u^r(x) = \sum_{i=1}^n (W_i \cdot L^r(x, X_i) \cdot Y_i)$, with

$$L^r(x, y) = (2\pi)^{-1/2} (x - y)^r \exp\left[-0.5\left\{h^{-1}(x - y)\right\}^2\right] (r = 0, 1, 2).$$

The smoothing bandwidth, h, was selected automatically by minimizing the following weighted cross-validation error criterion

$$CV = \sum_{i=1}^{n} W_i \left\{\hat{\psi}^{(-i)}(X_i) - Y_i\right\}^2,$$

where $\hat{\psi}^{(-i)}(X_i)$ indicates the fit at X_i leaving out the i-th data point.

Bidimensional Weighted Local Linear Kernel Estimators

Let the sample be $\{\mathbf{X}_i, Y_i\}_{i=1}^{n}$, with $\mathbf{X}_i = (X_{i1}, X_{i2})$, and a set of weights, $\{W_i\}_{i=1}^{n}$. The bidimensional weighted local linear kernel estimator $\hat{\psi}_{2D}(\mathbf{x}) = \hat{\psi}_{2D}(\mathbf{x}, \{\mathbf{X}_i, Y_i, W_i\}_{i=1}^{n}, h)$ at a localization $\mathbf{x} = (x_1, x_2)$ is defined as:

$$\hat{\psi}_{2D}(x_1, x_2) = (1, 0, 0) \begin{pmatrix} s^{00}(x_1, x_2) & s^{10}(x_1, x_2) & s^{01}(x_1, x_2) \\ s^{10}(x_1, x_2) & s^{20}(x_1, x_2) & s^{11}(x_1, x_2) \\ s^{01}(x_1, x_2) & s^{11}(x_1, x_2) & s^{02}(x_1, x_2) \end{pmatrix}^{-1} \times$$

$$\times \begin{pmatrix} t^{00}(x_1, x_2) \\ t^{10}(x_1, x_2) \\ t^{01}(x_1, x_2) \end{pmatrix},$$

with

$$s^{rt}(x_1, x_2) = \sum_{s=1}^{n} \hat{W}_s L^{rt}((x_1, x_2), (X_{sj}, X_{sk}))$$
$$t^{rt}(x_1, x_2) = \sum_{s=1}^{n} \hat{W}_s L^{rt}((x_1, x_2), (X_{sj}, X_{sk})) Y_s$$
$$L^{rt}((x, y), (u, v)) = (x - u)^r (y - v)^t K_2\left(\mathbf{H}^{-1/2}(x - u, y - v)^t\right),$$

$(r, t \in \{0, 1, 2\})$ and $K_2(\cdot)$ being the two-dimensional normal density function with mean zero and the same covariance matrix as the set $\{(X_{i1}, X_{i2})\}_{i=1}^{n}$ in the sample data. In this way, the contour curves of K_2 are "isobars" in the sample space, in the sense that sample points on the same contour have the same weight in the estimations, $\hat{\psi}$.

In the same way as the unidimensional case, the 2×2 matrix $\mathbf{H}_{jk}$ is selected by minimizing $CV = \sum_{i=1}^{n} \hat{W}_i \left(\hat{\psi}^{(-i)}(X_{i1}, X_{i2}) - Y_i\right)^2$ where $\hat{\psi}^{(-i)}(X_{i1}, X_{i2})$ indicates the fit at (X_{i1}, X_{i2}) leaving out the ith data point. For computational simplicity we set $\mathbf{H}_{jk} = \text{diag}(h_{j1}, h_{j2})$.

Bibliography

Coull, B., Ruppert, D. and Wand, M. (2001). Simple incorporation of interactions into additive models. *Biometrics*, **57**, 539-45.

Fan, J. and Marron, J.S. (1994). Fast implementation of nonparametric curve estimators. *Journal of Computational and Graphical Statistics*, **3**, 35-56.

Figueiras, A. and Cadarso-Suárez, C. (2001). Application of nonparametric models for calculating odds ratios and their confidence intervals for continuous exposures. *American Journal of Epidemiology*, **154**, 264-75.

Hastie, T. J. and Tibshirani, R. J. (1990). *Generalized Additive Models*. Vol. 43 of *Monographs on Statistics and Applied Probability*, Chapman and Hall, London.

Härdle, W. and Scott, D. W. (1992). Smoothing in Low and High Dimensions by Weighted Averaging Using Rounded Points. *Computational Statistics*, **1**, 97-128.

Kauermann, G. and Opsomer, J.D. (2003). Local Likelihood Estimation in Generalized Additive Models. *Scandinavian Journal of Statistics*, **30**, 317-37.

Linton, O.B. and Nielsen, J.B. (1995). A kernel method of estimating structured nonparametric regression based on marginal integration. *Biometrika*, **82**, 93-100.

Opsomer, J.D. (2000). Asymptotic properties of backfitting estimators. *Journal of Multivariate Analysis*, **73**, 166-79.

Roca-Pardiñas, J. (2003). *Aportaciones a la inferencia no paramétrica en Modelos Aditivos Generalizados and extensiones. Aplicaciones en Medioambiente y Salud.* Ph.D. Thesis, University of Santiago de Compostela, Spain.

Ruppert, D. and Wand, M.P. (1994). Multivariate locally weighted least squares regression. *Annals of Statistics*, **22**, 1346-70.

Ruppert, D., Wand, M.P. and Carroll, R.J. (2003). *Semiparametric Regression. Cambridge Series in Statistical and Probabilistic Mathematics*, University of Cambridge, Cambridge.

Sperlich, S., Tjøsteim D. and Yang, L. (2002). Nonparametric Estimation and Testing of Interaction in Additive Models. *Econometric Theory*, **18**, 197-251.

Tjøsteim, D. and Auestad, B.H. (1994). Nonparametric identification of non-linear time series: projections. *J. Amer. Stat. Assoc.*, **89**, 1398-1409.

Wand, M.P. (1994). Fast Computation of Multivariate Kernel Estimators. *Journal of Computational and Graphical Statistics*, **3**, 433-45.

Wand, M.P. and Jones, M.C. (1995). *Kernel Smoothing.* Vol. 60 of *Monographs on Statistics and Applied Probability*, Chapman and Hall, London.

9 Survival Trees

Carmela Cappelli and Heping Zhang

9.1 Introduction

Survival trees are a useful regression tool to model the relationship between a survival time and a set of covariates. Survival or censored data are particularly common in medical research, and they also arise from many different areas of scientific and clinical research. For example, in the social sciences, we may be interested in the school drop-out rates and the turnover in a labor market. Tree based methods, due to their nonparametric nature and flexibility, have become very popular in the last two decades as an alternative to the traditional proportional hazard model.

The term *survival data* refers to any data that deal with time to the occurrence of an event of interest. Although the methods developed to cope with survival data are primarily related to medical and biological research, they have their root in insurance statistics and, in general, they are widely used in the social and economic sciences, as well as in engineering. In economics we may study the "survival" of firms or the "survival" of products. For quality control purposes it is a common practice to study the "survival" of electronic components (reliability data analysis, failure time analysis, see Meeker and Escobar (1998)).

In medical research, the event of interest is usually the time to death of a patient after the diagnosis but it might be the time to recovery or remission as well. The main feature of survival data is the presence of incomplete data, which are referred to as *censored observations* and often provide the most relevant information about the phenomenon under study. Censoring can arise from several reasons: the observation time is limited and the study ends before the event is observed for all the subjects, some of the subjects may be lost to follow up the study, subjects are entered at fixed times and the event occurred before recording. In all these cases, the exact time of the event is not observed. Depending on the direction of the censoring, censored data can be classified into *right censored* when the survival time exceeds the observed one, and *left censored* when the survival time is less than the observed one. Left censoring is particularly important in studies on infectious diseases such hepatitis or HIV (human immunodeficiency) but it will not be discussed here. In the realm of right censored data, a distinction can be made among three different types of censoring:

- Type I censoring: the subjects enter the study at the same time, at a given date the study ends and some of them are lost to follow up or the event is not occurred;

- Type II censoring: the subjects enter the study at the same time, the end of the study is not initially fixed and it is carried on until the event occurs for a certain proportion of subjects;

- Type III censoring: the subjects enter the study at different times.

Figure 9.1 depicts these situations.

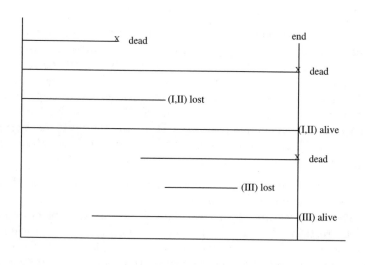

Figure 9.1: The various types of censor data

Note that Type II is *nonrandom censoring*, whereas Type I and III are *random censoring*.

The circumstance that the survival time cannot be fully observed for all the subjects under study can be formally expressed as follows. Let Y be the observed time and T be the survival time. Without censoring, $Y = T$, i.e., the observed time is the true survival time. With censoring, the observed time is the censoring time denoted by U. A censoring indicator δ takes into account the time being censored, so that $\delta = 1$ if $Y = T$ and $\delta = 0$ otherwise. For the latter, $Y = \min(T, U)$.

There are several important issues involved in the analysis of survival data. They include the comparison of the survival distributions among two or more groups and the identification of predictive variables of survival time. To these ends, parametric, semiparametric and nonparametric methods have been developed. Briefly, parametric methods require specifying a distribution for the survival times (for example Exponential or Weibull). The semi-parametric methods make no assumptions concerning the distributions of the survival times but assume a known form for the effects of the covariates on survivorship. Non-parametric methods make no assumptions on distributions of the survival times. General discussions on various methods can be found in textbooks such as Lee (1992) and Miller (1998).

Among nonparametric methods, tree based methods have become a very popular tool for survival data analysis thanks to the fact that multiple covariates may be associated with the survival time and researchers are commonly interested in identifying subgroups of subjects with similar survival distributions as determined by the covariates.

The XploRe quantlib `hazreg` provides a number of quantlets for the analysis of survival data. We will describe here the quantlet `stree`, which implements the tree based regression method for survival data developed by Zhang (1995) and Zhang and Singer (1999), providing a complete tool to grow, prune and display survival trees.

This chapter is a tutorial for the XploRe `stree` quantlet in the XploRe quantlib `hazreg` Grund and Yang (2000, Chapter 5), which represent the XploRe implementation of the methodology decribed by Zhang (1995) and Zhang and Singer (1999) and a modification of Heping Zhang's program called STREE. In Section 1, we describe censored survival data. In Section 2, the survival tree methodology is presented. In Section 3, the syntax of the quantlets `stree` is illustrated with some examples.

9.2   Methodology

Any tree based method involves two main steps:

1. *growing* the tree, i.e., partitioning the data (internal nodes) according to a splitting criterion which allows to select the best covariate and cut point along it to split any node;

2. *pruning* the tree, i.e, removing retrospectively some of the branches in order to get a shorter and more accurate tree.

With censored data the survival time is not completely observed for all the subjects and therefore it involves two response variables: the observed time and the censoring indicator defined above. As a consequence, the data are triplets $\{y_i, \delta_i, \mathbf{x}_i\}$, $i = 1, \ldots, n$ where y_i is the observed time for the i-th subjects, δ_i indicates whether y_i is censored and $\mathbf{x}_i = (x_{i1}, \ldots, x_{ip})$ is the vector of the p covariates associated with the i-th subject. The events $y_i = t_i$ are called *event times* or *failure times*. It is noteworthy that in this approach, the censoring is assumed to be random (Type I and Type III), so that, given the values of the covariates, the conditional distributions of the survival time and the censoring time are independent.

9.2.1   Splitting Criteria

The growing phase is led by the objective of forming a number of homogeneous subsets with respect to the response variable. In order to achieve this aim, the quantlet `stree` allows three splitting criteria as described by Zhang (1995). Two of them are based on an extension of the *impurity measure* introduced by Breiman, Friedman, Olshen and Stone (1984) and the other one is based on the log-rank test statistic.

Impurity based criteria   In order to discuss the impurity-based splitting criteria, it is useful to recall some basic concepts and notation in the classification of a multi-class response. Consider a candidate split s of a node t into two offsprings t_l and t_r and let $p(t_l)$ and $p(t_r)$ be the proportions of observations sent by s into node t_l and t_r, respectively. The impurity at node t, denoted by $i(t)$, measures the impurities based on the within-class probabilities. Then, a natural way to evaluate the performances of a candidate split is the change in impurity given by:

$$\Delta i(s,t) = i(t) - \{p(t_l)i(t_l) + p(t_r)i(t_r)\} \qquad (9.1)$$

The quantity $\Delta i(s,t)$ is used as a partitioning criterion. This notion of impurity in the case of censored survival data cannot be used as it stands because, although the outcome we are interested in is the survival time, this involves two response variables: the observed time y_i (continuous) and the censoring indicator δ_i (binary). In this respect, a pure node would contain subjects whose observed times are similar and who are in most part censored or uncensored. In other words, a suitable impurity measure for censored data must take account of both observed time and censoring. Therefore the impurity of a node can be expressed as:

$$i(t) = w_1 i_y(t) + w_2 i_\delta(t), \qquad (9.2)$$

where w_1 and w_2 are pre-specified weights and $i_y(t)$ and $i_\delta(t)$ denote the impurity of node t for the observed time and censoring, respectively. In particular, the impurity for the time is given by

$$i_y(t) = \sum_{i=1}^{n(t)} \frac{\{y_i - \bar{y}(t)\}^2}{\sum y_i^2} \qquad (9.3)$$

where $n(t)$ is the number of observations in node t and $\bar{y}(t)$ is the average of the observed times. The denominator is needed to be normalized with respect to the other component of the impurity. When the summation in the denominator is over node t observations the criterion is called *adaptive normalization*. When it is over the whole sample it is called *global normalization*.

For the impurity of the censoring indicator, it is measured by the entropy measure:

$$i_\delta(t) = -p_t \log(p_t) - (1 - p_t) \log(1 - p_t), \qquad (9.4)$$

where p_t denotes the proportion of censored data in node t. Among all the candidate splits at a given node, one split is chosen to maximize the reduction in impurity as measured by (9.1). This simple adaptation of the impurity criterion provides a straightforward way to combine the continuous and categorical outcomes that characterize censored data.

Log-rank statistic criterion   The log-rank test statistic is commonly used in the analysis of censored survival data to compare the survival distributions of different groups. For a given covariate and a split point, a 2×2 contingency table is created of the form

Table 9.1: Contingency table for the log-rank statistic

	Event	
	Yes	No
$x_{ij} \leq s$	a_i	n_i
$x_{ij} > s$	d_i	K_i

where x_{ij} is the value of the j-th covariate for the i-th observation, s is a split point, and K_i is the risk set at time y_i. The log-rank test statistic is defined as:

$$LR(s) = \frac{\sum_i (a_i - E_i)}{\sqrt{\sum_i V_i}} \tag{9.5}$$

where

$$E_i = \frac{d_i n_i}{K_i} \tag{9.6}$$

and

$$V_i = \left\{ \frac{d_i (K_i - n_i) n_i}{K_i (K_i - 1)} \right\} \left(1 - \frac{d_i}{K_i}\right). \tag{9.7}$$

Given that the log-rank statistic testes the significance of the difference between two survival distributions, it represents, in a way, a natural choice for splitting the data into two groups with different survivals and it is widely adopted as the splitting criterion Segal (1998), LeBlanc and Crowley (1993), Ciampi and Thiffault (1986).

At a given node t, for every covariate and split point, the log-rank test statistic is computed and the best split s^* is chosen if

$$LR(s^*, t) = \max LR(s, t). \tag{9.8}$$

9.2.2 Pruning

Tree growing, or recursive partitioning, is only one aspect of the tree construction. Tree pruning generally follows tree growing, because of the following two concerns:

1. **complexity** – the long resulting structure tends to be very large; this is especially the case with binary trees since an attribute may reappear (although in a restricted form) many times down the tree;

2. **overfitting** – several branches, especially the terminal ones, reflect particular features of the data arising from the sampling procedure rather than modeling the underlying relationship between the response variable and the covariates.

Therefore, after a large tree T_{max} is grown, a pruning step is carried out in order to simplify the structure and avoid overfitting as discussed in Cappelli, Mola and Siciliano (2002). The quantlet `stree` implements a practical bottom up pruning procedure following the proposal suggested by Segal (1998), which can be described as follows. A statistic S_t (say the log-rank test statistic) is assigned to each internal node t of T_{max}. These statistics are ordered in an increasing order. A threshold is then selected and any internal node whose statistic does not reach the threshold is changed into a terminal node.

The threshold can be fixed by simply considering a significance level. Cutting off the branches stemming from the internal nodes that do not reach the threshold results in a single final pruned tree. A more effective approach that allows insights into the pruning process is to generate a sequence of nested pruned subtrees of T_{max} in the spirit of the pruning procedure proposed in the CART book (see the XploRe CART tutorial). The sequence is created by iterating the process of locating the minimum value of the statistic and pruning the offsprings of the node(s) that reaches this minimum value. The threshold and therefore the final tree, is selected by plotting the minimal statistics against the size (number of terminal nodes) of the corresponding subtree.

The inspection of the plot allows to select the final tree, in particular, usually the plot shows a "kink" where the pattern changes suggesting that the corresponding tree could be the final one. An important point in the pruning process concerns the assignment of the statistic to the internal nodes. This assignment involves two steps: first, the statistic is computed for all internal nodes; next, the assigned value is replaced with the maximum over the node offsprings if the latter is greater. The sequence, therefore, is created considering the maximized values. In this way the pruning process tends to retain branches that contain sub-branches with higher values of the statistic.

9.3   The Quantlet stree

9.3.1   Syntax

The quantlet stree has the following syntax:

    streeout = stree (covars, time, censor, covartypes, method)

with input variables:

covars : A $n \times p$ matrix containing observations of covariates,

time : A $n \times 1$ vector containing observations of survival time

censor : A $n \times 1$ vector containing the censoring indicator,

covartypes : specifies the type of covariates

method : indicates the splitting criterion.

The arbitrary name streeout has been used to indicate the output which includes the following output variables:

nodenum : the node number,

cases : the number of observations falling into the node,

dnleft : the left descendant node number,

dnright : the right descendant node number,

median : the median survival time,

splitvar : the splitting variable chosen to split the node

splitval, splitting values or categories; observations having the variable splitvar larger than the value in splitval are sent to the right daughter node, otherwise to the left daughter node. For categorical variables splitval reports the categories for cases sent into the right descendant.

Optional parameters allows to modify the output presentation. Note that the output of stree is shown both in the form of a table and a graphical display.

9.3.2   Example

In order to illustrate the quantlet stree the Early Lung Cancer Detection data has been considered; this data set is available at the *Statlib* archive (http://lib.stat.cmu.edu/datasets/csb).

The following variables were recorded:

Table 9.2: Recorded variables

Variable name	Possible values
patient ID	integer
institution	0 = Memorial Sloan Kettering, 1 = Mayo Clinic, 2 = John Opkins
group	0 = study, 1 = controls
means of detection	0 = routine cytology, 1 = routine X-ray, 2 = both X-ray and cytology, 3 = interval
cell type	0 = epidermoid, 1 = adenocarcinoma, 2 = large cell, 3 = oat cell, 4 = other
stage	involves four covariates: overall stage, tumor, lymph nodes and distant metastases
overall stage	three levels
tumor	three levels
lymph nodes	three levels
distant metastases	two levels
operated	0 = no, 1 = yes
survival	days from detection to last date known alive
survival category	0 = alive, 1 = dead of lung cancer, 2 = dead of other causes

The analysis has been restricted to the study group, discarding the controls; also, in the study group, patients dead for other causes than the lung cancer has not been considered so that the subset consist of $n = 475$ patients. The following XploRe code reads the original data (file lung.dat), deletes the patient ID, creates the subset and the input variables for the quantlet stree and runs the quantlet considering as splitting criterion the global normalization.

The results are displayed in Table 9.3 and 9.4, moreover the pruned tree is displayed in Figure 9.2.

Q XCSstree01.xpl

Table 9.3: Global Normalization before Prune

node #	cases	left nodes	right nodes	median value	split var #	split value
1	475	2	3	805.00	4	3,2
2	183	4	5	1719.00	1	2,1
3	292	6	7	516.50	1	2
4	47	8	9	2282.00	5	2
5	136	10	11	1339.50	8	1
6	78	12	13	1479.50	2	3,2
7	214	14	15	415.50	4	3
8	25	16	17	2772.00	3	4,3
9	22	18	19	1586.00	2	3,2
10	23	20	21	1208.00	5	2
11	113	22	23	1343.00	3	4
12	31	24	25	1336.00	6	2
13	47	26	27	1617.00	6	2
14	28	28	29	490.00	5	2
15	186	30	31	405.00	3	4,1
22	56	32	33	1002.00	2	3,2
23	57	34	35	1720.00	1	2
25	17	36	37	1331.00	3	3
27	36	38	39	1826.50	3	3,2

XCSstree01.xpl

Table 9.4: Global Normalization after Prune

node #	cases	left nodes	right nodes	median value	split var #	split value
1	475	2	3	805.00	4	3,2
2	183	4	5	1719.00	1	2,1
3	292	6	7	516.50	1	2
4	47	8	9	2282.00	5	2
5	136	10	11	1339.50	8	1
7	214	14	15	415.50	4	3
11	113	22	23	1343.00	3	4
23	57	34	35	1720.00	1	2

Q XCSstree01.xpl

The first discriminant variable selected by the global normalization splitting criterion is the overall stage of the lung cancer, followed by the institution at both nodes 2 and 3. For example, the split of node 2 separates patients of the Mayo Clinic and of John Hopkins, who are sent to node 5, from patients of The Memorial Sloan Kittering. By setting in the above code the input variable method=``adaptnorm'' and method=``logrank'' , the other available criteria are used to grow the survival tree, adaptive normalization and log-rank statistic, respectively. Since the different splitting criteria affect the structure of the tree, it is advisable to try them all, selecting the final tree on the basis of scientific judgement.

Global normalization

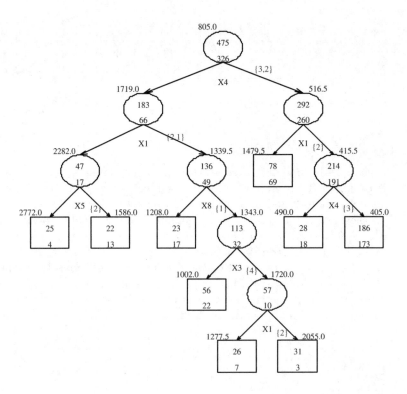

Figure 9.2: The survival tree for Early Lung Cancer Detection Data

Bibliography

Breiman L., Friedman J. H., Olshen R. A. and Stone C. J. (1984). *Classification and Regression Trees*, Wadsworth, Belmont CA.

Cappelli C., Mola F.and Siciliano R.(1984), A statistical approach to growing a honest reliable tree. *Computational Statistics and Data Analysis*, **38** (3), pp. 285–299.

Ciampi, A.and Thiffault, J. (1986), Stratification by stepwise regression, correspondence analysis and recursive partitioning: a comparison of three methods of analysis for survival data with covariates. *Computational Statistics and Data Analysis*, vol **4**, pp. 185–204.

Grund, B. and Yang, L. (2000), Hazard Regression in XploRe, in Härdle, Hlávka and Klinke (eds), *XploRe Application Guide*, Springer.

LeBlanc, M. and Crowley, J. (1993), Survival Trees by Goodness of Split. *J. Amer. Stat. Assoc.*, vol **88**, pp. 457–467.

Lee, E.T. (1989). *Statistical Methods for Survival Data Analysis*. Wiley, New York.

Meeker, W.Q. and Escobar, L. A., (1998). *Statistical Methods for Reliability Data* . John Wiley and Sons, Inc.

Miller, R.G, (1998). *Survival Analysis*. Wiley.

Segal, M. (1998), Regression Trees for Censored Data. *Biometrics*, vol **44**, pp. 35–48.

Zhang, H.P. (1995), Splitting Criteria in Survival Trees, in *Proceedings of the 10-th International Workshop on Statistical Modelling, Innsbruck Austria, July 1995*, pp. 305–314.

Zhang, H.P., and Singer, B. (1999). *Recursive Partitioning in the Health Science*, Springer.

10 A Semiparametric Approach to Estimate Reference Curves for Biophysical Properties of the Skin

Saracco Jérôme, Gannoun Ali, Guinot Christiane and Liquet Benoît

Reference curves which take one covariable into account such as the age, are often required in medicine, but simple systematic and efficient statistical methods for constructing them are lacking. Classical methods are based on parametric fitting (polynomial curves). In this chapter, we describe a new methodology for the estimation of reference curves for data sets, based on nonparametric estimation of conditional quantiles. The derived method should be applicable to all clinical or more generally biological variables that are measured on a continuous quantitative scale. To avoid the curse of dimensionality when the covariate is multidimensional, a new semiparametric approach is proposed. This procedure combines a dimension-reduction step (based on sliced inverse regression) and kernel estimation of conditional quantiles step. The usefulness of this semiparametric estimation procedure is illustrated on a simulated data set and on a real data set collected in order to establish reference curves for biophysical properties of the skin of healthy French women.

10.1   Introduction

The reference intervals are an important tool in clinical and medical practice. They provide a guideline to clinicians or clinical chemists seeking to interpret a measurement obtained from a new patient. Many experiments, in particular in biomedical studies, are conducted to establish the range of values that a variable of interest, say Y whose values are in $\mathbb{R}$, may normally take in a target population. Here "normally" refers to values that one can expect to see with a given probability under normal conditions or for typical individuals, and the corresponding ranges are often referred to as norms or reference values. Hence, a *reference interval* is the range of values bounded by a pair of quantiles which are symmetric about the median on the probability scale, such as the 5th and 95th centiles for a 90%-reference interval. Values which lie outside the limits of the reference interval are regarded as unusual or extreme and may indicate the presence of disease or disorder. To construct reference intervals, data (which are required to be continuous measurements) are collected from a reference population consisting of subjects who are believed healthy or "normal". Parametric methods are often used to calculate reference intervals. For this parametric approach, the data are generally assumed normally distributed. Nonparametric procedures have been developed to construct such intervals and do not require such a normality assumption.

When a covariable (or predictor) $\mathbf{X}$ (which can be p-dimensional) is simultaneously recorded with the variable of interest Y (assumed to be real at the moment), the notion of reference intervals is replaced by the one of *reference curves*. Conditional quantiles are widely used for building these curves. In medical or biomedical practice, the vector of covariables can be the measurement of the weight, height or age of the patient, while the dependent variable can be arterial pressure, cholesterol rate, etc. These reference curves are then constructed by estimating a set of conditional quantiles (also called regression quantiles). More details can be obtained from Cole (1988), Healy, Rasbash and Yang (1988), Goldstein and Pan (1992) or Royston and Altman (1992).

Mathematically speaking, for $\alpha \in (0, 1)$, when $\mathbf{X}$ and Y are $\mathbb{R}$-valued, the αth-conditional quantile of Y given $\mathbf{X} = \mathbf{x}$, denoted by $q_\alpha(\mathbf{x})$, is naturally defined as the root of the equation

$$F(y|\mathbf{x}) = \alpha, \tag{10.1}$$

where $F(y|\mathbf{x}) = P(Y \le y|\mathbf{X} = \mathbf{x})$ denotes the conditional distribution function of Y given $\mathbf{X} = \mathbf{x}$. For $\alpha > 0.5$, definition (10.1) allows us to define the $100(2\alpha - 1)\%$ reference curves, when $\mathbf{x}$ varies, by the following

$$I_\alpha(\mathbf{x}) = [q_{1-\alpha}(\mathbf{x}), q_\alpha(\mathbf{x})]. \tag{10.2}$$

So, estimating reference curves is reduced to estimating the conditional quantiles $q_{1-\alpha}(\mathbf{x})$ and $q_\alpha(\mathbf{x})$.

Note that there exists an alternative and direct characterization of the conditional quantile which does not use the conditional distribution function. It is well known, see for instance Fan, Hu and Truong (1994), that $q_\alpha(\mathbf{x})$ can be characterized as the value θ which minimizes the mathematical conditional expectation

$$\mathrm{E}\left[\rho_\alpha(Y - \theta)|\mathbf{X} = \mathbf{x}\right], \tag{10.3}$$

where ρ_α is the so-called "check" or "loss" function given by $\rho_\alpha(z) = (\alpha - 1)z$ if $z < 0$ and $\rho_\alpha(z) = \alpha z$ otherwise. Relevant theoretical background and details can be found for example in Basset and Koenker (1982), Jones and Hall (1990), Chaudhuri (1991a) and Yu (1997).

When n observations $\{(\mathbf{X}_i, Y_i)\}_{i=1}^n$ of $(\mathbf{X}, Y)$ are available, some basic estimation methods can be considered to estimate conditional quantiles. A typical parametric approach is the following. If $F(y|\mathbf{x})$ is assumed to be gaussian, an estimate of $q_\alpha(\mathbf{x})$ is given by $\hat{\mu}(\mathbf{x}) + \hat{\sigma}(\mathbf{x})N_\alpha$, where $\hat{\mu}(\mathbf{x})$ is the ordinary least square estimated regression of the conditional expectation $\mu(\mathbf{x}) = \mathrm{E}(Y|\mathbf{X} = \mathbf{x})$, $\hat{\sigma}(\mathbf{x})$ is an estimator of the conditional variance $\sigma(\mathbf{x}) = Var(Y|\mathbf{X} = \mathbf{x})$, and N_α is the αth-quantile of the standard normal distribution $N(0,1)$. Parametric assumptions (such as polynomial shape for $\mu(\mathbf{x})$ and $\sigma(\mathbf{x})$) are also usually added to reduce the number of parameters that are needed to be estimated. One simple nonparametric approach is to group data along the X-axis, estimate the αth-quantile value for each group and connect the values between groups by the use of a smoothing device. This method will usually be practical only for simple regressions where the data can be displayed as a two-dimensional scattergram. A more sophisticated nonparametric approach consists of estimating $q_\alpha(\mathbf{x})$ through a nonparametric estimator of $F(y|\mathbf{x})$.

In Section 10.2, we describe a kernel estimator of the conditional distribution which induces an estimator of corresponding quantiles. Theoretically, the extension of conditional quantiles to higher dimension p of $\mathbf{X}$ is obvious. But its practical success (as is the case for most nonparametric estimators) suffers from the so-called "*curse of dimensionality*". Furthermore, note that in this multivariate context, reference curves are a pair of p-dimensional hyper-surfaces. Their visual display is therefore rendered difficult, making it less directly useful for exploratory purposes (than the one-dimensional case). However, when $p \leq 2$, two-dimensional and three-dimensional plots can provide useful information on such changes. Though, it is now possible to view three-dimensional plots with most available software, it is very complicated to detect graphically if an individual is abnormal or not, even if we rotate the axis in the correct direction. When $p > 2$, graphical methods are more difficult, as viewing all the data in single $(p + 1)$-dimensional plot may no longer be possible. In Section 10.3, motivated by these practical and visual aspects, the key is to reduce the dimension of the predictor vector $\mathbf{X}$ without loss of information on the conditional distribution of Y given $\mathbf{X}$ and without requiring a prespecified parametric model. Sufficient dimension-reduction leads naturally to the idea of a sufficient summary plot that contains all information on the regression available from the sample. From a technical point of view, it would be a very helpful initial step in nonparametric estimation to circumvent the curse of dimensionality. In this chapter, we focus on linear projection method of reducing the dimensionality of the covariates in order to construct a more efficient estimator of conditional quantiles and consequently reference curves. The specific dimension reduction method used is based on Li's well known sliced inverse regression (SIR), see Duan and Li (1991) and Li (1991). A convergent semiparametric estimator of conditional quantiles based on this dimension-reduction method is then proposed. The method works in two steps: a dimension-reduction step based on SIR and a nonparametric estimation (of the conditional quantiles) step using a kernel method. The numerical performance of this estimator is illustrated with a simulated example. In Section 10.4, we describe a real-data application. The aim of the study is to establish 90%-reference curves for one biophysical property of the skin (the conductance of the skin) of healthy French women of Caucasian origin on the cheek area, using the age of the volunteer, the experimental conditions and other biophysical properties of the skin performed on this facial area as the multidimensional covariate $\mathbf{X}$. Finally, we give in Section 10.5 an extension of this semiparametric approach.

10.2   Kernel Estimation of Reference Curves

The nonparametric conditional quantile estimation approaches presented here yield consistent estimates of the corresponding conditional quantiles under general conditions, without requiring to specify the form of the distribution of Y.

Basic kernel estimation of reference curves. From (10.1), an estimator of the conditional distribution induces an estimator of corresponding quantiles. For instance, a Nadaraya-Watson estimator, $\hat{F}_n(y|\mathbf{x})$, can be affected to $F(y|\mathbf{x})$. If we write $Y^\star = \boldsymbol{I}\{Y \leq y\}$, then $F(y|\mathbf{x}) = E(Y^\star|\mathbf{X} = \mathbf{x})$, and then the estimation problem may be viewed as a regression of $Y^\star$ given $\mathbf{X}$.

The corresponding kernel estimator is given by

$$\hat{F}_n(y|\mathbf{x}) = \frac{\sum\limits_{i=1}^{n} K\{(\mathbf{x} - \mathbf{X}_i)/h_n\}Y_i^{\star}}{\sum\limits_{i=1}^{n} K\{(\mathbf{x} - \mathbf{X}_i)/h_n\}}, \tag{10.4}$$

where h_n and K are respectively a bandwidth and a bounded (kernel) function. The estimator $q_{n,\alpha}(\mathbf{x})$ of $q_\alpha(\mathbf{x})$ is naturally deduced from $\hat{F}_n(y|\mathbf{x})$ as the root of the equation

$$\hat{F}_n(y|\mathbf{x}) = \alpha. \tag{10.5}$$

Many authors have studied this estimator, Stute (1986), Samanta (1989), Gannoun (1990), Berlinet, Cadre and Gannoun (2001), Berlinet, Gannoun and Matzner-Løber (2001).

Then, the corresponding estimated $(2\alpha - 1)\%$ reference curves are given, as $\mathbf{x}$ varies, by the following

$$I_{n,\alpha}(\mathbf{x}) = [q_{n,1-\alpha}(\mathbf{x}), q_{n,\alpha}(\mathbf{x})]. \tag{10.6}$$

Two other nonparametric estimation of conditional quantiles. Various other nonparametric methods are explored in order to estimate $q_\alpha(\mathbf{x})$. Among them we can cite the local polynomial and the double kernel. For motivation, discussion and theoretical results on these estimation methods, the reader may also refer to Stone (1977), Tsybakov (1986), Lejeune and Sarda (1988), Bhattacharya and Gangopadhyay (1990), Fan, Hu and Truong (1994), Jones and Hall (1990), Chaudhuri (1991a), Chaudhuri (1991b), Yu and Jones (1998), Poiraud (2000), Mint el Mouvid (2000) and Cai (2002). Let us briefly discuss the first two.

Local constant kernel estimation of conditional quantiles. Using the formula (10.3), the idea of the local constant approach is to approximate the unknown $q_\alpha(\mathbf{x})$ by a constant function in a neighbourhood of $\mathbf{x}$. Then, the corresponding estimator of $q_\alpha(\mathbf{x})$ is defined as the value θ which minimizes the kernel estimate of the conditional expectation:

$$E_n[\rho_\alpha(Y - \theta)|\mathbf{X} = \mathbf{x}] = \frac{\sum_{i=1}^{n} \rho_\alpha(Y_i - \theta)K\left(\frac{\mathbf{x} - \mathbf{X}_i}{h_n}\right)}{\sum_{i=1}^{n} K\left(\frac{\mathbf{x} - \mathbf{X}_i}{h_n}\right)}. \tag{10.7}$$

Since the denominator of (10.7) does not depend on θ, the optimization problem is equivalent to the following minimization one : the local constant kernel estimatior of $q_\alpha(\mathbf{x})$ is defined as the value θ which minimizes

$$\sum_{i=1}^{n} \rho_\alpha(Y_i - \theta) K\left(\frac{\mathbf{x} - \mathbf{X}_i}{h_n}\right). \qquad (10.8)$$

Let us note that this estimator can be seen as a particular case of local linear or polynomial estimators, where estimating $q_\alpha(\mathbf{x})$ is equivalent to estimating the intercept. These methods have various advantages such as design adaptation and good boundary behavior, Chaudhuri (1991a), Chaudhuri (1991b), Fan, Hu and Truong (1994), Fan and Gijbels (1996), Koenker, Portnoy and Ng (1992), Mint el Mouvid (2000).

Double kernel estimation of conditional quantiles. A smoother version of the estimated conditional distribution function defined in (10.4) can be introduced by replacing the indicator function by a kernel density function ω. The corresponding estimator, called the double kernel estimator, is defined as follows:

$$\widetilde{F}_n(y|\mathbf{x}) = \frac{\sum_{i=1}^{n} K\left(\frac{\mathbf{x} - \mathbf{X}_i}{h_{1,n}}\right) \Omega\left(\frac{y - Y_i}{h_{2,n}}\right)}{\sum_{i=1}^{n} K\left(\frac{\mathbf{x} - \mathbf{X}_i}{h_{1,n}}\right)}, \qquad (10.9)$$

where Ω is the distribution function associated to the kernel ω. Mathematically, this estimator can be seen as the integrale of the kernel estimate of the conditional density function, Berlinet, Gannoun and Matzner-Løber (2001). So, the estimator of $q_\alpha(\mathbf{x})$, derived from (10.9), is defined as the root:

$$\widetilde{F}_n(y|\mathbf{x}) = \alpha.$$

This approach is attractive but suffers from the disadvantage of having to specify a second bandwidth $h_{2,n}$ as well as the bandwidth $h_{1,n}$ which plays much the same role as bandwidth h_n in (10.4).

Global remark on the bandwidths.   In order to get a maximum efficiency of the above nonparametric estimators, a good choice of the bandwidths is necessary. Unfortunately, there is no single and universal criterion to select optimal bandwidths.

Interesting proposals which address the crucial problem of bandwidth selection can be found in Fan and Gijbels (1992). Much literature has been written on automatic methods that attempt to minimize a lack-of-fit criterion such as integrated squared error. From a practical viewpoint, this is discarding much of the power of nonparametric regression. In the following, we only describe one particular choice of the bandwidth parameter h_n for the kernel estimator $q_{n,\alpha}(\mathbf{x})$ defined in (10.5).

For this estimator $q_{n,\alpha}(\mathbf{x})$, a data-driven bandwidth is derived by the cross-validation approach, Yao (1999). In other words, h_n minimizes

$$\sum_{i=1}^{n}\sum_{j=1}^{n}\{I\{Y_i \leq Y_j\} - F_n^{(-i)}(Y_j|\mathbf{x})\}^2, \tag{10.10}$$

where $F_n^{(-i)}$ is an estimator (depending on h_n) of F given as in (10.4) from the sample $\{(\mathbf{X}_k, Y_k), \ 1 \leq k \leq n, \ k \neq i\}$.

For the local constant kernel estimator or the double kernel estimator, note that one or two bandwiths are necessary. A bandwidth selection process, based on the usual rule-of-thumb calculations, has been explored recently by Yu and Jones (1998). Let us precise that, for these two estimators, this particular choice of bandwidths, relying on normality assumption on the conditional distribution, should be used with care. If this underlying assumption fails, there is theoretically no guarantee that such selected bandwidths are valid. The corresponding bandwidths can lead to over-smoothed or under-smoothed estimates in some cases, see Gannoun, Girard, Guinot and Saracco (2002a) and Gannoun, Girard, Guinot and Saracco (2002b) for numerical studies.

10.3 A Semiparametric Approach Via Sliced Inverse Regression

In this section, let Y_i denote the i-th observation on the univariate response Y and let $\mathbf{X}_i$ denote the corresponding $p \times 1$ vector of observed covariate values. The data $\{(\mathbf{X}_i^\top, Y_i)\}_{i=1}^{n}$ are assumed to be independent and identically distributed observations from the $(p+1)$-dimensional random vector $(\mathbf{X}^\top, Y)$ with finite moments.

10.3.1 Dimension Reduction Context

A convenient data reduction formulation is to assume there exists a $p \times r$ matrix B such that

$$F(y|\mathbf{x}) = F(y|B^\top\mathbf{x}), \tag{10.11}$$

where $F(.|.)$ is the conditional distribution function of the response Y given the second argument. Such matrix always exists because (10.11) is trivially true when $B = I_p$ the $p \times p$ identity matrix. This assumption implies that the

$p \times 1$ predictor vector $\mathbf{X}$ can be replaced by the $r \times 1$ predictor $B^\top \mathbf{X}$ without loss of regression information. Most importantly, if $r < p$, then sufficient reduction in the dimension of the regression is achieved. The linear subspace $S(B)$ spanned by the columns of B is a dimension reduction subspace, see Li (1991), and its dimension denotes the number of linear components of $\mathbf{X}$ needed to model Y. When (10.11) holds, then it also holds with B replaced by any matrix whose columns form a basis for $S(B)$. Clearly, knowledge of the smallest dimension reduction subspace would provide the most parsimonious characterization of Y given $\mathbf{X}$, as it provides the greatest dimension reduction in the predictor vector. Let $S_{Y|\mathbf{X}}$ denote the unique smallest dimension reduction subspace, referred to the central dimension reduction subspace in Cook (1994), Cook (1996) and Cook (1998). Let $d = \dim(S_{Y|\mathbf{X}})$, be the dimension of this subspace, note that d is such that $d \leq r$. Let β be the $p \times d$ matrix whose columns form a basis of $S_{Y|\mathbf{X}}$, that is $S(\beta) = S_{Y|\mathbf{X}}$. Then, from (10.11), we have

$$q_\alpha(\mathbf{x}) = q_\alpha(\beta^\top \mathbf{x}). \tag{10.12}$$

In the following, let Σ be the covariance matrix of $\mathbf{X}$, supposed to be positive-definite.

Characterization of the dimension reduction subspace.   A characterization fo the subspace $S(\beta)$ has been proposed by Li (1991) and Duan and Li (1991) via an inverse regression approach. This approach needs to assume that:

the marginal distribution of the predictors $\mathbf{X}$ satisfies the following linearity condition: (LC)   For all $b \in \mathbb{R}^p$, $E(b^\top \mathbf{X} | \beta^\top \mathbf{X})$ is linear in $\beta^\top \mathbf{X}$.

REMARK 10.1 *This condition (LC) is required to hold only for the basis β of the central subspace. Since β is unknown, in practice we may require that it holds for all possible β, which is equivalent to elliptical symmetry of the distribution of $\mathbf{X}$, Eaton (1986). This condition holds for instance when $\mathbf{X}$ is normally distributed. Li (1991) mentioned that the linearity condition is not a severe restriction, since most low-dimensional projections of high-dimensional data clouds are close to being normal, Diaconis and Freedman (1984), Hall and Li (1993). Experience indicates that linearizing predictor transformations often result in relatively simple models. In addition, it is possible to use the reweighting procedure proposed by Cook and Nachtsheim (1994) after predictor transformations to remove gross nonlinearities.*

Under **(LC)**, Li (1991) showed that the centered inverse regression curve fall in the linear subspace spanned by the columns of $\Sigma\beta$, that is $E(\mathbf{X}|Y) - E(\mathbf{X}) \in$

$S(\Sigma\beta)$. Thus,

$$S_{E(\mathbf{X}|Y)} \subseteq S(\Sigma\beta) = \Sigma S_{Y|\mathbf{X}}, \tag{10.13}$$

where $S_{E(\mathbf{X}|Y)}$ denote the subspace spanned by $\{E(\mathbf{X}|Y) - E(\mathbf{X}) : Y \in \Omega_Y\}$ and $\Omega_Y \in \mathbb{R}$ is the sample space of Y.

In order to simplify the calculus, a standardized version of this result can be used. Let $\mathbf{Z}$ denote the standardized version of the predictor $\mathbf{X}$ defined by $\mathbf{Z} = \Sigma^{-1/2}\{\mathbf{X} - E(\mathbf{X})\}$, where $\Sigma^{-1/2}$ is the symmetric positive-definite square root of Σ^{-1}. There is no loss of generality working on the $\mathbf{Z}$-scale, because any basis for $S_{Y|\mathbf{Z}}$ can be back-transformed to a basis for $S_{Y|\mathbf{X}}$ since $S_{Y|\mathbf{X}} = \Sigma^{-1/2}S_{Y|\mathbf{Z}}$. Therefore, from (10.13), we have

$$S_{E(\mathbf{Z}|Y)} \subseteq S(\eta) = S_{Y|\mathbf{Z}}, \tag{10.14}$$

where $\eta = \Sigma^{1/2}\beta$. This does not guarantee equality between $S_{E(\mathbf{Z}|Y)}$ and $S_{Y|\mathbf{Z}}$ and, thus, inference about $S_{E(\mathbf{Z}|Y)}$ possibly covers only part of $S_{Y|\mathbf{Z}}$. Moreover, it is clear that

$$S\{V[E(\mathbf{Z}|Y)]\} = S_{E(\mathbf{Z}|Y)}, \tag{10.15}$$

except on a set of measure zero, Cook (1998).

Using results (10.14) and (10.15), the estimation of the inverse regression curve $E(\mathbf{Z}|Y)$ serves to estimate the central dimension-reduction subspace by estimating the covariance matrix $V[E(\mathbf{Z}|Y)]$. Methods are available for estimating portions of the central subspace. In the next paragraph, we mainly focus on the classical Sliced Inverse Regression (SIR) method introduced by Duan and Li (1991), Li (1991) which is a simple non-smooth nonparametric estimation method for $S_{Y|\mathbf{Z}}$.

Sliced Inverse Regression Approach. The idea is based on partitionning the range of the one-dimensional response variable Y into a fixed number H of slices denoted $\mathcal{S}_1,\ldots,\mathcal{S}_H$. Then, the p components of $\mathbf{Z}$ are regressed on $\widetilde{Y}$, the discrete version of Y resulting from slicing its range, giving p one-dimensional regression problems, instead of the high-dimensional forward regression of Y on $\mathbf{Z}$. Let M denote the covariance matrix $V\left[E(\mathbf{Z}|\widetilde{Y})\right]$. Note that, using the slicing $\mathcal{S}_1,\ldots,\mathcal{S}_H$, M is written

$$M = \sum_{h=1}^{H} p_h m_h m_h^{\top}, \tag{10.16}$$

where $p_h = P(Y \in S_h)$ and $m_h = E[\mathbf{Z}|Y \in S_h]$. From (10.14) and (10.15), it is clear that

$$S(M) = S_{E(\mathbf{Z}|\widetilde{Y})} \subseteq S_{\widetilde{Y}|\mathbf{Z}} \subseteq S_{Y|\mathbf{Z}}. \tag{10.17}$$

The last inclusion in (10.17) holds because $\widetilde{Y}$ is a function of Y, which implies that $S_{Y|\mathbf{Z}}$ is a dimension-reduction subspace for the regression of $\widetilde{Y}$ on $\mathbf{Z}$. Let $\lambda_1 \geq \cdots \geq \lambda_p$ denote the eigenvalues of M, and $u_1, \ldots, u_p$ denote the corresponding eigenvectors. Assuming that $d = \dim\{S(M)\}$, it follows that $S(M) = S(u_1, \ldots, u_d)$. Transforming back to the $\mathbf{X}$-scale, the vectors $\{b_k = \Sigma^{-1/2} u_k\}_{k=1}^d$ form a basis of $S(\beta)$. Following SIR vocabulary, the dimension reduction subspace $S(\beta)$ is called the *effective dimension-reduction* (EDR) space, and the vectors b_k are named EDR directions. As we focus our dimension reduction approach on the SIR method, we will use this terminology from now on.

REMARK 10.2 *Pathological cases for the SIR approach have been identified. Li (1991), Li (1992), Cook and Weisberg (1991) mention that SIR can miss EDR directions even if the* (**LC**) *condition is valid. The reason is that it is "blind" for symmetric dependencies. In this case, the inverse regression curve does not contain any information about the EDR directions. For handling such cases, in order to recover the EDR directions, a natural extension is to consider higher moments of the conditional distribution of* $\mathbf{X}$ *given* Y. *Various methods based on second moments for estimating the EDR space have been developped: for example, SIR-II and SIR$_\alpha$ by Li (1991), SAVE by Cook and Weisberg (1991), the pooled slicing version of these methods and the choice of α by Saracco (2001), Gannoun and Saracco (2003a) and Gannoun and Saracco (2003b), and Principal Hessian directions by Li (1992). These methods may help, at least for completeness, when SIR fails to capture all the EDR directions.*

REMARK 10.3 *More details and comments on the SIR estimation procedure can be found in Li (1991), Chen and Li (1998). SIR has been discussed in several articles with emphasis on its asymptotic properties, see for example, Hsing and Carroll (1992), Kotter (1996), Zhu and Fang (1996), Saracco (1997) or Saracco (1999) among others. Carroll and Li (1992) used SIR in a nonlinear regression model with measurement error in the covariates. The situation of small sample sizes has been studied by Aragon and Saracco (1997). Bura (1997) used a multivariate linear model for the inverse regression curve. The case of censored regression data is considered by Li, Wang and Chen (1999).*

10.3.2   Estimation Procedure

We first describe here the practical implementation of the dimension-reduction step. Then, in a second step, we present the kernel method for estimating the conditional quantiles.

SIR estimation step. Let $\overline{\mathbf{X}}$ and $\widehat{\Sigma}$ be the sample mean and the sample covariance matrix of the $\mathbf{X}_i$'s. Let $\widehat{\mathbf{Z}}_i$ be the estimated standardized predictor defined by $\widehat{\mathbf{Z}}_i = \widehat{\Sigma}^{-1/2}(\mathbf{X}_i - \overline{\mathbf{X}})$, $i = 1, \ldots, n$. Then the SIR estimate of M defined in (10.16) is given by $\widehat{M} = \sum_{h=1}^{H} \widehat{p}_h \widehat{m}_h \widehat{m}_h^\top$, where H is the fixed number of slices, $\widehat{p}_h = n_h/n$ with n_h being the number of observations in the hth slice, and $\widehat{m}_h$ is the p-vector of the average of $\widehat{\mathbf{Z}}$ within slice h. Let $\widehat{\lambda}_1 \geq \cdots \geq \widehat{\lambda}_p$ denote the eigenvalues of $\widehat{M}$, and $\widehat{u}_1, \ldots, \widehat{u}_p$ denote the corresponding eigenvectors. Assuming that the dimension d of $S(M)$ is known, $S(\widehat{M}) = S(\widehat{u}_1, \ldots, \widehat{u}_d)$ is a consistent estimate of $S(M)$. In practice, the dimension d is replaced with an estimate $\widehat{d}$ equal to the number of eigenvalues that are inferred to be nonzero in the population, see for example, Li (1991), Schott (1994) or Ferré (1998).

When $\dim\{S(\eta)\} = d$, an estimated basis of $S(\eta)$ is clearly provided by the eigen-decomposition of $\widehat{M}$. Transforming back to the original scale, an estimated basis of $S(\beta)$ is formed by the vectors $\{\widehat{b}_k = \widehat{\Sigma}^{-1/2}\widehat{u}_k\}_{k=1}^d$ forms. Similarly to the population version, the vectors $\widehat{b}_k$ are the estimated EDR directions and they span the estimated EDR space.

Conditional quantile estimation step. Using the SIR estimates obtained in the previous subsection, we now give an estimator of the conditional distribution function from which we derive an estimator of the conditional quantile. For the sake of convenience, we assume that $d = 1$. Let us recall that, in the present dimension-reduction context, we have

$$F(y|\mathbf{x}) = F(y|\beta^\top \mathbf{x}) = F(y|b^\top \mathbf{x}) \quad \text{and} \quad q_\alpha(\mathbf{x}) = q_\alpha(\beta^\top \mathbf{x}) = q_\alpha(b^\top \mathbf{x}).$$

Using the notation $\widehat{b} = \widehat{b}_1$, $\widehat{b}$ is an estimated EDR direction, that is an estimated basis of $S(\beta)$. Then, the corresponding estimated index values of $\mathbf{X}_i$ and $\mathbf{x}$ are defined as follows: $\{\widehat{v}_i = \widehat{b}^\top \mathbf{X}_i\}_{i=1}^n$ and $\widehat{v} = \widehat{b}^\top \mathbf{x}$. Following (10.4), from the data $\{(Y_i, \widehat{v}_i)\}_{i=1}^n$, we define a kernel estimator of $F(y|\mathbf{x})$ by

$$F_n(y|\widehat{b}^\top \mathbf{x}) = F_n(y|\widehat{v}) = \frac{\sum_{i=1}^n K\{(\widehat{v} - \widehat{v}_i)/h_n\}\mathbf{I}\{Y_i \leq y\}}{\sum_{i=1}^n K\{(\widehat{v} - \widehat{v}_i)/h_n\}}. \tag{10.18}$$

Then, as in (10.5), we derive from (10.18) an estimator of $q_\alpha(\mathbf{x})$ by

$$q_{n,\alpha}(\hat{b}^\top \mathbf{x}) = q_{n,\alpha}(\hat{v}) = F_n^{-1}(\alpha|\hat{v}). \qquad (10.19)$$

As a consequence of the above result, for $\alpha > 0.5$, the corresponding estimated $100 \times (2\alpha - 1)\%$ reference curves are given, as $\mathbf{x}$ varies, by

$$I_{n,\alpha}(\mathbf{x}) = [q_{n,1-\alpha}(\hat{v}); q_{n,\alpha}(\hat{v})] = [q_{n,1-\alpha}(\hat{b}^\top \mathbf{x}); q_{n,\alpha}(\hat{b}^\top \mathbf{x})].$$

REMARK 10.4 *The above definitions have been presented in the context of single index $(d = 1)$. A natural extension is to consider the general multiple indices $(d > 1)$ context and to work with $\{\hat{b}_j\}_{j=1}^d$ and $\{\hat{v}_i = (\hat{b}_1^T \mathbf{X}_i, \ldots, \hat{b}_d^T \mathbf{X}_i)\}_{i=1}^n$. Then we follow the multi-kernel estimation can be used to get $q_{n,\alpha}(\hat{b}_1^T \mathbf{x}, \ldots, \hat{b}_d^T \mathbf{x})$ as in (10.19), the corresponding kernel K used in (10.18) can be the d-dimensional normal density.*

10.3.3   Asymptotic Property

The following theorem gives the weak convergence of the estimator $q_{n,\alpha}(\hat{b}^T \mathbf{x})$. Let us assume the following assumptions:

(A1) The random vectors $(\mathbf{X}_i, Y_i), i \geq 1$, are defined on probability space $(\Omega, \mathcal{A}, P)$ and constitute a strictly stationary process.

(A2) The kernel $K : \mathbb{R} \longrightarrow \mathbb{R}$ is a probability density function such that: K is bounded; $|v|K(v) \longrightarrow 0$ as $|v| \longrightarrow \infty$; $\int vK(v)dv = 0$ and $\int v^2 K(v)dv < \infty$.

(A3) The sequence of bandwidth h_n tends to zero such that $nh_n/\log n \longrightarrow \infty$.

(A4) The variable $\mathbf{X}$ admits a continuous marginal density.

(A5) $F(.|b^\top \mathbf{x})$ and $F(y|.)$ are both continuous.

(A6) For $\alpha \in (0,1)$ and $\mathbf{x} \in \mathbb{R}^p$, $F(.|b^\top \mathbf{x})$ has a unique αth-quantile.

THEOREM 10.1 *Under Assumptions (A1)-(A6) and Condition (LC), for a fixed $\mathbf{x}$ in $\mathbb{R}^p$,*

$$\sup_{y \in \mathbb{R}} \left| F_n(y|\hat{b}^\top \mathbf{x}) - F(y|\mathbf{x}) \right| \xrightarrow{\mathcal{P}} 0 \quad \text{as } n \to \infty,$$

and

$$q_{n,\alpha}(\hat{b}^\top \mathbf{x}) \xrightarrow{\mathcal{P}} q_\alpha(\mathbf{x}), \quad \text{as } n \to \infty.$$

Comments on the Assumptions. Asumptions **(A2)** and **(A3)** are quite usual in kernel estimation. As a direct consequence of Assumption **(A4)**, the variable $b^T X$ admits a continuous marginal density. Assumption **(A5)** is used to prove the uniform convergence (in probability) of $F_n(.|\hat{b}^T x)$ to $F(.|b^T x)$. Assumption **(A6)** is used in the proof of the convergence of $q_{n,\alpha}(\hat{b}^T x)$ to $q_\alpha(x)$. Note that if there is no unicity, we can define $q_\alpha(x) = \inf\{y : F(y|b^T x) \geq \alpha\}$.

Comments on the Theorem. This weak convergence is enough to make application. The proof of this theorem can be found in Gannoun, Girard, Guinot and Saracco (2004). Note that in order to get the uniform convergence, one can also suppose that $\mathbf{X}$ is defined on compact set of $\mathbb{R}^p$, and proceed by the same manner as in Berlinet, Cadre and Gannoun (2001).

10.3.4 A Simulated Example

We illustrate the numerical performance of the proposed semiparametric estimation method on simulated data. We consider the following regression model with $p = 10$:

$$Y = 1 + \exp(2\beta^\top \mathbf{X}/3) + \varepsilon,$$

where $\mathbf{X}$ follows the standard multinormal distribution $N_p(0, I_p)$, the error term ε is normally distributed from $N(0,1)$ and is independent of $\mathbf{X}$, and $\beta = 3^{-1}(1,1,1,1,1,-1,-1,-1,-1,0)^\top$. Note that, when $\mathbf{X} = \mathbf{x}$, the true corresponding αth-conditional quantile can be written: $q_\alpha(\mathbf{x}) = 1 + \exp(2\beta^\top \mathbf{x}/3) + N_\alpha$, where N_α is the αth-quantile of the standard normal distribution.

A sample of size $n = 300$ has been generated from this model. The conditional quantiles have been estimated for $\alpha = 5\%$ and $\alpha = 95\%$ on a grid. For the computational implementation, the kernel used is the normal density. Each reference curve is evaluated on 50 points equidistributed on the range of the (true or estimated) index. For each point of the grid, the bandwidth parameter h_n has been obtained with the cross-validation criterion 10.10. Note that the estimated eigenvalue of the SIR matrix $\widehat{M}$ are: 0.436,0.096,0.088,0.050,0.037,0.032,0.019, 0.011,0.009,0.003. Clearly, we only keep one estimated EDR direction:

$$\hat{b} = (0.348, 0.241, 0.272, 0.353, 0.375, -0.353, -0.358, -0.216, -0.386, -0.182)^\top$$

which is very close to β (with $\cos^2(\beta, \hat{b}) \simeq 0.94$).

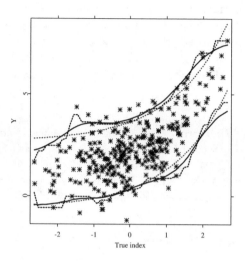

Figure 10.1: Comparison of the true 90%-reference curves (red dotted lines)
and the corresponding kernel estimated 90%-reference curves
(blue dashed lines for the non smoothed version and blue solid
lines for the smoothed version) using the true index $\beta^\top \mathbf{x}$

Q XCSSARGGLprog.xpl

An example of graphical representation of the 90%-reference curves is given
on figures 10.1 and 10.2. In the first one, we present the scatterplot of the
"true" reduced data $\{(\beta^\top \mathbf{X}_i, Y_i), \ i = 1, \ldots, n\}$ and the "true" 90%-reference
curves are plotted (with red dotted lines) as well as the corresponding es-
timated reference curves (which have no practical interest since they are
based on the estimated conditional quantile $q_{n,\alpha}(\beta^\top \mathbf{x})$ using the theoretical dimension-reduction direction β). Let $\{\tilde{v}_t, \ t = 1, \ldots, T\}$ be the set of
the "true" index values on which the nonparametric estimates of conditional
quantiles are evaluated. Then, we use the pairs $\{(\tilde{v}_t, q_{n,\alpha}(\tilde{v}_t)), \ t = 1, \ldots, T\}$
to get reference curves. A common approach to connect different quantiles,
is to use the well-known linear interpolation (this is done with blue dashed
lines). Although this method is practical, the visual aspect is not smooth. To
make up for this imperfection, we can use the Nadaraya-Watson method to
obtain the wanted smoothed curves (see the corresponding blue solid lines).
The superimposition of the theoretical and estimated 90%-reference curves

shows the accuracy of the nonparametric kernel estimation of the conditional quantiles. In Figure 10.2, the horizontal axis is now the estimated index, the scatterplot of the "estimated" reduced data $\{(\hat{b}^T \mathbf{X}_i, Y_i),\ i = 1, \ldots, n\}$ is plotted as well as the corresponding estimated 90%-reference curves (based on the estimated conditional quantile $q_{n,\alpha}(\hat{b}^\top \mathbf{x})$). The resulting curves are visually similar to the theoretical ones.

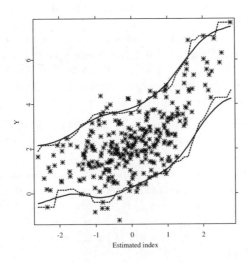

Figure 10.2: Semiparametric estimation of the 90%-reference curves using the SIR estimated index $\hat{b}^\top \mathbf{x}$ (blue dashed lines for the non smoothed version and blue solid lines for the smoothed version)

      Q XCSSARGGLprog.xpl

10.4   Case Study on Biophysical Properties of the Skin

When studying biophysical skin properties of healthy women, knowledge about the reference curves of certain parameters is lacking. Information concerning biophysical skin properties is limited to few studies. The aim of a global study managed by the CE.R.I.E.S. ("CEntre de Recherches et d'Investigations Epidermiques et Sensorielles" or Epidermal and Sensory Research and Investigation Centre) is to establish reference curves for biophysical parameters of the skin reflecting human variability among healthy subjects without any skin disease. These variables are measured in conditions that minimize physiological stress. The reference curves could be used in dermatology to detect an abnormal condition, even if unlabelled as a specific disease, which should be examined and corrected. In cosmetology, they could be used for product development in order to select specific group of subjects. In a previous study described in Gannoun, Girard, Guinot and Saracco (2002a), the 90%-reference curves for biophysical properties of the skin of healthy Caucasian women have been established. The biophysical properties of the skin of healthy Caucasian women have been performed on two facial areas and one forearm area. The biophysical skin properties have been studied one after the other as the variable of interest Y and the only covariate was the age of the volunteer.

The aim of the current study is to establish 90%-reference curves for one biophysical property of the skin (the conductance of the skin) of healthy Caucasian women on the cheek area, using the age and a set of covariates (experimental conditions and other biophysical properties of the skin performed on this facial area). In the next subsection, we describe more precisely the corresponding study and we give an brief overview of these biophysical parameters. Then, we present the methodological procedure used with an additional step in order to simplify the EDR indices. Finally, we describe the results and give a brief biophysical interpretation.

10.4.1   Overview of the Variables

The study was conducted from November 1998 to March 1999 on 287 Caucasian women between the age of 20 and 80 with apparently healthy skin (i.e. without any sign of ongoing skin disease or general disease with proven cutaneous manifestations), and living in the Ile de France area. Each healthy volunteer was examined at CE.R.I.E.S. ("CEntre de Recherches et d'Investigations Epidermiques et Sensorielles" or Epidermal and Sensory Research and Investigation Centre) in a controlled environment (temperature $22.9 \pm 0.3°C$ and a relative humidity of $48.4 \pm 2.4\%$).

As the CERIES (which is the investigator) is located in Paris, the present study concerns women living in Ile de France (which is an area around Paris). Moreover, to keep homogeneity, the statistical sample contains only women having the same skin characteristics (namely Caucasian woman). Similarly, other studies have been conducted (for instance on Japenese women) but are not presented here.

This evaluation included self-administered questionnaires on skin-related habits, a medical examination and a biophysical evaluation of the skin. The biophysical investigation was performed on two areas of the face (forehead and cheek) and on the left volar forearm.

Within the framework of the subsection 10.4.3, the variable of interest is the conductance of the skin performed on the cheek area and denoted by KCHEEK. The available covariates included in the study are the following.

- Other biophysical properties of the skin performed on the cheek area: the skin temperature (denoted by TCHEEK), the transepidermal water loss (denoted by CHEEK1), the skin pH (denoted by PCHEEK), the skin hydration given by the capacitance (denoted by C2CHEEK), the skin colour which is was expressed using L* a* b* for the standard CIE 1976 colour system (denoted by LCHEEK, ACHEEK and BCHEEK), and the sebum excretion rate (denoted by SCHEEK).

- One components concerns the volunteer: AGE (age of volunteer).

- Two covariates concern the experimental conditions: HYGRO (relative humidity of the controlled environment) and TEMP (temperature of the controlled environment).

The goal is to estimate the 90%-reference curves for the variable of interest KCHEEK using the corresponding set of the $p = 11$ covariates.

10.4.2   Methodological Procedure

The following methodology is applied in the practical case study. For convenience, let us denote by $\mathcal{X}$ the set of the p covariates ($p = 11$ in the current study). Three steps are necessary to describe the estimation procedure.

- **Step 1: application of SIR on the set $\mathcal{X}$.** We apply the SIR method using the variable of interest Y and all the covariates of $\mathcal{X}$. From the eigenvalues scree plot, we determine the number $\hat{d}$ of EDR directions to keep, that is the number of eigenvalues significantly different from zero in theory. From a practical point of view, we look for a visible jump in the scree plot and $\hat{d}$ is then the number of the eigenvalues located before this jump. Note that if no jump is detected, no dimension reduction is possible. The eigenvalues scree plot approach used here is a useful explanatory tool in determining d. Of course testing procedure could be also used to identify d, see for instance, Schott (1994) or Ferré (1998). For simplicity of notation, we continue to write d for $\hat{d}$ in the following.

The corresponding estimated EDR directions are therefore $\hat{b}_1, \ldots, \hat{b}_d$. We can visualize the structure of the "reduced" data $\{(Y_i, \hat{b}_1^\top \mathbf{X}_i, \ldots, \hat{b}_d^\top \mathbf{X}_i)\}_{i=1}^n$.

- **Step 2: study and simplification of the EDR indices.** The aim here is to "simplify" the indices $\hat{b}_k^\top \mathbf{x}$ in order to obtain an simpler interpretation. To this end, for each index, we make a forward-selected linear regression model of $\hat{b}_k^\top \mathbf{x}$ on the covariates of $\mathcal{X}$ (based on the AIC criterion for instance). We then obtain $\mathcal{X}_1, \ldots, \mathcal{X}_d$, the corresponding subsets of selected covariates. The final subset is then $\widetilde{\mathcal{X}} = \cup_{k=1}^d \mathcal{X}_k$. Let us remark that the selection of covariates is effective if $\widetilde{\mathcal{X}}$ is strictly included in $\mathcal{X}$. We apply SIR again with the covariates of $\widetilde{\mathcal{X}}$ and we obtain the corresponding d estimated EDR directions $\widetilde{b}_1, \ldots, \widetilde{b}_d$. Finally, we graphically check that each plot $\{(\hat{b}_k^\top \mathbf{X}_i, \widetilde{b}_k^\top \widetilde{\mathbf{X}}_i)\}_{i=1}^n$ has a linear structure. The corresponding Pearson correlation R^2 can be also calculated.

- **Step 3: estimation of the conditional quantiles with the simplified indices.** We are now able to estimate the reference "curves" (which are hypersurfaces when $d > 1$) on the sample $\{(Y_i, \widetilde{b}_1^\top \widetilde{\mathbf{X}}_i, \ldots, \widetilde{b}_d^\top \widetilde{\mathbf{X}}_i)\}_{i=1}^n$, by the kernel method described in subsection 10.3.2.

10.4.3   Results and Interpretation

We apply the previous methodology in order to construct the 90%-reference curves for the variable KCHEEK. Following the step 1, from the eigenvalues scree plot (see Figure 10.3), we straighfordly select the dimension $\hat{d} = 1$. We estimate the corresponding EDR direction $\hat{b}_1 \in \mathbb{R}^{11}$.

Step 2 is summarized in Table 10.1 which gives the selected covariates (first column), the value of the AIC criterion in the corresponding single term addition step of the forward selection step (secon column). Finally, only 6 covariates have been selected. The corresponding estimated EDR direction $\widetilde{b}_1 \in \mathbb{R}^6$ is provided in the last column.

In Figure 10.4, the indices computed at the first step with all the covariates $(\hat{b}_1^\top \mathbf{X}_i, \ i = 1, \ldots, n)$ are plotted versus the indices computed at the second step with the selected covariates $(\widetilde{b}_1^\top \widetilde{\mathbf{X}}_i, \ i = 1, \ldots, n)$. Since this plot reveals a linear structure (with $R^2 = 0.984$ close to one), there is no loss of infor-

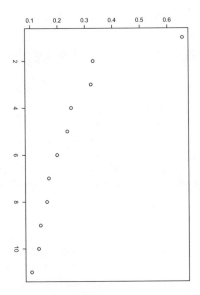

Figure 10.3: Eigenvalues scree plot for SIR of step 1

mation working with only the subset of the remaining selected covariates. In the third step, we construct the 90%-reference curves for KCHEEK using the estimated index $\widetilde{b}_1^\top \widetilde{\mathbf{X}}_i$, with the kernel method, see Figure 10.5. Regarding the cheek area, the results of this analysis show that, apart from AGE, five covariates enter in the model. The environmental conditions are represented only by room temperature in the model (which is to be expected). The sebum casual level SCHEEK plays a major role on skin hydration. The three other covariates are directly related with skin hydration: skin pH (PCHEEK), capacitance and transepidermal water loss (C2CHEEK and CHEEK1). This results lead to a slightly different model than those obtain for the forearm or the forehead (not given here), which is perfectly consistent with the anatomo-physiological topographic specificity of the skin area studied. These reference curves indicatin skin hydration assessed by conductance gives physiological consistent results.

Table 10.1: Results of the forward-selection step and final estimated EDR direction for the cheek area

Covariate	AIC	final EDR direction
AGE	301.85	-0.003
C2CHEEK	29.56	-0.102
SCHEEK	25.67	0.004
TEMP	23.51	0.439
CHEEK1	20.07	-0.036
PCHEEK	18.48	0.273

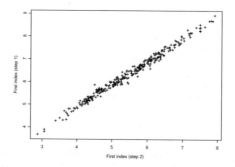

Figure 10.4: Graphical validation of the covariate selection step (step 2)

10.5 Conclusion

We can deal with a more general multivariate case for the variable of interest. From now on, we assume that the variable of interest **Y** belongs to $\mathbb{R}^q$ and the covariable **X** takes its values in $\mathbb{R}^p$. Based on the dimension-reduction motivation described above, we propose to reduce simultaneously the dimension of **Y** and **X** with the Alternating SIR method as a first step, see for instance Li, Aragon, Shedden and Thomas-Agnan (2003) for a description of Alternating SIR approach which allows to estimate EDR direction in the space of **X** and also interesting directions in the space of **Y**, these directions are called MP (for most predictable) directions. As previously, a nonparametric estimation of univariate conditional quantiles (if only one MP direction is

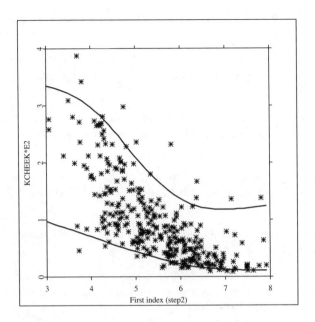

Figure 10.5: Estimated 90%-reference curves for the variable KCHEEK

retained) or a nonparametric estimation of spatial conditional quantiles (if two or more than two MP directions are retained) based on a kernel method can be used as a second step. This multivariate approach is described in Gannoun, Guinot and Saracco (2004) and is applied on a biomedical example using the data set on the biophysical properties of the skin of healthy French women.

Bibliography

Aragon, Y. and Saracco, J. (1997). Sliced Inverse Regression (SIR): An Appraisal of Small Sample Alternatives to Slicing. *Computational Statistics*, **12**, 109-130.

Basset, G. and Koenker, R. (1982). An empirical quantile function for linear models with iid errors. *J. Amer. Stat. Assoc.*, **77**, 407-415.

Berlinet, A., Cadre, B. and Gannoun, A. (2001). Estimation of conditional

L_1-median from dependent observations. *Statistics & Probability Letters*, **55**, 353-358.

Berlinet, A., Gannoun, A. and Matzner-Løber, E. (2001). Asymptotic Normality of Convergent Estimates of Conditional Quantiles. *Statistics*, **35**, 139-169.

Bhattacharya, P.K. and Gangopadhyay, A.K. (1990). Kernel and nearest-neighbor estimation of a conditional quantile. *Annals of Statistics*, **18**, 1400-1415.

Bura, E. (1997). Dimension Reduction via Parametric Inverse Regression. *L_1-Statistical procedures and related topics*, MS Lecture Notes, **31**, 215-228.

Cai, Z. (2002). Regression Quantiles for Time Series. *Econometric Theory*, **18**, 169-192.

Carroll, R. J. and Li, K. C. (1992). Measurement Error Regression with Unknown Link: Dimension Reduction and Data Visualization. *J. Amer. Stat. Assoc.*, **87**, 1040-1050.

Chaudhuri, P. (1991a). Nonparametric estimates of regression quantiles and their local Bahadur representation. *Annals of Statistics*, **19**, 760-777.

Chaudhuri, P. (1991b). Global nonparametric estimation of conditional quantile functions and their derivative. *Journal of Multivariate Analysis*, **39**, 246-269.

Chen, C. H. and Li, K. C. (1998). Can SIR Be as Popular as Multiple Linear Regression? *Statistica Sinica*, **8**, 289-316.

Cole, T. J. (1988). Fitting Smoothed Centile Curves to Reference Data. *Journal of the Royal Statistical Society, Series B*, **151**, 385-418.

Cook, R. D. (1994). On the Interpretation of the Regression Plots. *J. Amer. Stat. Assoc.*, **89**, 177-189.

Cook, R. D. (1996). Graphics for Regressions with a Binary Response. *J. Amer. Stat. Assoc.*, **91**, 983-992.

Cook, R. D. (1998). *Regression Graphics: Ideas for Studying the Regressions Through Graphics*. New York: Wiley.

Cook, R. D. and Nachtsheim, C. J. (1994). Reweighting to Acheive Elliptically Contoured Covariates in Regression. *J. Amer. Stat. Assoc.*, **89**, 592-599.

Cook, R. D. and Weisberg, S. (1991). Comment on "sliced inverse regression for dimension reduction". *J. Amer. Stat. Assoc.*, **86**, 328-332.

Diaconis, P. and Freedman, D. (1984). Asymptotic of Graphical Projection Pursuit. *Annals of Statistics*, **12**, 793-815.

Eaton, M. L. (1986). A Characterization of Spherical Distributions. *Journal of Multivariate Analysis*, **20**, 272-276.

Duan, N. and Li, K. C. (1991). Slicing regression: a link-free regression method. *Annals of Statistics*, **19**, 505-530.

Fan, J. and Gijbels, I. (1992). Variable bandwidth and local linear regression smoothers. *Annals of Statistics*, **20**, 2008-2036.

Fan, J. and Gijbels, I. (1996). *Local Polynomial Modelling and Its Applications*. Vol. 66 of *Monographs on Statistics and Applied Probability*, Chapman and Hall, New York.

Fan, J., Hu, T. and Truong, Y. K. (1994). Robust non-parametric function estimation. *Scandinavian Journal of Statistics*, **21**, 433-446.

Ferré, L. (1998). Determining the Dimension in Sliced Inverse Regression and Related Methods. *J. Amer. Stat. Assoc.*, **93**, 132-140.

Gannoun, A. (1990). Estimation Non Paramétrique de la Médiane Conditionnelle, Médianogramme et Méthode du Noyau. *Revue de l'Institut de Statistique de Université de Paris*, **45**, 11-22.

Gannoun, A., Girard, S., Guinot, C. and Saracco, J. (2002a). Reference curves based on nonparametric quantile regression. *Statistics in Medicine*, **21**, 3119-3155.

Gannoun, A., Girard, S., Guinot, C. and Saracco, J. (2002b). Trois méthodes non paramétriques pour l'estimation de courbes de référence. Application à l'analyse des propriétés biophysiques de la peau. *Revue de Statistique appliquée*, **1**, 65-89.

Gannoun, A., Girard, S., Guinot, C. and Saracco, J. (2004). Sliced Inverse Regression In Reference Curves Estimation. *Computational Statistics and Data Analysis*, **46**, 103-122.

Gannoun, A., Guinot, C. and Saracco, J. (2004). Reference curves estimation via alternating sliced inverse regression. *Environmetrics*, **15**, 81-99.

Gannoun, A. and Saracco, J. (2003a). A cross validation criteria for SIR_α and $PSIR_\alpha$ methods in view of prediction. *Computational Statistics*, **18**, 585-603.

Gannoun, A. and Saracco, J. (2003b). An asymptotic theory for SIR_α method. *Statistica Sinica*, **13**, 297-310.

Goldstein, H. and Pan, H. (1992). Percentile Smoothing using Piecewise Polynomials, with Covariates. *Biometrics*, **48**, 1057-1068.

Hall, P. and Li, K. C. (1993). On Almost Linearity of Low-Dimensional Projections from High-Dimensional Data. *Annals of Statistics*, **21**, 867-889.

Healy, M. J. R., Rasbash, J. and Yang, M. (1988). Distribution-Free Estimation of Age-Related Centiles. *Annals of Human Biology*, **15**, 17-22.

Hsing, T. and Carroll, R. J. (1992). An Asymptotic Theory for Sliced Inverse Regression. *Annals of Statistics*, **20**, 1040-1061.

Jones, M. C. and Hall, P. (1990). Mean Squared Error Properties of Kernel Estimates of Regression Quantiles. *Statistics & Probability Letters*, **10**, 283-289.

Koenker, R., Portnoy, S. and Ng, P. (1992). Nonparametric estimation of conditional quantile functions. L_1- *statistical analysis and related methods*, ed Y. Dodge, Elsevier: Amsterdam; 217-229.

Kötter, T. (1996). An Asymptotic Result for Sliced Inverse Regression. *Computational Statistics*, **11**, 113-136.

Lejeune, M. and Sarda, P. (1988). Quantile regression: a nonparametric approach. *Computational Statistics and Data Analysis*, **6**, 229-239.

Li, K. C. (1991). Sliced Inverse Regression for Dimension Reduction (with discussion). *J. Amer. Stat. Assoc.*, **86**, 316-342.

Li, K. C. (1992). On Principal Hessian Direction for Data Visualization and Dimension Reduction: Another Application of Stein's Lemma. *J. Amer. Stat. Assoc.*, **87**, 1025-1039.

Li, K. C., Aragon Y., Shedden, K. and Thomas-Agnan, C. (2003). Dimension reduction for multivariate response data. *J. Amer. Stat. Assoc.*, **98**, 99-109.

Li, K. C., Wang J. L. and Chen, C. H. (1999). Dimension Reduction for Censored Regression Data. *Annals of Statistics*, **27**, 1-23.

Mint el Mouvid, M. (2000). *Sur l'estimateur linéaire local de la fonction de répartition conditionnelle*. Ph.D. thesis, Montpellier II University (France).

Poiraud-Casanova, S. (2000). *Estimation non paramétrique des quantiles conditionnels*. Ph.D. thesis, Toulouse I University (France).

Royston, P. and Altman, D. G. (1992). Regression Using Fractional Polynomials of Continuous Covariates: Parsimonious Parametric Modelling (with discussion). *Applied Statistics*, **43**, 429-467.

Samanta, T. (1989). Non-parametric Estimation of Conditional Quantiles. *Statistics & Probability Letters*, **7**, 407-412.

Saracco, J. (1997). An Asymptotic Theory for Sliced Inverse Regression. *Communications in Statistics - Theory and methods*, **26**, 2141-2171.

Saracco, J. (1999). Sliced Inverse Regression Under Linear Constraints. *Communications in Statistics - Theory and methods*, **28**, 2367-2393.

Saracco, J. (2001). Pooled Slicing Methods Versus Slicing Methods. *Communications in Statistics - Simulations and Computations*, **30**, 499-511.

Schott, J. R. (1994). Determining the Dimensionality in Sliced Inverse Regression. *J. Amer. Stat. Assoc.*, **89**, 141-148.

Stone, C. J. (1977). Consistent Nonparametric Regression (with discussion). *Annals of Statistics*, **5**, 595-645.

Stute, W. (1986). Conditional Empirical Processes. *Annals of Statistics*, **14**, 638-647.

Tsybakov, A. B. (1986). Robust reconstruction of functions by the local approximation method. *Problems of Information Transmission*, **22**, 133-146.

Yao, Q. (1999). *Conditional predictive regions for stochastic processes*. Technical repport, University of Kent at Canterbury, UK.

Yu, K. (1997). *Smooth regression quantile estimation*. Ph.D. thesis, The Open University (UK).

Yu, K. and Jones, M. C. (1998). Local linear quantile regression. *J. Amer. Stat. Assoc.*, **93**, 228-237.

Zhu, L. X. and Fang, K. T. (1996). Asymptotics for kernel estimate of Sliced Inverse Regression. *Annals of Statistics*, **24**, 1053-1068.

11 Survival Analysis

Makoto Tomita

11.1 Introduction

This chapter explains the method of fundamental survival time analysis employing XploRe. Kaplan-Meier estimator (Kaplan, 1958) is mentioned as the typical method of non-parametric survival time analysis. The most common estimate of the survival distribution, the Kaplan-Meier estimate, is a product of survival proportions. It produces non-parametric estimates of failure probability distributions for a single sample of data that contains exact time of failure or right censored data. It calculates surviving proportion and survival time, and then plots a Kaplan-Meier survival curve.

Some methods are proposed for approval of the difference in survival time between two groups. Log-rank test (Peto, 1977) is the approval method in which Kaplan-Meier estimation is applied. This tests the difference of survival proportions as a whole.

Lastly, Cox's regression (Cox, 1972) using proportional hazard rate is indispensable in this latest field. It belongs to the group of semi-parametric survival time analyzing methods. Cox's proportional hazard model is based on multiple linear regression analysis considered by survival time which can be taken to response variable Y and explanatory variable X and hazard rate is applied to variable Y. Treatment effect is shown with coefficient β on multiple linear regression analysis. Then, β is evaluated.

11.2   Data Sets

Two data sets will be studied with survival time analysis in this chapter. Both were gathered from April 1, 2001 to September 30, 2004 at the Riumachi Center, Tokyo Women's University of Medicine. We have analyzed survival time of the two data sets here. The first is data on the period whose symptoms are shown again, after prescribing a steroid and CY (Cyclophosphamide) agent for the rheumatic patient, and on how the disease settles down. It does not identify the span of time until symptoms occurs again. The second is data on the period until aseptic necrosis, a side effect that occurs with the quantity of steroid used as medication. It does not identify the time when aseptic necrosis occurs. Although we analyzed the data using three popular techniques, Kaplan-Meier estimation, log-rank test and Cox's regression, we have omitted explanations of these techniques and focused on the interesting results.

11.3   Data on the Period up to Sympton Recurrence

Tanaka (2003) have studied pulmonary hypertension associated with collagen tissue disease. They investigated into the difference in the length of time until symptom recurs, after prescribing a steroid and CY agent. Next, we decided to analyze survival time. The data is shown in Table 11.1.

11.3.1   Kaplan-Meier Estimate

Easy quantlet called kaplanmeier is prepared to identify the survival rate of Kaplan-Meier with XploRe. If we want to ask for the survival rate about CY agent of the above data, for instance, it is necessary to process data as x of output as shown below, so that the quantlet kaplanmeier may be suited. It is named "tanakacy.dat" and is saved. Then, the rest should just typed in the command as follows.

```
library("stats")
x=read("tanakacy.dat")
x
h = kaplanmeier(x)
h
```

Table 11.1: Data on the period up to sympton recurrence (Tanaka, 2003)

Medicine	months	occurred again
CY	2	occurred
CY	5	occurred
CY	24	not occurred
CY	28	not occurred
CY	33	not occurred
CY	46	not occurred
CY	57	not occurred
CY	84	not occurred
steroid	0.5	occurred
steroid	1	occurred
steroid	1	occurred
steroid	1	not occurred
steroid	5	occurred
steroid	11	occurred
steroid	20	not occurred
steroid	21	occurred
steroid	60	not occurred

Then, output is produced as follows.

Contents of x

```
[1,]            1             2
[2,]            1             5
[3,]            0            24
[4,]            0            28
[5,]            0            33
[6,]            0            46
[7,]            0            57
[8,]            0            84
```

Contents of h

```
[1,]            2      0.125       0.875
[2,]            5    0.14286        0.75
```

Therefore, 0.75 is the survival rate.
Next, a Kaplan-Meier survival curve will created for plotting in a graph.

Then, the graphic is obtained as Figure 11.1.

The graph for steroid can also be plotted similarly as Figure 11.2.

11.3.2   log-rank Test

Finally, log-rank test compares these two. The test statistical data is as
follows.

$$\chi_0^2 = \frac{(O_{CY} - E_{CY})^2}{E_{CY}} + \frac{(O_{steroid} - E_{steroid})^2}{E_{steroid}} \sim \chi_1^2$$

where, O_x is observation of occurrence, and E_x is expectation of occurrence.
The result was obtained as follows.

```
chi-square: 2.559262603
p-value: 0.109649747
```

Although small sample size may have been a factor, the result was unfortunately not significant. However, in the experiment team, it decided to study
continuously, because p-value is about 10%.

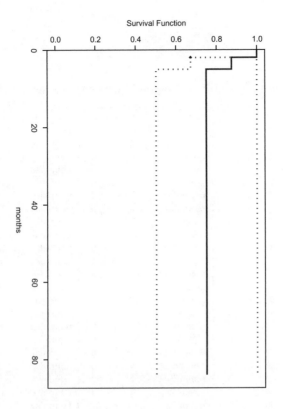

Figure 11.1: Kaplan-Meier survival curve of CY

Q XCSKMscurve01.xpl

11.4 Data for Aseptic Necrosis

Steroid is sometimes often prescribed for a rheumatic patient. However, if excessive steroid is prescribed, aseptic necrosis occurs at a joint as side effect. A patient has to perform an operation on this by seemingly being very painful. A method called pulse treatment is employed in the medication method of steroid, and medication is given at once and in large quantity. Table 11.2 is the data which was obtained from the group of patients who were administered pulse treatment, and the group of the patient who were performed the non-pulse treatment.

Table 11.2: Data for Aseptic Necrosis (Fukasawa, 2001)

Steroid	months	AN*	Steroid	months	AN	Steroid	months	AN
nonpulse	3	0	pulse	6	1	nonpulse	3	0
pulse	2	0	nonpulse	18	0	nonpulse	9	0
nonpulse	3	0	nonpulse	7	0	nonpulse	2	0
nonpulse	5	0	nonpulse	23	0	nonpulse	3	0
nonpulse	3	0	pulse	17	0	pulse	10	1
nonpulse	6	0	nonpulse	7	0	nonpulse	6	0
nonpulse	3	0	nonpulse	7	0	nonpulse	12	0
nonpulse	11	0	pulse	5	0	nonpulse	7	0
nonpulse	6	1	nonpulse	12	0	nonpulse	4	0
nonpulse	3	0	nonpulse	3	0	nonpulse	7	0
nonpulse	2	0	pulse	7	1	nonpulse	6	0
pulse	8	0	nonpulse	7	0	nonpulse	31	0
nonpulse	7	1	nonpulse	15	0	pulse	3	0
pulse	9	0	nonpulse	21	0	pulse	9	0
nonpulse	10	0	pulse	6	0	pulse	7	0
nonpulse	8	0	nonpulse	18	0	nonpulse	6	0
nonpulse	16	0	pulse	6	0	pulse	12	1
nonpulse	10	0	nonpulse	3	0	nonpulse	8	0
nonpulse	22	0	pulse	6	0	nonpulse	4	0
nonpulse	11	0	nonpulse	4	0	pulse	5	1
nonpulse	18	0	pulse	3	0	nonpulse	14	0
pulse	4	1	nonpulse	13	1	nonpulse	10	0
nonpulse	6	0	nonpulse	6	0	nonpulse	9	0
nonpulse	11	1	nonpulse	4	0	nonpulse	13	0
nonpulse	22	0	nonpulse	7	0	nonpulse	21	0
pulse	8	0	nonpulse	4	0	pulse	4	1
pulse	4	0	nonpulse	19	0	nonpulse	9	0
pulse	22	0	nonpulse	5	0	pulse	26	0
pulse	2	1	nonpulse	10	0	nonpulse	7	0
nonpulse	4	0	nonpulse	9	0	nonpulse	4	0
nonpulse	6	0	nonpulse	9	0	pulse	11	1
pulse	8	0	pulse	14	0	pulse	5	1
nonpulse	17	0	nonpulse	10	0	nonpulse	5	0
pulse	3	0	nonpulse	7	0	nonpulse	7	0
nonpulse	9	0	nonpulse	10	0	pulse	6	0
nonpulse	4	0	nonpulse	19	0	nonpulse	7	0

AN: aseptic necrosis

Steroid	months	AN	Steroid	months	AN	Steroid	months	AN
pulse	5	0	nonpulse	3	0	nonpulse	16	0
nonpulse	16	1	pulse	5	0	nonpulse	6	0
nonpulse	8	0	nonpulse	6	0	pulse	6	0
nonpulse	12	0	pulse	4	0	nonpulse	13	0
nonpulse	15	0	nonpulse	4	0	nonpulse	7	0
nonpulse	15	0	pulse	4	0	nonpulse	9	1
nonpulse	7	0	nonpulse	12	0	pulse	6	1
nonpulse	17	0	pulse	8	0	nonpulse	17	0
nonpulse	3	0	nonpulse	6	0	pulse	11	0
pulse	10	0	nonpulse	12	0	nonpulse	9	1
nonpulse	10	0	pulse	11	0	pulse	9	0
nonpulse	8	0	nonpulse	2	0	nonpulse	7	
pulse	6	0	nonpulse	9	0	pulse	5	0
pulse	4	0	nonpulse	5	0	pulse	9	0
pulse	5	0	nonpulse	8	0	nonpulse	5	0
pulse	7	0	pulse	8	0	pulse	7	0
pulse	9	0	nonpulse	4	0	pulse	6	0
nonpulse	4	0	nonpulse	5	0	nonpulse	7	0
pulse	8	0	nonpulse	10	1	nonpulse	9	0
pulse	6	0	nonpulse	11	0	pulse	11	0
pulse	14	0	nonpulse	8	0	pulse	19	0
pulse	6	1	nonpulse	5	0	pulse	6	1
nonpulse	4	0	nonpulse	10	0	pulse	8	0
pulse	6	0	nonpulse	3	0	nonpulse	6	0
pulse	8	0	pulse	5	0	pulse	4	0
nonpulse	12	0	pulse	4	0	nonpulse	1	0
pulse	6	0	nonpulse	7	0	nonpulse	4	0
nonpulse	9	0	nonpulse	9	1	pulse	10	0
pulse	8	0	pulse	11	0	nonpulse	7	0
nonpulse	9	0	nonpulse	9	0			

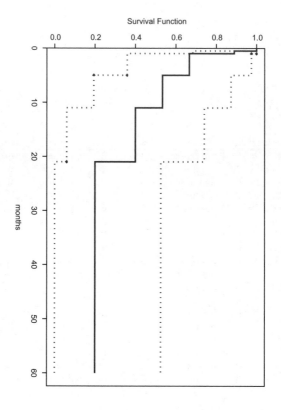

Figure 11.2: Kaplan-Meier survival curve of steroid

11.4.1   Kaplan-Meier Estimate

Kaplan-Meier survival curves were plotted for these two groups. Since it is
identical to that described in the foregoing paragraph, the method has been
omitted. (What is necessary is just to use the library `hazreg`).

If Figure 11.3 and Figure 11.4 are compared, a clear difference is likely.

11.4.2   log-rank Test

We performed log-rank test. The result is as follows.

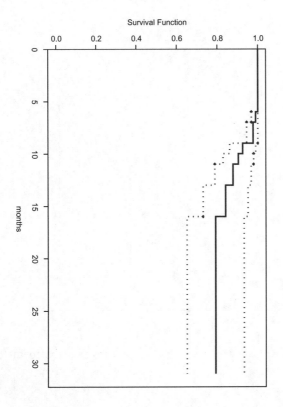

Figure 11.3: Kaplan-Meier survival curve of nonpulse treatment for steroid

```
chi-square: 9.486524263
p-value: 0.002069866
```

The advanced significant difference was accepted in two treatments.

11.4.3 Cox's Regression

Although data could not be shown in addition to this, there were sex, age, and hyperlipemia included in the data. Cox's regression can be used to investiage into how much variables other than steroid, and relationship with

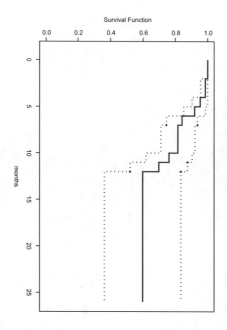

Figure 11.4: Kaplan-Meier survival curve of pulse treatment for steroid

aseptic necrosis.

$$\lambda(months; sex, age, hyperlipemia, steroid) = \lambda_0(months) \exp\left(\beta^\top \mathbf{Z}\right)$$
$$(11.1)$$

where λ_0 is baseline hazard function. In XploRe, it can be analyzed using library **hazreg** with functions **hazdat** and **haztest** used. Since data could not be exhibited and commands are puzzling, the result is shown without describing input for details.

On the result (Table 11.3), sex and age are almost unrelated to aseptic necrosis. As expected, steroid (pulse treatment) resulted in significant result, and hyperlipemia led to suggestive result. By above results, it decided to need sufficient cautions for pulse treatment, and not to treatment it as much as possible.

Table 11.3: Result of Cox's regression

	$\exp(\beta)$	lower .95	upper .95	p-value
sex	0.461	0.151	1.40	0.170
age	1.005	0.968	1.04	0.810
hyperlipemia	2.484	0.896	6.88	0.080
steroid	1.829	1.143	2.93	0.012

Bibliography

Cox, D. R.(1972). Regression models and life tables. *J. Amer. Stat. Assoc.*, **34**, 187-220.

Fukasawa, C., Uesato, M., Katsumata, Y., Hara, M., Kamatani, N.(2001). Aseptic Necrosis in patients with Systemic Lupus Erythematosus. *Riumachi*, **41**(2), 419.

Kaplan, E. L. and Meier, P(1958). Nonparametric estimation from incomplete observations. *J. Amer. Stat. Assoc.*, **53**, 457-481.

Peto, R., Pike, M.C., Armitage, P., Breslow, N.E., Cox, D.R., Howard, S.V., Mantel, N., McPherson, K., Peto, J., and Smith, P.G. (1977). Design and analysis of randomized clinical trials requiring prolonged observation of each patient. II. Analysis and examples. *Br. J. Cancer*, **35**, 1-39.

Tanaka, E., Harigai, M., Yago, T., Ichikawa, N., Kawaguchi, Y., Hara, M. and Kamatani, N.(2003). Pulmonary hypertension associated with collagen tissue disease - early diagnosis and treatment. *Riumachi*, **43**(2), 195.

Part II

Related Sciences

12 Ozone Pollution Forecasting Using Conditional Mean and Conditional Quantiles with Functional Covariates

Hervé Cardot, Christophe Crambes and Pascal Sarda

12.1 Introduction

Prediction of Ozone pollution is currently an important field of research, mainly in a goal of prevention. Many statistical methods have already been used to study data dealing with pollution. For example, Ghattas (1999) used a regression tree approach, while a functional approach has been proposed by Damon and Guillas (2002) and by Aneiros-Perez, Cardot, Estevez-Perez and Vieu (2004). Pollution data often consist now in hourly measurements of pollutants and meteorological data. These variables are then comparable to curves known in some discretization points, usually called *functional data* in the literature, Ramsay and Silverman (1997). Many examples of such data have already been studied in various fields, Franck and Friedman (1993), Ramsay and Silverman (2002), Ferraty and Vieu (2002). It seems then natural to propose some models that take into account the fact that the variables are functions of time.

The data we study here were provided by the ORAMIP ("Observatoire Régional de l'Air en Midi-Pyrénées"), which is an air observatory located in the city of Toulouse (France). We are interested in a pollutant like Ozone. We consider the prediction of the maximum of pollution for a day (maximum of Ozone) knowing the Ozone temporal evolution the day before. To do this, we consider two models. The first one is the functional linear model introduced by Ramsay and Dalzell (1993). It is based on the prediction of the conditional mean. The second one is a generalization of the linear model for quantile regression introduced by Koenker and Bassett (1978) when the covariates are curves. It consists in forecasting the conditional median. More generally, we introduce this model for the α-conditional quantile, with $\alpha \in (0,1)$. This allows us to give prediction intervals. For both models, a spline estimator of the functional coefficient is introduced, in a way similar to Cardot, Ferraty and Sarda (2003).

This work is divided into four parts. First, we give a brief statistical description and analysis of the data, in particular by the use of principal components analysis (PCA), to study the general behaviour of the variables. Secondly, we present the functional linear model and we propose a spline estimator of the functional coefficient. Similarly, we propose in the third part a spline estimator of the functional coefficient for the α-conditional quantile. In both models, we describe the algorithms that have been implemented to obtain the spline estimator. We also extend these algorithms to the case where there are several functional predictors by the use of a *backfitting* algorithm. Finally, these approaches are illustrated using the real pollution data provided by the ORAMIP.

12.2   A Brief Analysis of the Data

12.2.1   Description of the Data

The data provided by ORAMIP consist in hourly measurements during the period going from the 15th May to the 15th September for the years 1997, 1998, 1999 and 2000, of the following variables:

- Nitrogen Monoxide (noted NO),

- Nitrogen Dioxide (noted N2),

- Ozone (noted O3),

- Wind Direction (noted WD),

- Wind Speed (noted WS).

These variables were observed in six different stations in Toulouse. There are some missing data, mainly because of breakdowns. There were also other variables (such as the temperature) for which the missing data were too numerous and we could not use them, so, in the following, we just consider the five variables mentioned above. We first noticed that these variables take values which are very similar from one station to another. Thus, for each variable, we consider the mean of the measurements in the different stations. This approach is one way to deal with missing values.

A descriptive analysis of the variables can show simple links between them. For example, we can see that the mean daily curves of the first three variables NO, N2 and O3 (cf. Figure 12.1) have a similar evolution for NO and N2 (at least in the first part of the day). On the contrary, the curves for NO and O3 have opposite variations. These observations are also confirmed by the correlation matrix of the variables NO, N2 and O3.

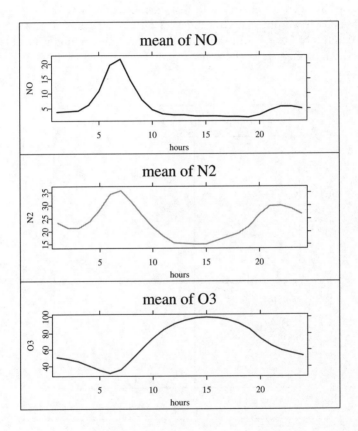

Figure 12.1: Daily mean curves for the variables NO (blue curve), N2 (green curve and O3 (red curve).

12.2.2   Principal Component Analysis

A first PCA has been done on the matrix whose columns are the different
daily mean variables. As these variables have different units, we also consider
the reduced matrix. The first two components allow to explain more than
80% of the variance. To visualize the results of this PCA, we have represented
the mean hours (Figure 12.2) and the variables (Figure 12.3) in the plane
formed by the two first principal axes. We notice on Figure 12.2 that the
first axis separates the morning and the afternoon evolution while the second
axis separates the day and the night. Concerning Figure 12.3, the first axis
separates Nitrogen Monoxide and Nitrogen Dioxide of Ozone. We can also
remark that, if we put the Graphic 12.2 on the Graphic 12.3, we find that
the maximum of Ozone is in the afternoon and that the quantity of Ozone is
low in the morning. It is the contrary for Nitrogen Monoxide and Nitrogen
Dioxide.

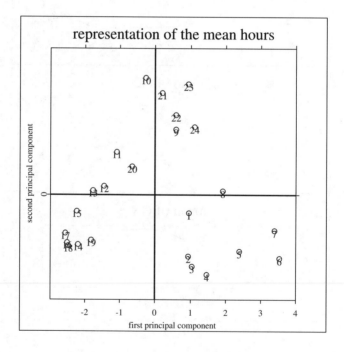

Figure 12.2: Representation of the mean hours 1, ..., 24 in the plane generated by the two first principal components.

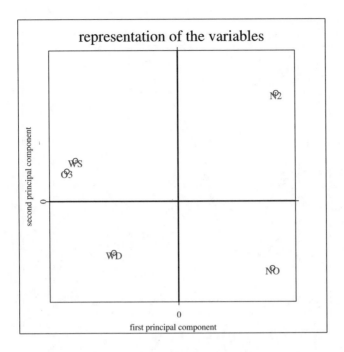

Figure 12.3: Representation of the variables NO, N2, O3, WD and WS in the plane generated by the two first principal components.

12.2.3 Functional Principal Component Analysis

We also performed a functional PCA of the different variables. We come back here to the functional background where we consider each variable as a curve discretized in some points. We can look at the variations of each variable around its mean by representing the functions μ, $\mu + C\xi$ and $\mu - C\xi$, where μ is the mean curve of the variable, C is a constant and ξ is a principal component. For example, for Ozone, we make this representation for the first principal component (that represents nearly 80% of the information) on Figure 12.4. The constant C has been fixed arbitrarily in this example equal to 10, to obtain a figure easily interpretable. We can see that the first principal component highlights variations around the mean at 3:00 pm. It is the time of the maximum of Ozone in the middle of the afternoon.

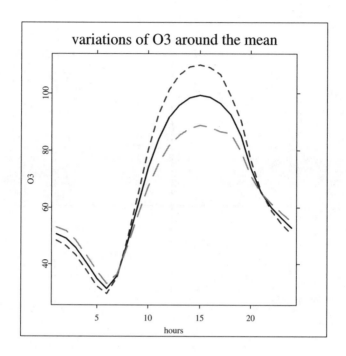

Figure 12.4: Variations of O3 around the mean. The blue solid curve represents the mean curve μ of Ozone, the red dotted curve represents
$\mu + 10\xi$ where ξ is the first principal component, and the green
dashed curve represents $\mu - 10\xi$.

12.3   Functional Linear Model

We describe now the functional linear model presented for example by Ramsay and Silverman (1997). Let us consider a sample $\{(X_i, Y_i)\}_{i=1}^{n}$ of pairs
of random variables, independent and identically distributed, with the same
distribution as (X, Y), with X belonging to the functional space $L^2(D)$ of
the integrable square functions defined on a bounded interval D of $\mathbb{R}$, and Y
belonging to $\mathbb{R}$. We center each function X_i by introducing $\widetilde{X_i} = X_i - E(X_i)$.
The functional linear model is then defined by

$$Y_i = \mu + \int_D \alpha(t) \widetilde{X_i}(t) \, dt + \epsilon_i, \tag{12.1}$$

with $E(\epsilon_i|X_i) = 0$. We have $E(Y_i) = \mu$ and $E(Y_i|X_i) = \mu + \int_D \alpha(t)\widetilde{X}_i(t)\, dt$.

In practice, each function X_i is known in $p = 24$ equispaced discretization points $t_1, \ldots, t_p \in D$ (with $t_1 \leq \ldots \leq t_p$). So, the integral above is approximated by

$$\int_D \alpha(t)\widetilde{X}_i(t)\, dt \approx \frac{\lambda(D)}{p} \sum_{j=1}^{p-1} \alpha(t_j)\widetilde{X}_i(t_j),$$

where $\lambda(D)$ stands for the length of the interval D. More generally, when the discretization points are not equispaced, the integral can be easily approximated by

$$\int_D \alpha(t)\widetilde{X}_i(t)\, dt \approx \sum_{j=1}^{p-1} (t_{j+1} - t_j)\alpha(t_j)\widetilde{X}_i(t_j).$$

12.3.1   Spline Estimation of α

We choose to estimate the functional coefficient of regression $\alpha : D \longrightarrow \mathbb{R}$ by a spline function (see de Boor (1978) for details). Let us consider $k \in \mathbb{N}^*$ and $q \in \mathbb{N}$. We split D into k intervals of the same length. A spline function is a piecewise polynomial function of degree $q \in \mathbb{N}^*$ on each sub-interval, $(q - 1)$ times differentiable on D. The extremities of the sub-intervals are called knots. It is known that the space of such splines functions is a vectorial space of dimension $k + q$. We consider the basis $\mathbf{B}_{k,q}$ of this space called B-splines basis and that we write $\mathbf{B}_{k,q} = (B_1, \cdots, B_{k+q})^\top$.

We estimate α by a linear combination of the functions B_l, $l = 1, \ldots, k + q$, that leads us to find $\widehat{\mu} \in \mathbb{R}$ and a vector $\widehat{\boldsymbol{\theta}} \in \mathbb{R}^{k+q}$ such that

$$\widehat{\alpha} = \sum_{l=1}^{k+q} \widehat{\theta}_l B_l = \mathbf{B}_{k,q}^\top \widehat{\boldsymbol{\theta}},$$

with $\widehat{\mu}$ and $\widehat{\boldsymbol{\theta}}$ solutions of the following minimization problem

$$\min_{\mu \in \mathbb{R}, \boldsymbol{\theta} \in \mathbb{R}^{k+q}} \left\{ \frac{1}{n} \sum_{i=1}^{n} (Y_i - \mu - \langle \mathbf{B}_{k,q}^\top \boldsymbol{\theta}, \widetilde{X}_i \rangle)^2 + \rho \parallel (\mathbf{B}_{k,q}^\top \boldsymbol{\theta})^{(m)} \parallel^2 \right\}, \qquad (12.2)$$

where $(\mathbf{B}_{k,q}^\top \boldsymbol{\theta})^{(m)}$ is the mth derivative of $\mathbf{B}_{k,q}^\top \boldsymbol{\theta}$ and ρ is a penalization parameter that allows to control the smoothness of the estimator, see Cardot, Ferraty and Sarda (2003). The notation $\langle .,. \rangle$ refers to the inner product of $L^2(D)$ and $\|.\|$ is the norm induced by this inner product.

If we set $\boldsymbol{\beta} = \begin{pmatrix} \mu \\ \boldsymbol{\theta} \end{pmatrix} \in \mathbb{R}^{k+q+1}$, then, the solution of the minimization problem (12.2) above is given by

$$\widehat{\boldsymbol{\beta}} = \frac{1}{n}(\frac{1}{n}\mathbf{D}^\top\mathbf{D} + \rho\mathbf{K})^{-1}\mathbf{D}^\top\mathbf{Y},$$

with

$$\mathbf{D} = \begin{pmatrix} 1 & \langle B_1, X_1 \rangle & \cdots & \langle B_{k+q}, X_1 \rangle \\ \vdots & \vdots & & \vdots \\ 1 & \langle B_1, X_n \rangle & \cdots & \langle B_{k+q}, X_n \rangle \end{pmatrix} \quad \text{and} \quad \mathbf{K} = \begin{pmatrix} 0 & 0 \\ 0 & \mathbf{G} \end{pmatrix},$$

where $\mathbf{G}$ is the $(k+q) \times (k+q)$ matrix with elements $\mathbf{G}_{jl} = < B_j^{(m)}, B_l^{(m)} >$. It also satisfies

$$\boldsymbol{\theta}^\top \mathbf{G} \boldsymbol{\theta} = \| (\mathbf{B}_{k,q}^\top \boldsymbol{\theta})^{(m)} \|^2 .$$

The computation of the matrices $\mathbf{D}$ and $\mathbf{G}$ is performed with the functions XCSbspline and XCSbsplineini.

Q XCSbspline.xpl

Q XCSbsplineini.xpl

Let us notice that a convergence result for this spline estimator is given by Cardot, Ferraty and Sarda (2003).

12.3.2   Selection of the Parameters

The estimator defined by (12.2) depends on a large number of parameters: the number of knots k, the degree q of splines, the order m of derivation in the penalization term, and the smoothing parameter ρ. It seems that only the penalization parameter ρ is really important provided that the number of knots is large enough, see Marx and Eilers (1999), Besse, Cardot and Ferraty (1997).

The parameter ρ is chosen by the generalized cross validation criterion, see Wahba (1990), which is described below.

Consider the "hat matrix" $\mathbf{H}(\rho) = \frac{1}{n}\mathbf{D}(\frac{1}{n}\mathbf{D}^\top\mathbf{D} + \rho\mathbf{K})^{-1}\mathbf{D}^\top$. It satisfies $\widehat{\mathbf{Y}} = \mathbf{H}(\rho)\mathbf{Y}$. The generalized cross validation criterion is then given by

$$GCV(\rho) = \frac{\frac{1}{n}\sum_{l=1}^{n}(Y_l - \widehat{Y}_l)^2}{\left[1 - \frac{1}{n}\operatorname{tr}\{\mathbf{H}(\rho)\}\right]^2}. \tag{12.3}$$

We select the optimal parameter ρ_{GCV} as the one that minimizes the GCV criterion (12.3). Let us notice that we do not have to compute the matrix $\mathbf{H}(\rho)$ (whose size is $n \times n$) since we have $\operatorname{tr}(\mathbf{H}(\rho)) = \operatorname{tr}(\frac{1}{n}\mathbf{D}^\top\mathbf{D}(\frac{1}{n}\mathbf{D}^\top\mathbf{D} + \rho\mathbf{K})^{-1})$.

The XploRe function XCSsflmgcv uses this GCV criterion and gives the estimations of μ, θ and α.

Q XCSsflmgcv.xpl

12.3.3 Multiple Functional Linear Model

We now want to generalize the model (12.1) to the case where there are several (centered) functional covariates $\widetilde{X}^1, \ldots, \widetilde{X}^v$. We consider the following additive model

$$Y_i = \mu + \int_D \alpha_1(t)\widetilde{X}_i^1(t)\, dt + \ldots + \int_D \alpha_v(t)\widetilde{X}_i^v(t)\, dt + \epsilon_i. \tag{12.4}$$

To get the estimates of $\mu, \alpha_1, \ldots, \alpha_v$, we used the *backfitting* algorithm, see Hastie and Tibshirani (1990), which principle is described below. It allows us to avoid inverting large scale matrices and leads to a faster estimation procedure. The XploRe function giving the estimates of $\mu, \alpha_1, \ldots, \alpha_v$ using the backfitting algorithm for v covariates is XCSsflmgcvmult.

Q XCSsflmgcvmult.xpl

- **Step 1**
  We initialize $\widehat{\alpha_1}^{(1)}, \ldots, \widehat{\alpha_{v-1}}^{(1)}$ to 0 and $\widehat{\mu}$ to $\frac{1}{n}\sum_{i=1}^{n} Y_i$. Then, we

determine $\widehat{\mu}^{(1)}$ and $\widehat{\alpha_v}^{(1)}$ by using the spline estimation procedure for the functional linear model with one covariate.

- **Step 2**
  For $r = 1, \ldots, v$, we consider

$$Y_i^{r,2} = Y_i - \sum_{l=1}^{r-1} \int_D \widehat{\alpha_l}^{(2)}(t)\widetilde{X_i^l}(t)\,dt - \sum_{l=r+1}^{v} \int_D \widehat{\alpha_l}^{(1)}(t)\widetilde{X_i^l}(t)\,dt,$$

and we make a simple functional regression

$$Y_i^{r,2} = \mu + \int_D \alpha_r^{(2)}(t)\widetilde{X_i^r}(t)\,dt + \epsilon_i.$$

Then, we obtain $\widehat{\mu}^{(2)}$ and $\widehat{\alpha_r}^{(2)}$, for $r = 1, \ldots, v$. The optimal penalization parameter is determined for each estimator with generalized cross validation.

- **Step $j + 1$**
  While $\max_{r=1,\ldots,v}(\|\widehat{\alpha_r}^{(j)} - \widehat{\alpha_r}^{(j-1)}\|) > \xi$ (where ξ is an error constant to be fixed), we consider

$$Y_i^{r,j+1} = Y_i - \sum_{l=1}^{r-1} \int_D \widehat{\alpha_l}^{(j+1)}(t)\widetilde{X_i^l}(t)\,dt - \sum_{l=r+1}^{v} \int_D \widehat{\alpha_l}^{(j)}(t)\widetilde{X_i^l}(t)\,dt,$$

and we make a simple functional regression

$$Y_i^{r,j+1} = \mu + \int_D \alpha_r^{(j+1)}(t)\widetilde{X_i^r}(t)\,dt + \epsilon_i,$$

by using the estimator defined for the functional linear model with one covariate. We then deduce $\widehat{\mu}^{(j+1)}$ and $\widehat{\alpha_r}^{(j+1)}$, for $r = 1, \ldots, v$. The optimal penalization parameter is determined for each estimator with generalized cross validation.

12.4 Functional Linear Regression for Conditional Quantiles Estimation

Our goal is now to find the Ozone threshold value such that the conditional probability to exceed this value is equal to a certain given risk $\alpha \in (0,1)$. More precisely, if Y is a real random value, we define its α-quantile by the real number q_α such that

$$P(Y \leq q_\alpha) = \alpha.$$

Koenker and Bassett (1978) use the following property to define quantile estimators (which can be naturally generalized to conditional quantiles):

$$q_\alpha = \arg\min_{a \in \mathbb{R}} E(l_\alpha(Y - a)),$$

with

$$l_\alpha(u) = |u| + (2\alpha - 1)u.$$

Let us now come back to our functional case. We still consider the sample $\{(X_i, Y_i)\}_{i=1}^n$ of pairs of random variables, independent and identically distributed, with the same distribution as (X, Y), with X belonging to the functional space $L^2(D)$, and Y belonging to $\mathbb{R}$. Without loss of generality, we suppose that X is a centered variable, that is to say $E(X) = 0$. Let α be a real number in $(0,1)$ and x a function in $L^2(D)$. We suppose that the *conditional α-quantile* of Y given $[X = x]$ is the unique scalar $g_\alpha(x)$ such that

$$P[Y \leq g_\alpha(x)|X = x] = \alpha, \qquad (12.5)$$

where $P(.|X = x)$ is the conditional probability given $[X = x]$.

Let us remark that $g_\alpha(x)$ can be defined in an equivalent way as the solution of the minimization problem

$$\min_{a \in \mathbb{R}} E[l_\alpha(Y - a)|X = x]. \qquad (12.6)$$

We assume now that there exists a unique function $\Psi_\alpha \in L^2(D)$ such that g_α can be written in the following way

$$g_\alpha(X) = c + \langle \Psi_\alpha, X \rangle = c + \int_D \Psi_\alpha(t) X(t) \, dt. \qquad (12.7)$$

This condition can be seen as a direct generalization of the model introduced by Koenker and Bassett (1978), the difference being that here, the covariates are functions.

12.4.1 Spline Estimator of Ψ_α

Our goal is now to give a nonparametric estimator of the function Ψ_α. In the case where the covariate X is real, many nonparametric estimators have already been proposed, see for example Bhattacharya and Gangopadhyay (1990), Fan, Hu and Truong (1994), Lejeune and Sarda (1988) or He and Shi (1994).

As for the spline estimator described in Section 12.3.1, we consider the vectorial space of spline functions with $k - 1$ interior knots and of degree q, and its B-splines basis $\mathbf{B_{k,q}} = (B_1, \ldots, B_{k+q})^\top$. We estimate Ψ_α by a linear combination of the B_l functions for l going from 1 to $k + q$. This leads us to find a vector $\widehat{\boldsymbol{\theta}} = (\widehat{\theta}_1, \ldots, \widehat{\theta}_{k+q})^\top$ in $\mathbb{R}^{k+q}$ such that

$$\widehat{\Psi}_\alpha = \sum_{l=1}^{k+q} \widehat{\theta}_l B_l = \mathbf{B_{k,q}}^\top \widehat{\boldsymbol{\theta}}. \qquad (12.8)$$

The vector $\widehat{\boldsymbol{\theta}}$ will be solution of the following minimization problem, which is the penalized empirical version of (12.6),

$$\min_{c \in \mathbb{R}, \theta \in \mathbb{R}^{k+q}} \left\{ \frac{1}{n} \sum_{i=1}^n l_\alpha(Y_i - c - \langle \mathbf{B_{k,q}}^\top \boldsymbol{\theta}, X_i \rangle) + \rho \parallel (\mathbf{B_{k,q}}^\top \boldsymbol{\theta})^{(m)} \parallel^2 \right\}, \qquad (12.9)$$

where $(\mathbf{B_{k,q}}^\top \boldsymbol{\theta})^{(m)}$ is the m-th derivative of the spline function $\mathbf{B_{k,q}}^\top \boldsymbol{\theta}$ and ρ is a penalization parameter which role is to control the smoothness of the estimator, as for the minimization problem (12.2) considered in Section 12.3.1. This criterion is similar to (12.2), the quadratic function being here replaced by the loss function l_α. In this case, we have to deal with an optimization problem that does not have an explicit solution, contrary to the estimation of the conditional mean. That is why we adopted the strategy proposed by Lejeune and Sarda (1988). It is based on an algorithm that consists in performing iterative weighted least squares, see Ruppert and Caroll (1988)). Let us consider the function δ_i defined by

$$\delta_i(\alpha) = 2\alpha \boldsymbol{I}\{Y_i - c - \langle \mathbf{B}_{k,q}^\top \boldsymbol{\theta}, X_i \rangle \geq 0\} + 2(1 - \alpha)\boldsymbol{I}\{Y_i - c - \langle \mathbf{B}_{k,q}^\top \boldsymbol{\theta}, X_i \rangle < 0\}.$$

The minimization problem (12.9) is then equivalent to

$$\min_{c \in \mathbb{R}, \boldsymbol{\theta} \in \mathbb{R}^{k+q}} \left\{ \frac{1}{n} \sum_{i=1}^n \delta_i(\alpha) \mid Y_i - c - \langle \mathbf{B}_{k,q}^\top \boldsymbol{\theta}, X_i \rangle \mid + \rho \parallel (\mathbf{B}_{k,q}^\top \boldsymbol{\theta})^{(m)} \parallel^2 \right\}. \quad (12.10)$$

Then, we can approximate this criterion by replacing the absolute value by a weighted quadratic term, hence we can obtain a sequence of explicit solutions. The principle of this Iterative Reweighted Least Squares algorithm is described below.

- **Initialization**

  We determine $\boldsymbol{\beta}^1 = (c^1, \boldsymbol{\theta}^1)^\top$ solution of the minimization problem

$$\min_{c \in \mathbb{R}, \boldsymbol{\theta} \in \mathbb{R}^{k+q}} \left\{ \frac{1}{n} \sum_{i=1}^n (Y_i - c - \langle \mathbf{B}_{k,q}^\top \boldsymbol{\theta}, X_i \rangle)^2 + \rho \parallel (\mathbf{B}_{k,q}^\top \boldsymbol{\theta})^{(m)} \parallel^2 \right\},$$

  which solution $\boldsymbol{\beta}^1$ is given by $\boldsymbol{\beta}^1 = \frac{1}{n}(\frac{1}{n}\mathbf{D}^\top \mathbf{D} + \rho \mathbf{K})^{-1}\mathbf{D}^\top \mathbf{Y}$, with $\mathbf{D}$ and $\mathbf{K}$ defined in Section 12.3.1.

- **Step j+1**

  Knowing $\boldsymbol{\beta}^j = (c^j, \boldsymbol{\theta}^j)^\top$, we determine $\boldsymbol{\beta}^{j+1} = (c^{j+1}, \boldsymbol{\theta}^{j+1})^\top$ solution of the minimization problem

$$\min_{c \in \mathbb{R}, \boldsymbol{\theta} \in \mathbb{R}^{k+q}} \left\{ \frac{1}{n} \sum_{i=1}^n \frac{\delta_i^j(\alpha)(Y_i - c - \langle \mathbf{B}_{k,q}^\top \boldsymbol{\theta}, X_i \rangle)^2}{[(Y_i - c - \langle \mathbf{B}_{k,q}^\top \boldsymbol{\theta}, X_i \rangle)^2 + \eta^2]^{1/2}} + \rho \parallel (\mathbf{B}_{k,q}^\top \boldsymbol{\theta})^{(m)} \parallel^2 \right\},$$

  where $\delta_i^j(\alpha)$ is $\delta_i(\alpha)$ on step j of the algorithm, and η is a strictly positive constant that allows us to avoid a denominator equal to zero.

Let us define the $n \times n$ diagonal matrix $\mathbf{W}_j$ with diagonal elements given by

$$[\mathbf{W}_j]_{ll} = \frac{\delta_1^j(\alpha)}{n[(Y_l - c - \langle \mathbf{B}_{k,q}^\top \boldsymbol{\theta}, X_l \rangle)^2 + \eta^2]^{1/2}}.$$

Then, $\beta^{j+1} = (\mathbf{D}^\top \mathbf{W}_j \mathbf{D} + \rho \mathbf{K})^{-1} \mathbf{D}^\top \mathbf{W}_j \mathbf{Y}$.

Remark: Since our algorithm relies on weighted least squares, we can derive a generalized cross validation criterion to choose the penalization parameter value ρ at each step of the algorithm. Indeed, the "hat matrix" defined by $\mathbf{H}(\rho) = \mathbf{D}(\mathbf{D}^\top \mathbf{W} \mathbf{D} + \rho \mathbf{K})^{-1} \,{}^t\mathbf{D} \mathbf{W}$ satisfies $\widehat{\mathbf{Y}} = \mathbf{H}(\rho)\mathbf{Y}$, where $\mathbf{W}$ is the weight matrix obtained at the previous step of the algorithm. The generalized cross validation criterion is then given by

$$GCV(\rho) = \frac{\dfrac{1}{n}(\mathbf{Y} - \widehat{\mathbf{Y}})^\top \mathbf{W}(\mathbf{Y} - \widehat{\mathbf{Y}})}{\left[1 - \dfrac{1}{n}\mathrm{tr}\{\mathbf{H}(\rho)\}\right]^2}, \qquad (12.11)$$

where $\mathrm{tr}(\mathbf{H}(\rho)) = \mathrm{tr}\{\mathbf{D}^\top \mathbf{W}(\mathbf{D}^\top \mathbf{W} \mathbf{D} + \rho \mathbf{K})\}$.

We select the optimal parameter ρ_{GCV} as the one that minimizes the GCV criterion (12.11). The XploRe function XCSsquantgcv uses this GCV criterion and gives the estimations of c, θ and Ψ_α.

Q XCSsquantgcv.xpl

A convergence result of the estimator $\widehat{\Psi}_\alpha$ is also available in Cardot, Crambes and Sarda (2004)

12.4.2   Multiple Conditional Quantiles

Assuming we have now v functional covariates $X^1, \ldots, X^v$, this estimation procedure can be easily extended. We consider the following model

$$P\left[Y_i \le g_\alpha^1(X_i^1) + \ldots + g_\alpha^v(X_i^v) | X_i^1 = x_i^1, \ldots, X_i^v = x_i^v\right] = \alpha. \qquad (12.12)$$

Similarly as before, we assume that $g_\alpha^1(X_i^1) + \ldots + g_\alpha^v(X_i^v) = c + \langle \Psi_\alpha^1, X_i^1 \rangle + \ldots + \langle \Psi_\alpha^v, X_i^v \rangle$ with $\Psi_\alpha^1, \ldots, \Psi_\alpha^v$ in $L^2(D)$. The estimation of each function

Ψ_α^r is obtained using the iterative backfitting algorithm combined with the Iterative Reweighted Least Squares algorithm. The XploRe function giving the estimates of $c, \Psi_\alpha^1, \ldots, \Psi_\alpha^v$ is:

Q XCSsquantgcvmult.xpl

12.5 Application to Ozone Prediction

We want to predict the variable maximum of Ozone one day i, noted Y_i, using the functional covariates observed the day before until 5:00 pm. We consider covariates with length of 24 hours. We can assume that beyond 24 hours, the effects of the covariate are negligible knowing the last 24 hours, so each curve X_i begins at 6:00 pm the day $i - 2$.

We ramdomly splitted the initial sample $(X_i, Y_i)_{i=1,\ldots,n}$ into two sub-samples:

- a learning sample $(X_{a_i}, Y_{a_i})_{i=1,\ldots,n_l}$ whose size is $n_l = 332$, used to compute the estimators $\widehat{\mu}$ and $\widehat{\alpha}$ for the functional linear model and the estimators $\widehat{c}$ and $\widehat{\Psi}_\alpha$ for the model with quantiles,

- a test sample $(X_{t_i}, Y_{t_i})_{i=1,\ldots,n_t}$ whose size is $n_t = 142$, used to evaluate the quality of the models and to make a comparison between them.

We also have chosen to take $k = 8$ for the number of knots, $q = 3$ for the degree of spline functions and $m = 2$ for the order of the derivative in the penalization.

To predict the value of Y_i, we use the conditional mean and the conditional median (*i.e.* $\alpha = 0.5$). To judge the quality of the models, we give a prediction of the maximum of Ozone for each element of the test sample,

$$\widehat{Y_{t_i}} = \widehat{\mu} + \int_D \widehat{\alpha}(t) X_{t_i}(t)\, dt$$

for the prediction of the conditional mean, and

$$\widehat{Y_{t_i}} = \widehat{c} + \int_D \widehat{\Psi}_\alpha(t) X_{t_i}(t)\, dt$$

for the prediction of the conditional median.

Then, we consider three criteria given by

$$C_1 = \frac{n_t^{-1} \sum_{i=1}^{n_t} (Y_{t_i} - \widehat{Y_{t_i}})^2}{n_t^{-1} \sum_{i=1}^{n_t} (Y_{t_i} - \overline{Y}_l)^2},$$

$$C_2 = n_t^{-1} \sum_{i=1}^{n_t} |\, Y_{t_i} - \widehat{Y_{t_i}}\, |,$$

$$C_3 = \frac{n_t^{-1} \sum_{i=1}^{n_t} l_\alpha(Y_{t_i} - \widehat{Y_{t_i}})}{n_t^{-1} \sum_{i=1}^{n_t} l_\alpha(Y_{t_i} - q_\alpha(Y_l))},$$

where $\overline{Y}_l$ is the empirical mean of the learning sample $(Y_{a_i})_{i=1,\ldots,n_l}$ and $q_\alpha(Y_l)$ is the empirical α-quantile of the learning sample $(Y_{a_i})_{i=1,\ldots,n_l}$. This last criterion C_3 is similar to the one proposed by Koenker and Machado (1999). We remark that, the more these criteria take low values (close to 0), the better is the prediction. These three criteria are all computed on the test sample.

12.5.1   Prediction of the Conditional Mean

The values of the criteria C_1 and C_2 are given in the Table 12.5.1. It appears that the best model with one covariate to predict the maximum of Ozone is the one that use the curve of Ozone the day before. We have also built multiple functional linear models, in order to improve the prediction. The errors for these models are also given in Table 12.5.1. It appears that the best model is the one that use the four covariates Ozone, Nitrogen Monoxide, Wind Direction and Wind Speed. So, adding other covariates allows to improve the prediction, even if the gain is low.

12.5.2   Prediction of the Conditional Median

Table 12.5.2 gathers the prediction errors of the different models. As for the functional linear model, the best prediction using one covariate is the one obtained by using the Ozone curve the day before. Moreover, the prediction is slightly improved by adding other covariates. The best prediction for the criterion C_3 is obtained for the model using the covariates Ozone, Nitrogen Monoxide, Nitrogen Dioxide and Wind Speed. For this model with these four covariates, we have represented on Figure 12.5 the GCV criterion versus $-\log(\rho)$ for the different values of ρ from 10^{-5} to 10^{-10}. The minimum value of the FP criterion is reached for $\rho = 10^{-8}$, see Härdle, Müller, Sperlich and Werwatz (2004). Figure 12.6 represents the predicted maximum of Ozone

Table 12.1: Prediction error criteria C_1 and C_2 for the different functional linear models

Models	Variables	C_1	C_2
models with 1 covariate	NO	0.828	16.998
	N2	0.761	16.153
	O3	**0.416**	**12.621**
	WD	0.910	18.414
	WS	0.796	16.756
models with 2 covariates	O3, NO	0.409	12.338
	O3, N2	0.410	12.373
	O3, WD	0.405	12.318
	O3, WS	0.400	12.267
models with 3 covariates	O3, NO, N2	0.408	12.305
	O3, NO, WD	0.394	11.956
	O3, NO, WS	0.397	12.121
	O3, N2, WD	0.397	12.003
	O3, N2, WS	0.404	12.156
	O3, WD, WS	0.397	12.101
models with 4 covariates	**O3, NO, WD, WS**	**0.391**	**11.870**
	O3, NO, N2, WD	0.395	11.875
	O3, NO, N2, WS	0.398	12.069
	O3, N2, WD, WS	0.394	11.962
model with 5 covariates	O3, NO, N2, WD, WS	0.392	11.877

(with this model of 4 covariates) versus the measured maximum of Ozone for the test sample. We see on this graphic that the points are quite close to the straight line of equation $y = x$.

Another interest of the conditional quantiles is that we can build some prediction intervals for the maximum of Ozone, which can be quite useful in the context of prevention of Ozone pollution. Coming back to the initial sample (that is to say when the days are chronologically ordered), we have plotted on Figure 12.7 the measures of the maximum of Ozone during the first 40 days of our sample, that is to say from the 17th May of 1997 to the 25th June of 1997 (blue solid curve). The red dotted curve above represents the values of the 90% quantile and the green dashed curve below represents the values of the 10% quantile predicted for these measures. The prediction model used is again the quantile regression model with the 4 covariates O3, NO, N2 and WS.

Table 12.2: Prediction error criteria C_1, C_2 and C_3 for the different functional quantile regression models

Models	Variables	C_1	C_2	C_3
models with 1 covariate	NO	0.826	16.996	0.911
	N2	0.805	16.800	0.876
	O3	**0.425**	**12.332**	**0.661**
	WD	0.798	18.836	0.902
	WS	0.885	18.222	0.976
models with 2 covariates	O3, NO	0.412	12.007	0.643
	O3, N2	0.405	11.936	0.640
	O3, WD	0.406	12.109	0.649
	O3, WS	0.406	11.823	0.633
models with 3 covariates	O3, NO, N2	0.404	11.935	0.639
	O3, NO, WD	0.404	12.024	0.644
	O3, NO, WS	0.407	11.832	0.638
	O3, N2, WD	0.402	11.994	0.642
	O3, N2, WS	0.403	12.108	0.641
	O3, WD, WS	0.403	12.123	0.640
models with 4 covariates	O3, NO, WD, WS	0.399	11.954	0.641
	O3, NO, N2, WD	0.397	11.921	0.639
	O3, NO, N2, WS	**0.397**	**11.712**	**0.634**
	O3, N2, WD, WS	0.398	11.952	0.640
model with 5 covariates	O3, NO, N2, WD, WS	0.397	11.864	0.638

12.5.3   Analysis of the Results

Both models, the functional linear model and the model with conditional quantiles for functional covariates, give satisfying results concerning the maximum of Ozone prediction. Concerning Figure 12.6, it seems that few values are not well predicted. This highlights a common problem for statistical models, which get into trouble when predicting extreme values (outliers). The interval of prediction given by the 90% and 10% conditional quantiles can be an interesting answer to that problem, as seen on Figure 12.7.

In spite of the lack of some important variables in the model, such as temperature for example, we can produce good estimators of maximum of pollution knowing the data the day before. The most efficient variable to estimate the maximum of Ozone is the Ozone curve the day before; however, we noticed

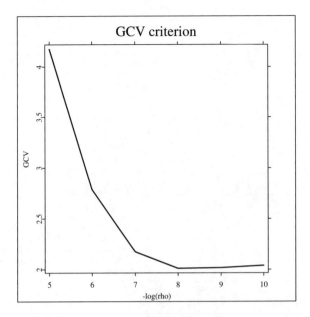

Figure 12.5: Generalized Cross Validation criterion for different values of ρ in the quantile regression model using the covariates O3, NO, N2, WS.

that prediction accuracy can be improved by adding other variables in the model. We can suppose that it will be possible to improve again these results when other covariates will be available from ORAMIP, such as temperature curves.

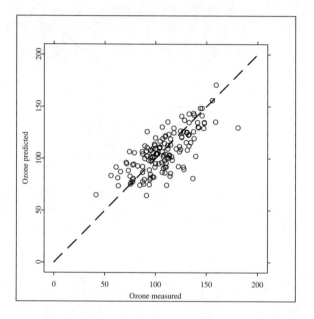

Figure 12.6: Predicted Ozone versus measured Ozone for the test sample, using the prediction quantile regression model with the covariates
O3, NO, N2, WS.

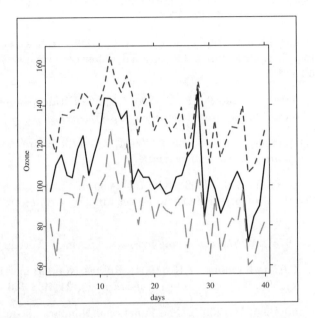

Figure 12.7: Prediction interval of the measures of maximum of Ozone for the period going from the 17th May of 1997 to the 25th June of 1997 (blue solid curve). The red dotted curve and the green dashed curve represent respectively the values of the 90% and 10% quantiles predicted for these measures.

Bibliography

Aneiros-Perez, G., Cardot, H., Estevez-Perez, G. and Vieu, P. (2004). Maximum Ozone Concentration Forecasting by Functional Nonparametric Approaches. *Environmetrics*, to appear.

Besse, P.C., Cardot, H. and Ferraty, F. (1997). Simultaneous Nonparametric Regression of Unbalanced Longitudinal Data. *Computational Statistics and Data Analysis*, **24**, 255-270.

Bhattacharya, P.K. and Gangopadhyay, A.K. (1990). Kernel and Nearest-Neighbor Estimation of a Conditional Quantile. *Annals of Statistics*, **18**, 1400-1415.

Cardot, H., Ferraty, F. and Sarda, P. (2003). Spline Estimators for the Functional Linear Model. *Statistica Sinica*, **13**, 571-591.

Cardot, H., Crambes, C. and Sarda, P. (2004). Quantile Regression when the Covariates are Functions. *Preprint*.

Damon, J. and Guillas, S. (2002). The Inclusion of Exogenous Variables in Functional Autoregressive Ozone Forecasting. *Environmetrics*, **13**, 759-774.

de Boor, C. (1978). *A Practical Guide to Splines*. Springer-Verlag, New-York.

Fan, J., Hu, T.C. and Truong, Y.K. (1994). Robust Nonparametric Function Estimation. *Scandinavian Journal of Statistics*, **21**, 433-446.

Ferraty, F. and Vieu, P. (2002). The Functional Nonparametric Model and Application to Spectrometric Data. *Computational Statistics and Data Analysis*, **17**, 545-564.

Frank, I.E. and Friedman, J.H. (1993). A statistical View of some Chemometrics Regression Tools (with discussion). *Technometrics*, **35**, 109-148.

Ghattas, B. (1999). Prévisions des Pics d'Ozone par Arbres de Régression Simples et Agrégés par Bootstrap. *Revue de Statistique Appliquée*, **XLVII**, 2, 61-80.

Härdle W., Müller M., Sperlich S. and Werwatz A. (2004). *Nonparametric and Semiparametric Models*, Springer.

Hastie, T.J. and Tibshirani, R.J. (1990). *Generalized Additive Models*. Vol. 43 of *Monographs on Statistics and Applied Probability*. Chapman and Hall, London.

He, X. and Shi, P. (1994). Convergence Rate of B-Spline Estimators of Non-parametric Conditional Quantile Functions. *Nonparametric Statistics*, **3**, 299-308.

Koenker, R. and Bassett, G. (1978). Regression Quantiles. *Econometrica*, **46**, 33-50.

Koenker, R. and Machado, J. (1999). Goodness of Fit and Related Inference Processes for Quantile Regression. *J. Amer. Stat. Assoc.*, **94**, 1296-1310.

Lejeune, M. and Sarda, P. (1988). Quantile Regression: A Nonparametric Approach. *Computational Statistics and Data Analysis*, **6**, 229-239.

Marx, B.D. and Eilers P.H. (1999). Generalized Linear Regression on Sampled Signals and Curves: A *P*-Spline Approach. *Technometrics*, **41**, 1-13.

Ramsay, J.O. and Dalzell, C.J. (1993). Some Tools for Functional Data Analysis. *Journal of the Royal Statistical Society, Series B*, **3**, 539-572.

Ramsay, J.O. and Silverman, B.W. (1997). *Functional Data Analysis*. Springer-Verlag.

Ramsay, J.O. and Silverman, B.W. (2002). *Applied Functional Data Analysis*. Springer-Verlag.

Ruppert, D. and Caroll, J. (1988). *Transformation and Weighting in Regression*. Chapman and Hall.

Wahba, G. (1990). *Spline Models for Observational Data*. Society for Industrial and Applied Mathematics, Philadelphia.

13 Nonparametric Functional Methods: New Tools for Chemometric Analysis

Frédéric Ferraty, Aldo Goia and Philippe Vieu

13.1 Introduction

The aim of this contribution is to look at two recent advances in nonparametric study of curve data. Firstly we will look at some regression type problem, for which the objective is to predict a (real) response variable from a (continuous) curve data. Secondly, we will look at the question of discrimination inside of a set of curve data. These two problems have been selected among the numerous statistical problems for curve data that have been attacked by the recent methodology on functional data. So, even if we will concentrate our purposes on these two problems, we will give several bibliographical supports all along the contribution in order to allow the reader to have a larger view on the state of art in Nonparametric Functional Statistics. A special attention will be paid to the problem of the dimension, which is known to play a great role in (high) finite-dimensional setting and therefore expected to be a key point for our infinite-dimensional purposes, and which is solved here by means of semi-metric spaces modelization.

The choice of these two problems (regression and discrimination) has been done because these questions appear quite often in the chemometrical context that we wish to deal with. Indeed, in chemometric analysis curve data appearing naturally by means of spectrometric curves. This work will be centered around one spectrometric data set, coming from food industry quality control. Along the contribution, we will provide two XploRe quantlets (one for regression and one for discrimination). Even if our applied purpose here is on chemometrical applications, these quantlets are obviously utilisable in many other fields of applied statistics for which curve data are involved (medicine, econometry, environmetrics, ...).

This chapter is organized as follows. In Section 13.2 we discuss generalities about functional statistics and spectrometric curve data. Then, in Sections 13.3 and 13.4, we present respectively the nonparametric functional regression problem and the curves discrimination problem. Note that, to help the reader, each of these sections can be followed independently of the other. For both of these sections, we present the statistical backgrounds (model, estimate and XploRe quantlets) in a general way to make possible the utilization of the procedure in any setting (and not only for chemometrical purpose), and then we present the results obtained by our approaches on one spectrometric data set.

13.2   General Considerations

13.2.1   A Short Introduction to Spectrometric Data

Spectrometry is a usual technique for chemometric analysis. Spectrometric data consist in continuous spectra of some components to be analysed. From a statistical point of view these data are of functional (continuous) nature. We will center our purpose around a food industry spectrometric real data set, which is a set of absorbances spectra observed on several pieces of meat. These data are presented in Figure 13.1 below.

These data are composed by 215 spectra of absorbance (which is defined to be $-\log_{10}$ of the light transmittance) for a channel of wavelenghts varying from $\lambda = 850$ up to $\lambda = 1050$, and observed on 215 finely chopped pure meat food samples. These data have been recorded on a Tecator Infratec Food and Feed Analyzer by the NIR (near infrared) usual transmission principle. Because of the fineness of the discretisation, and because of the quite smooth aspect of spectrometric data, they are to be considered and treated as functional data. From now on, we will denote these curve data by:

$$X_i = \{X_i(\lambda),\ \lambda \in (850, 1050)\},\ i = 1, \ldots 215.$$

Usually going with such kind of spectrometric data, is the measurement of some chemical characteristic of interest. For instance, in our food quality problem we have at hand the measurements of the percentages of fatness:

$$Y_i,\ i = 1, \ldots 215.$$

In such a situation, one is interested in knowing the relation between the curve X and the scalar response Y, in order to be able to predict the corresponding

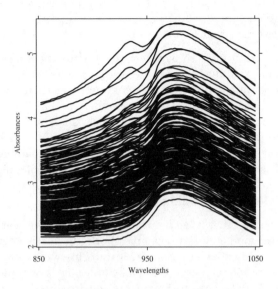

Figure 13.1: The spectrometric data set

percentage of fatness for a future new sample of meat just looking at its spectrum (this is, of course, considerably less expensive, in time and in costs, than doing a full chemical analysis of this new sample of meat). This is indeed a regression type problem for functional (curve) data and with scalar (real) response variable, which will be investigated later on in Section 13.3.

Another case of interest is when, rather than some quantitative response variable, we have at hand some categorical variable (let say T) that may correspond to different groups of spectra. For instance, in the food industry example discussed beforewe will deal with the measurements of the dichotomous variable

$$T_i, \ i = 1, \ldots 215,$$

which is defined to be $T_i = 1$ if the sample of meat contains less than 20% of fatness, and to be $T_i = 2$ otherwise. The question here is to understand the link between the continuous spectrum and the categorical response, in order to be able to assign a new piece of meat in some of the groups just by looking at its spectrum (which is, again, less expensive in time and in costs than doing a new chemical analysis). This is known as a curves discrimination problem (also called supervised curves classification problem) which will be investigated later on Section 13.4.

The aim of our contribution is to show how the recent nonparametric methodology for functional data may provide interesting results in this setting. Concretely, we will present two functional nonparametric methods, corresponding to both different statistical problems discussed before. The first one is a Nonparametric Functional Regression method, which is adapted to the problem of predicting the percentage of fatness Y corresponding to some given continuous absorbance spectra X. The second one is a Nonparametric Curves Discrimination method, which is adapted to the question of assigning a new spectrum X in one among both groups defined by both values of T. For each method, an XploRe quantlet will be given.

It is worth being noted that, even if our presentation will be centered around this spectrometric food industry example, both the methodology and the programs will be presented in a general way. This will allow for possible application of the proposed methods in many other fields of applied statistics in which functional data have to be treated (environmetrics, econometrics, biometrics, ...). Other cases that can be analysed by our procedures are climatologic data (Ramsay and Silverman, 1997), speech recognition data (Ferraty and Vieu, 2003b), pollution data (Aneiros-Pérez et al., 2003) or (Damon and Guillas, 2002), econometric time series (Ferraty, Goia and Vieu, 2002a), satellite measurements data (Dabo-Niang et al., 2004), medical data (Gasser, Hall and Presnell, 1998), signal data (Hall, Poskitt and Presnell, 2001).

13.2.2   A Short Introduction to Nonparametric Statistics for Curve Data

The infatuation for developping statistical procedures has considerably increased in the last decade. At the beginning the literature was concentrated on linear statistical procedures. Nice monographies in this direction include Ramsay and Silverman (1997), Bosq (2000) and Ramsay and Silverman (2002). Since a few years, nonparametric approaches are available, most of them being based on adaptation of usual kernel smoothing ideas to infinite-dimensional settings. These approaches are now covering a wide scope of statistical problems, including regression from functional explanatory variables (Ferraty and Vieu, 2002), density estimation of functional variables (Dabo-Niang, 2003a) and its direct applications for diffusion processes (Dabo-Niang, 2003b) and for unsupervised curves classification (Dabo-Niang et al., 2004), conditional distribution estimation (Ferraty, Laksaci and Vieu, 2003) and its direct application in nonparametric functional conditional mode/quantiles estimation, curves discrimination (Ferraty and Vieu, 2003b), or time series forecasting from continuous past values (Ferraty, Goia and Vieu, 2002a). Indeed, all these recent developments are part of a large infatuation around different aspects of Functional Statistics, Ferraty (2003) and (Boudou et al., 2003).

In this contribution, we will look specially at the functional regression problem (see Section 13.3) and at the curves discrimination problem (see Section 13.4). For each of them, we will present the methodology in a general framework, we will provide a corresponding XploRe quantlet and each technique will be applied to the spectrometric data set presented before.

13.2.3   Notion of Proximity Between Curves

Before starting to develop any nonparametric methodology for curve data (that is for variables taking values in some infinite-dimensional space), one should keep in mind what is known in finite-dimensional setting. More specifically, one should remind that most of nonparametric techniques are local and are therefore very sensitive to the sparseness of data. This is the reason why, in (high) finite dimensional settings the pure nonparametric approaches have a bad behaviour (see for instance Stone (1985) for discussion, references and alternative methods). This is known as the *curse of dimensionality*, and it is natural to have (at least at the first attempt) strong interrogations about the possibility of developping nonparametric methods in infinite-dimensional setting, since now it can be viewed as a *curse of infinite dimension*. Anyway, because this *curse of dimensionality* is completely linked with the sparseness of the data, one can hope to get round it by using a "suitable" measure of proximity between curves, (Ferraty and Vieu, 2003a).

Of course, the relevant measure of proximity between curves has to be driven by the knowledge on the practical problem. To be more convinced on this point, let us look at Figure 13.2 below which the derivatives of the spectrometric curves are displayed while the curves themselves have already been presented in Figure 13.1.

Comparing Figures 13.1 and 13.2, it appears clearly that higher order derivatives of the spectrometric curves are more accurate than the curves themselves. The second derivatives concentrate the data but are less sensitive to some vertical shift than the first derivatives or the curves themselves are. On the other hand, higher order (3 or 4) derivatives exhibit too much variability.

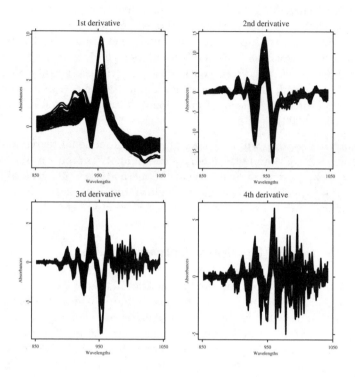

Figure 13.2: Derivatives of the spectrometric curves

So in our situation, there is real evidence for using a measure of proximity based on the second derivatives of the curves. The reader can find more insight, both from statistical and chemometrical points of view, about the interest of dealing with second order derivatives in Ferraty and Vieu (2002).

That means concretely that in our functional purpose here, we will use the following quantity as a measure of proximity between two spectrometric curves X_i and X_j:

$$d_{der,2}(X_i, X_j) = \sqrt{\int_{850}^{1050} \left\{ X_i''(\lambda) - X_j''(\lambda) \right\}^2 d\lambda}.$$

Note that, such a measure of quality is not a metric but only a semi-metric. This is the case for most of proximity measures for curve data, and this explains why most of theoretical developments available for nonparametric functional statistics are modelling the functional variable X as an element of some abstract semi-metric space $(E, d(\cdot; \cdot))$ (see Section 13.3.1).

13.2.4   XploRe Quantlets for Proximity Between Curves

Let $\mathcal{A} = \{X_1, \ldots X_p\}$ and $\mathcal{B} = \{Z_1, \ldots Z_q\}$ be two sets of curves. In practice, $\mathcal{A}$ will be the learning sample (for which the scalar response is known), while $\mathcal{B}$ corresponds to the new curves for which we have to predict the response. Distances are computed with a semi-metric. A semi-metric on a vector space E is a function $d(\cdot, \cdot)$ from $E \times E$ to $\mathbb{R}^+$ such that:

for all $(x, y, z) \in E \times E \times E$, $d(x, y) = d(y, x) \le d(x, z) + d(z, y)$;
for all $x \in E$, $d(x, x) = 0$.

The following quantlet XCSSemiMetricDer2 computes the function

    XCSSemiMetricDer2(A, nknot, rangegrid, B)

                Q XCSSemiMetricDer2.xpl

which returns the following $p \times q$ matrix:

$$SM_{ij} = d_{der,2}(X_i, Z_j), \ X_i \in \mathcal{A}, Z_j \in \mathcal{B}.$$

More generally, the quantlet XCSSemiMetricDer computes the function

    XCSSemiMetricDer(A, m, nknot, rangegrid, B)

                Q XCSSemiMetricDer.xpl

which returns the following $p \times q$ matrix:

$$SM_{ij} = d_{der,2}(X_i, Z_j), \ X_i \in \mathcal{A}, Z_j \in \mathcal{B},$$

where

$$d_{der,m}(X, Z) = \sqrt{\int \left(X^{(m)}(t) - Z^{(m)}(t)\right)^2 dt}.$$

The parameter nknot is the number of interior knots needed to build the B-spline approximations of the curves in order to compute their successive derivatives. The vector `rangegrid` of length 2 specifies the range on which the curves are defined (for the spectrometric curves we have `rangegrid` $= (850, 1050)$). Note that our procedure is based on the quantlet `XSCbspline` written by Christophe Crambes and presented in Chapter 12 of this book.

Q `XCSbspline.xpl`

Of course, some other kind of semi-metrics could be used. The quantlet `XCSSemiMetricPCA` computes the function

`XCSSemiMetricPCA(A,B)`

using a functional semi-metric based on PCA ideas, as defined in Section 3.1 of Ferraty and Vieu (2003b).

Q `XCSSemiMetricPCA.xpl`

For the reasons explained before, for our spectrometric purpose, we will only deal here with the semi-metric $d_{der,2}$, but all the functional methods can be used with the alternative semi-metrics presented before (as well with any new semi-metric that the user could wish to program by himself).

13.3   Functional Nonparametric Regression

13.3.1   The Statistical Problem

Let us consider that we have a set of n independent realizations $X_1, \ldots X_n$ of some variable valued in a semi-metric space $(E, d(\cdot; \cdot))$ of possibly infinite dimension. In our spectrometric example, the space E could be the space of twice continuously differentiable functions on $(850, 1050)$ and the associated semi-metric would be the euclidian metric but for second derivatives, that is:

$$d(X_i, X_j) = d_{der,2}(X_i, X_j).$$

Assume that, associated with each X_i, we have at hand also some scalar (real) response variable Y_i. For instance, in the spectrometric example, the response is the percentage of fatness in the corresponding piece of meat. Finally, one is interested in predicting fatness from the absorbance spectrum, and the statistical model consists in assuming the following regression relation:

$$Y_i = R(X_i) + \epsilon_i, \tag{13.1}$$

where the ϵ_i are zero-mean real random variables, each ϵ_i being uncorrelated with X_i. The aim is therefore to estimate the functional operator R, without assuming any linearity (or other parametric form) for it. A nice presentation of alternative ideas based on linear assumptions can be found in Ramsay and Silverman (1997) while the most recent advances in this direction are in Cardot et al. (2003).

The statistical model defined by (13.1) is a Functional Nonparametric Regression model. It is called Functional because of the infinite dimensional nature of the data, and it is called Nonparametric because we just wish to state smoothing restriction on the operator R to be estimated. We will present below some nonparametric estimate of the functional (non linear) operator R.

13.3.2 The Nonparametric Functional Estimate

Based on the usual finite-dimensional smoothing ideas, Ferraty and Vieu (2002) have proposed the following estimate of the functional operator R:

$$\hat{R}(x) = \sum_{i=1}^{n} Y_i W_{n,i}(x), \tag{13.2}$$

where $W_{n,i}(x)$ is a sequence of local weights. From this regression estimate, given new functional data (i.e. given a new spectrometric curve) x_{new} the response (i.e. the % of fatness) will be predicted by

$$\hat{y}_{new} = \hat{R}(x_{new}).$$

Even if it is not our main purpose here, it is worth giving some ideas about the asymptotic properties of this estimate. Of course, the asymptotic behaviour depends on the smoothness of the nonparametric model. For instance, one may assume a regression model of Lipschitz type:

$$\text{for all } (u, v), \ |R(u) - R(v)| \leq C|u - v|^{\beta}.$$

As discussed before, the concentration of the distribution of X in a small ball is a crucial point for insuring a good behaviour of the method, and so the asymptotic rate will depend on the following function:

$$\phi_x(\epsilon) = P(d(X, x) \leq \epsilon).$$

By constructing weights from a kernel function K and from a sequence of bandwidths $h_{n,x}$ in way that

$$W_{n,i}(x) = \frac{K\left(\frac{d(x,X_i)}{h_{n,x}}\right)}{\sum_{j=1}^{n} K\left(\frac{d(x,X_j)}{h_{n,x}}\right)}, \tag{13.3}$$

the following result can be shown.

THEOREM 13.1 *Under suitable conditions on the kernel function K and on the bandwidth sequence $h_{n,x}$, we have:*

$$\hat{R}(x) - R(x) = \mathcal{O}\left(h_{n,x}^{\beta}\right) + \mathcal{O}_p\left(\sqrt{\frac{\log n}{n\phi_x(h_{n,x})}}\right).$$

It is out of purpose to give here neither the proof nor the technical assumptions. Let us just note that a proof is given by Ferraty and Vieu (2002) in the very much simpler situation when the function $\phi_x(\epsilon)$ is of fractal form (i.e. $\phi_x(\epsilon) \sim C_x\epsilon^{\alpha}$). This proof was extended to dependent samples in Ferraty, Goia and Vieu (2002a). The general proof of Theorem 13.1 can be found in Ferraty and Vieu (2004). Note also that some of these above mentionned papers are also giving uniform (over x) versions of Theorem 13.1. Finally, it is worth being noted that a recent extension of the methodology has been propoosed by Dabo-Niang and Rhomari (2003) to the case when the response variable Y_i is functional.

13.3.3   Prediction of Fat Percentage from Continuous Spectrum

The above described kernel methodology is applied to the fat content prediction problem. To do that, we choose as kernel function the following parabolic one:

$$K(u) = \begin{cases} 1 - u^2 & \text{if } 0 \le u \le 1 \\ 0 & \text{otherwise} \end{cases} \tag{13.4}$$

and as explained before the semi-metric is:

$$d = d_{der,2}.$$

For this presentation, and in order to be able to highlight the good behaviour of our method, we have separated the sample of 215 pairs (X_i, Y_i) into two subsamples. A first subsample, denoted by $\mathcal{A}$ and of size 165 is the learning sample that allows for the computation of $\hat{R}(x)$ for any curve x. A second one, denoted by $\mathcal{B}$ and of size 50 is the sample for which the Y_k's are ignored and predicted by the $\hat{Y}_k = \hat{R}(X_k)$. Of course, in real prediction problems, we do not have at hand the measurements of the Y_k's corresponding to the sample $\mathcal{B}$. Here we wish to give to the reader an idea on the behaviour of the method, and so we constructed this subsample $\mathcal{B}$ in such a way that we know the true corresponding Y_k's.

Using the XploRe quantlet `XCSFuncKerReg` described in Section 13.3.4, we computed the 50 predicted values $\hat{Y}_k$ corresponding to the X_k of the second sample. We present in left-hand side of Figure 13.3 the scatter plot of these predicted values versus the true values Y_i. Even if our objective here is not to compare the method with existing alternative ones, in the right-hand side of Figure 13.3 we also present the same results but when using a usual L_2 metric in our procedure.

Undoubtly, Figure 13.3 shows both the good behaviour of our procedure and the interest of a semi-metric modelization rather than a simple metric approach. More insight on these data, including comparisons of this kernel functional approach with competitive alternative techniques, can be found in Ferraty and Vieu (2002).

13.3.4   The XploRe Quantlet

Assume that we have at hand one sample $\mathcal{A}$ of curves and the corresponding sample $\mathcal{Y}$ of real response values. Assume that we have another sample $\mathcal{B}$ of new curves for which we want to predict the corresponding response values. The quantlet `XCSFuncKerReg` computes the function

```
XCSFuncKerReg(Y, A, B,param, semi)
```

Q XCSFuncKerReg.xpl

The argument `semi` corresponds to the semi-metric that has been used (`semi` = "pca" or "der" as described in Section 13.2.3). The argument `param` contains all the corresponding arguments needed by the quantlet involved in the choice of `semi` (see again Section 13.2.3).

This function returns the predicted values (in the vector `PredictedValues`) for the unobserved response variable corresponding to all the new curves in $\mathcal{B}$. The predictions are obtained by the kernel technique defined by (13.2)-(13.3),

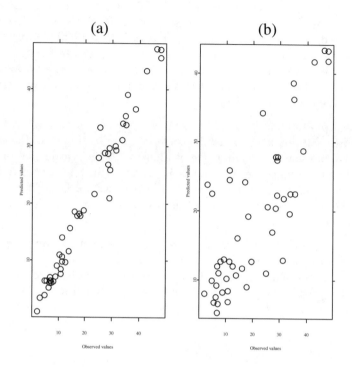

Figure 13.3: Functional kernel Predictions of Fatness: (a) with the semi-metric $d_{der,2}$; (b) with the usual L_2 metric.

with the semi-metric d and from the data $(X_i, Y_i) \in \mathcal{A} \times \mathcal{Y}$. This function returns also some other results such as estimated values of the observed scalar responses for the learning sample $\mathcal{A}$ (in the vector `EstimatedValues`), optimal bandwidth (in the vector `Band`) for each curve in $\mathcal{A}$ and mean squared error (`MSE`) for the curves in $\mathcal{A}$.

This function automatically selects the optimal bandwidths according to the method described in next section.

13.3.5   Comments on Bandwidth Choice

An important point, as always in nonparametric smoothing (either in functional or in finite-dimensional problems), is the choice of the smoothing parameter (i.e. the choice of the bandwidths $h_{n,x}$). Let us now describe how this bandwidth selection is performed by the quantlet `XCSFuncKerReg`. For computing the estimate $\hat{R}$ our algorithm randomly divides the dataset $\mathcal{A} \times \mathcal{Y}$ into two subsets. A first sub-subsample, denoted by $\mathcal{A}_1 \times \mathcal{Y}_1$ and of size $n = 2Card(\mathcal{A})/3$, is the one from which the estimate $\hat{R}$ is calculated. A second sub-subsample, denoted by $\mathcal{A}_2 \times \mathcal{Y}_2$ and of size $Card(\mathcal{A})/3$, is used to select the bandwidths.

The bandwidths $h_{n,x}$ are selected by some cross-validation procedure, to be the ones leading to the best predictions for the data x belonging to the testing curves $\mathcal{A}_2$. To make the computational aspects easier and faster, the optimization is performed over a discrete set of bandwidths

$$h_{n,X_j}(k),\ k = 1, \ldots, k_0$$

where, for each X_j in $\mathcal{A}_2$, $h_{n,X_j}(k)$ is such that there are exactly k data among all the X_i's $\in \mathcal{A}_1$ such that $d(x, X_i) \le h_{n,X_j}(k)$. This is a so-called k-nearest neighbour approach. At this stage, we have at hand the optimal bandwidth, denoted by h_{n,X_j}^{opt} corresponding to each $X_j \in \mathcal{A}_2$. What we need really, is to have a bandwidth $h_{n,x}$ associated with each $x \in \mathcal{B}$, and naturally we state:

$$\forall x \in \mathcal{B},\ h_{n,x} = h_{n,X_{j(x)}}^{opt},$$

where $X_{j(x)}$ is the element of $\mathcal{A}_2$ which is the closest to the new curve x:

$$X_{j(x)} = \arg\min_{X_j \in \mathcal{A}_2} d(x, X_j).$$

13.4 Nonparametric Curves Discrimination

13.4.1 The Statistical Problem

Let us consider again a set of n independent realizations $X_1, \ldots X_n$ of some variable valued in a semi-metric space $(E, d(\cdot, \cdot))$, and assume that, associated with each X_i, we have at hand also some categorical response variable T_i taking a finite number of values $t^1, \ldots t^\tau$. In other words, that means that our sample of curves $X_1, \ldots X_n$ is divided into τ (known) groups. For instance, in our spectrometric data, we have two groups (i.e. $\tau = 2$) and the categorical variable is defined to be $T_i = 1$ or 2, according to the fact that the percentage of fatness is smaller or greater than 20%. In Figure 13.4 below, both groups of spectrometric data set are displayed (we just present a randomly selected subsample of 20 curves of each group). The question is: can we assign a new curve x_{new} in some among the τ different groups?

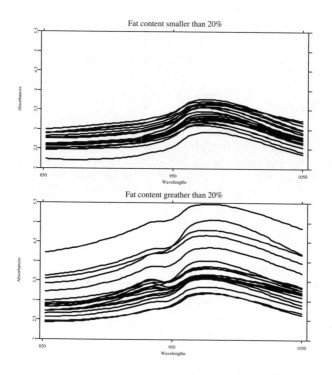

Figure 13.4: The two groups of spectrometric curves

In the spectrometric example, we have to decide if a new spetrometric curve
corresponds to a piece of meat having more or less than 20% of fatness. This
is known as a Discrimination problem, also called Supervised Curves Classification problem. For shortness reasons we only deal here with supervised
curves classification problems. Recent advances on unsupervised curves classification by functional approaches can be found in Abraham, C. et al. (2003),
Tarpey and Kinateder (2003) and Dabo-Niang et al. (2004).

13.4.2   A Nonparametric Curves Discrimination Method

Given a new curve x_{new}, the idea is to estimate the following posterior probabilities:

$$p_s(x_{new}) = P(T = t^s | X = x_{new}), \forall s \in \{1, \dots \tau\}.$$

Once these probabilities are estimated, for instance by means of some estimate $\hat{p}_s(x)$, we assign the new curve in the group with highest probability:

$$\hat{T}^{new} = \arg\max_{\{s=1,\dots,\tau\}} \hat{p}_s(x_{new}). \tag{13.5}$$

It remains now to construct an estimate of the $p_s(\cdot)$'s. As in the regression problem described before, kernel ideas can be used to estimate these probabilities. Concretely, by using the same notations as in Section 13.3, we define:

$$\hat{p}_s(x) = \sum_{i,\, T_i=t^s} \frac{K\left(\frac{d(x,X_i)}{h_{n,x}}\right)}{\sum_{j=1}^n K\left(\frac{d(x,X_j)}{h_{n,x}}\right)}. \tag{13.6}$$

These estimates are functional versions of usual finite-dimensional ones. They were previously introduced (in some more particular version) by Hall, Poskitt and Presnell (2001). It is important to note, that the underlying model is purely nonparametric in the sense that only smoothness assumptions on the true conditional probablities $p_s(\cdot)$ are needed. Some of the asymptotic properties of the estimate (13.6) are studied in Ferraty and Vieu (2004), under some nonparametric model defined by some Lipschitz type condition on posterior probabilities:

$$\exists\beta > 0,\ \forall s,\ \exists C_s < \infty,\ |p_s(x) - p_s(y)| \le C_s\, d(x,y)^\beta.$$

To fix the ideas, let us just mention one result issued from Ferraty and Vieu (2004). Indeed, this paper states a much more general version of this result, including for instance the case of dependant data, but it is out of the scope of this book to enter in these theoretical considerations.

THEOREM 13.2 *Under suitable conditions on the kernel function K and on the bandwidth sequence $h_{n,x}$, we have:*

$$\hat{p}_s(x) - p_s(x) = \mathcal{O}\left(h_{n,x}^\beta\right) + \mathcal{O}_p\left(\sqrt{\frac{\log n}{n\phi_x(h_{n,x})}}\right).$$

As in regression setting (see Theorem 13.1 above), the concentration of the distribution of the functional variable X plays a determinant role. In other words, because this concentration is exclusively linked with the semi-metric $d(\cdot,\cdot)$, we can say that the choice of the semi-metric will be a crucial point for practical applications of the method. Of course, this semi-metric has to be chosen by means of some practical considerations based on the knowledge on the curves. For the reasons described before in Section 13.2.3, in our spectrometric context there is a real motivation to use

$$d = d_{der,2},$$

as given by the quantlet `XCSSemiMetricDer2` presented before in Section 13.2.4.

Of course, one could perfectly think about other real curve data application for which this semi-metric is not the most appropriate. Ferraty and Vieu (2003b) proposed another example, based on phonetic data, and for which the noisy structure of the curves needs obviously another kind of functional semi-metric, that is the one based on PCA as given by the quantlet `XCSSemiMetricPCA` presented before in Section 13.2.4.

13.4.3 Discrimination of Spectrometric Curves

The treatment of the spectrometric curves by this curves classification procedure has been carried out by following the same steps as before in Section 13.3.3. We applied the above described kernel methodology to our fat content discrimination problem, by choosing again the same kernel as defined in (13.4) and the semi-metric $d = d_{der,2}$. We have separated the sample of 215 pairs (X_i, T_i) into two subsamples. A first subsample, denoted by $\mathcal{A}$ and of size 165 is the learning sample which conducts the estimation of the conditional probabilities $\hat{p}_s(\cdot)$. A second one, denoted by $\mathcal{B}$ and of size 50, for which the groups T_k are ignored and predicted by $\hat{T}_k = \arg\max_{\{s=1,...D\}} \hat{p}_s(X_k)$.

Of course, in real discrimination problems, we do not have at hand the measurements of the T_k corresponding to the sample $\mathcal{B}$. Here this subsample $\mathcal{B}$ (for which we know the corresponding values of the T_k) is only used to give the reader an idea on the behaviour of the method. Using the XploRe quantlet `XCSFuncKerDiscrim` to be decsribed in the next Section 13.4.4, we computed the 50 predicted assignment groups $\hat{T}_k$ corresponding to this sample $\mathcal{B}$.

More precisely, we randomly did the above mentionned splitting 50 times, and we present the results of the study in Figure 13.5 by means of the boxplots (over these 50 replications) of the missclassification rate

$$\frac{1}{Card(\mathcal{B})} \sum_{X_k \in \mathcal{B}} 1_{\{T_k \neq \hat{T}_k\}}.$$

Clearly, the method works well with this semi-metric $d = d_{der,2}$ since we have a percentage of misclassification which is mainly concentrated between 1% and 3%. To highlight the importance of the semi-metric we also did the same with other ones (see again Figure 13.5). However, it is not the purpose here to do extensive comparison of our method with alternative ones. Some elements in this direction are provided by Ferraty and Vieu (2003b).

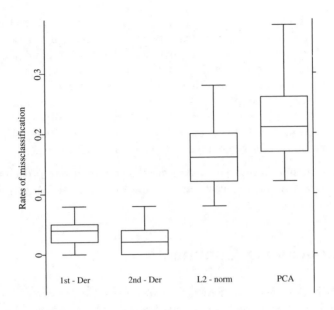

Figure 13.5: Boxplots of the rates of misclassification for spectrometric data

13.4.4   The XploRe Quantlet

Assume that we have at hand one sample $\mathcal{A}$ of curves and the corresponding
sample $\mathcal{T}$ of categorical responses. Assume that we have another sample $\mathcal{B}$
of new curves for which we want to predict the group membership.

The quantlet XCSFuncKerDiscrim computes the function

    XCSFuncKerDiscrim(T,A,B,param,semi)

                              Q XCSFuncKerDiscrim.xpl

The argument semi corresponds to the semi-metric that has been used
(semi = "pca" or "der" as described in Section 13.2.3). The argument param
contains all the corresponding arguments needed by the quantlet involved in

the choice of `semi` (see again Section 13.2.3).

This function returns the predicted groups (in the vector `PredictedValues`) for the unobserved categorical response variable corresponding to all the new curves in $\mathcal{B}$. The predictions are obtained by the kernel technique defined by (13.6)-(13.5), with the semi-metric d and from the data $(X_i, T_i) \in \mathcal{A} \times \mathcal{T}$. This function returns also some other results. The estimated groups for the curves in the learning sample $\mathcal{A}$ are in the vector `EstimatedValues`. The misclassification rates for the curves in the learning sample $\mathcal{A}$ are in the output `MAE`. The matrix `EstimatedProb` (resp. `PredictedProb`) stores the posterior probabilities for the curves in the sample $\mathcal{A}$ (resp. $\mathcal{B}$).

Once again, the smoothing parameters $h_{n,x}$ involved in our procedure are obtained by cross-validation over some training subsample of $\mathcal{A}$ as indicated before in Section 13.3.5.

13.5 Concluding Comments

In this contribution, we have shown how spectrometric data can be successfully analysed by considering them as curve data and by using the recent nonparametric methodology for curve data. However, note that all the statistical backgrounds are presented in a general way (and not only for spectrometric data). Similarly, the XploRe quantlets that we provided can be directly used in any other applied setting involving curve data. For reason of shortness, and because it was not the purpose here, we only presented the results given by the nonparametric functional methodology without discussing any comparison with alternative methods (but relevant references on these points are given all along the contribution).

Also for shortness reasons, we just presented two statistical problems (namely regression from curve data and curves discrimination) among the several problems that can be treated by nonparametric functional methods (on this point also, our contribution contains several references about other problems that could be attacked similarly). These two problems have been chosen by us for two reasons: first, these issues are highly relevant to many applied studies involving curve analysis and second, their theoretical and practical importance led to emergence of different computer automated procedures.

Bibliography

Abraham, C., Cornillon, P.A., Matzner-Lober, E. and Molinari, N. (2003). Unsupervised curve clustering using B-splines. *Scand. J. of Statist.*, **30**, 581-595.

Aneiros-Péez, G., Cardot, H., Estévez-Pérez, G. and Vieu, P. (2003). Maximum ozone forecasting by functional nonparametric approaches. *Environmetrics*. In print.

Boudou, A., Cardot, H., Ferraty, F., Romain, Y., Sarda, P., Viguier-Pla, S. and Vieu, P. (2003). Statistique Fonctionnelle et Opératorielle IV. (French) . *Techical Report, Labo. Statist. Proba., Toulouse, France.* Available on line at *http://www.lsp.ups-tlse.fr*

Bosq, D. (2000). *Linear process in function spaces*, Lecture Notes in Statistics, **149**, Springer-Verlag.

Cardot, H., Ferraty, F., Mas, A. and Sarda, P. (2003). Testing hypotheses in the functional linear model. *Scand. J. Statist.*, **30**(1), 241-255.

Dabo-Niang, S. (2003). Kernel density estimator in an infinite dimensional space with a rate of convergence in the case of diffusion processes. *Applied Mathematical Letters*, In print.

Dabo-Niang, S. (2003b). Density estimation by orthogonal series estimators in an infinite dimensional space. *Nonparametric Staisitics*, **16**(1-2), 171-186.

Dabo-Niang, S., Ferraty, F. and Vieu, P. (2004). Nonparametric unsupervised classification of satellite wave altimeters forms. *Preprint.*

Dabo-Niang, S. and Rhomari, N. (2003). Estimation non paramétrique de la régression avec variable explicative dans un espace métrique. (French) *C. R. Math. Acad. Sci. Paris*, **336**(1), 75-80.

Damon, J. and Guillas, S. (2002). The inclusion of exogeneous variables in functional autoregressive ozone forecasting. *Environmetrics*, **13**, 759-774.

Ferraty, F. (2003). Modélisation statistique pour variables aléatoires fonctionnelles: Théorie et Applications. (French) *HDR, Université Paul Sabatier Toulouse.* Available on line at *http://www.lsp.ups-tlse.fr/Fp/Ferraty*

Ferraty, F., Goia, A. and Vieu, P. (2002). Functional nonparametric model for time series: a fractal approach to dimension reduction. *Test*, **11**(2), 317-344.

Ferraty, F., Goia, A. and Vieu, P. (2002b). *Statistica funzionale: modeli di regressione non-parametrici.* (Italian). Franco-Angeli, Milano.

Ferraty, F., Laksaci, A. and Vieu, P. (2003). Estimating some characteristics of the conditional distribution in nonparametric functional models. *Statist. Inf. for Stoch. Proc.*, Submitted for publication.

Ferraty, F., Nunez-Antón, V. and Vieu, P. (2001). *Regresión no paramétrica: desde la dimensión uno hasta la dimensión infinita* (Spanish). Ed. Univ. del Pais Vasco, Bilbao.

Ferraty, F. and Vieu, P. (2001). *Statistique Fonctionnelle: Modéles de Régression pour Variables Aléatoires Uni Multi et Infini-Dimensionnées.* (French). Technical Report, Labo. Statist. Proba., Toulouse, France. Available on line at *http://www.lsp.ups-tlse.fr/Fp/Ferraty*

Ferraty, F. and Vieu, P. (2002). The functional nonparametric model and application to spectrometric data. *Computational Statistics*, **4**, 545-564.

Ferraty, F. and Vieu, P. (2003a). Functional Nonparametric Statistics: a double infinite dimensional framework. In *Recent adavances and trends in nonparametric statistics* (Ed. M. Akritas and D. Politis), 61-79. Elsevier.

Ferraty, F. and Vieu, P. (2003b). Curves discrimination: a Nonparametric Functional Approach. *Comp. Statist. Data Anal.*, **44**, 161-173.

Ferraty, F. and Vieu, P. (2004). Nonparametric models for functional data, with applications in regression, time series prediction and curves discrimination. *Nonparametric Statistics*, **16**(1-2), 11-126.

Gasser, T., Hall, P. and Presnell, B. (1998). Nonparametric estimation of the mode of a distribution of random curves. *J. R. Statist. Soc. B*, **60**(4), 681-691.

Hall, P., Poskitt, D. and Presnell, B. (2001). A functional data-analytic approach to signal discrimination. *Technometrics*, **43**, 1-9.

Ramsay, J. and Silverman, B. (1997). *Functional Data Analysis*, Springer-Verlag.

Ramsay, J. and Silverman, B. (2002). *Applied Functional Data Analysis*, Springer-Verlag.

Stone, C. (1985). Additive regression and other nonparametric models. *Annals of Statistics*, **22**, 118-144.

Tarpey, T. and Kinateder, K. (2003). Clustering functional data. *J. of Classification*, **20**, 93-114.

14 Variable Selection in Principal Component Analysis

Yuichi Mori, Masaya Iizuka, Tomoyuki Tarumi and Yutaka Tanaka

While there exist several criteria by which to select a reasonable subset of variables in the context of PCA, we introduce herein variable selection using criteria in Tanaka and Mori (1997)'s modified PCA (M.PCA) among others.

In order to perform such variable selection via XploRe, the quantlib `vaspca`, which reads all the necessary quantlets for selection, is first called, and then the quantlet `mpca` is run using a number of selection parameters.

In the first four sections we present brief explanations of variable selection in PCA, an outline of M.PCA and flows of four selection procedures, based mainly on Tanaka and Mori (1997), Mori (1997), Mori, Tarumi and Tanaka (1998) and Iizuka *et al.* (2002a). In the last two sections, we illustrate the quantlet `mpca` and its performance by two numerical examples.

14.1 Introduction

Consider a situation in which we wish to select items or variables so as to delete the redundant variables or to make a small dimensional rating scale to measure latent traits. Validity requires that all of the variables are to be included. On the other hand, practical application requires that the number of variables to be as small as possible.

There are two types of examples: a clinical test and a plant evaluation. As for the former case, a clinical test for ordinary persons is sometimes not suitable for handicapped persons because the number of checkup items is too large. It is desirable to reduce the number of variables (checkup items) and obtain global scores which can reproduce the information of the original test. As for the latter case, there is a large number of sensors (checkpoints) in a plant that are used to measure some quantity at each point and evaluate the performance of the entire plant. Exact evaluation requires evaluation based on data measured at all points, but the number of points may be too large to obtain the result within limited time for temporary evaluation. Therefore, appropriately reducing the number of points to be used in temporary analysis is helpful. For such cases, we meet the problem of variable selection in the context of principal component analysis (PCA).

Let us show another example. In Figure 14.1, the left-hand plot is a scatter plot of the first and second principal components (PCs) obtained based on all 19 original variables, and the right-hand plot is based on seven selected variables. There are not so many differences between the two configurations of PCs. This illustrates the meaningfulness of variable selection in PCA since selected variables can provide almost the same result as the original variables if the goal of the analysis is to observe the configuration of the PCs.

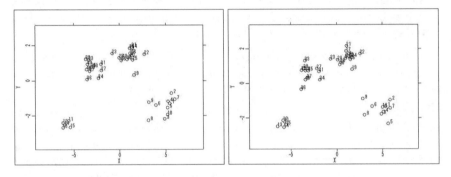

Figure 14.1: Scatter plots of principal component scores based on 19 variables (left) and based on 7 selected variables {3, 7, 13, 15, 16, 17, 18} (right).

XCSvaspca01.xpl

Furthermore we can perform variable selection in PCA as a prior analysis, for example, when the number of original variables is too large for the desired analysis, or as a posterior analysis, for example, when some clusters are obtained and typical variables must be selected from among those in each cluster.

Thus, specifying a subset of variables in the context of PCA is useful in many practical applications.

14.2   Variable Selection in PCA

The problem of variable selection in PCA has been investigated by Jolliffe (1972, 1973), Robert and Escoufier (1976), McCabe (1984), Bonifas *et al.* (1984), Krzanowski (1987a, 1987b), Falguerolles and Jmel (1993), and Mori, Tarumi and Tanaka (1994), among others. These studies sought to obtain ordinary principal components (PCs) based on a subset of variables in such a way that these PCs retain as much information as possible compared to PCs based on all the variables: the methods of Jolliffe (1972, 1973) consider PC loadings, and the methods of McCabe (1984) and Falguerolles and Jmel (1993) use a partial covariance matrix to select a subset of variables, which maintains information on all variables to the greatest extent possible. Robert and Escoufier (1976) and Bonifas *et al.* (1984) used the RV-coefficient and Krzanowski (1987a, 1987b) used Procrustes analysis to evaluate the closeness between the configuration of PCs computed based on selected variables and that based on all variables. Tanaka and Mori (1997) discuss a method called the "modified PCA" (M.PCA) to derive PCs which are computed using only a selected subset of variables but which represent all of the variables, including those not selected. Since M.PCA naturally includes variable selection procedures in the analysis, its criteria can be used directly to detect a reasonable subset of variables (e.g. see Mori (1997, 1998), and Mori, Tarumi and Tanaka (1998)). Furthermore, other criteria can be considered, such as criteria based on influence analysis of variables using the concept reported in Tanaka and Mori (1997) and criteria based on predictive residuals using the concept reported in Krzanowski (1987b), for details see Mori *et al.* (1999), Mori and Iizuka (2000) and Iizuka *et al.* (2003).

Thus, the existence of several methods and criteria is one of the typical characteristics of variable selection in multivariate methods without external variables such as PCA (here the term "external variable" is used as a variable to be predicted or to be explained using the information derived from other variables). Moreover, the existing methods and criteria often provide different results (selected subsets of variables), which is regarded as another typical characterirstic. This occurs because each criterion or PC procedure has its own reasonable purpose of selecting variables. Therefore, we can not say that one is better than the other. These characteristics are not observed in multivariate methods with external variable(s), such as multiple regression analysis.

In practical applications of variable selection, it is desirable to provide computation environment where those who want to select variables can apply a suitable method for their own purposes of selection without difficulties and/or they can try various methods and choose the best method by comparing the results. However, previously, we had no device by which to perform any method easily. In order to provide useful tools for variable selection in PCA, we have developed computation environments in which anyone can easily perform variable selection in PCA using any existing criteria. A windows package "VASPCA (VAriable Selection in PCA)" was initially developed (Mori, 1997) and has been converted to functions for use in general statistical packages, such as R and XploRe. In addition, we have also constructed web-based software using the functions as well as the document pages of variable selection in PCA, see Mori *et al.* (2000a), Iizuka *et al.* (2002a) and also either of the URLs, http://face.f7.ems.okayama-u.ac.jp/~masa/vaspca/indexE.html or http://mo161.soci.ous.ac.jp/vaspca/indexE.html.

14.3   Modified PCA

M.PCA (Tanaka and Mori, 1997) is intended to derive PCs which are computed using only a selected subset but which represent all of the variables, including those not selected. If we can find such PCs which represent all of the variables very well, we may say that those PCs provide a multidimensional rating scale which has high validity and is easy to apply practically. In order to find such PCs we can borrow the concepts of PCA of instrumental variables introduced in Rao (1964) and RV-coefficient-based approach presented in Robert and Escoufier (1976).

Suppose we obtain an $n \times p$ data matrix Y. If the original data set of Y consists of categorical variables, the data set should be quantified in an appropriate manner (Mori, Tanaka and Tarumi, 1997). Let Y be decomposed into an $n \times q$ submatrix Y_1 and an $n \times (p - q)$ submatrix Y_2 ($1 \leq q \leq p$). We denote the covariance matrix of $Y = (Y_1, Y_2)$ as $S = \begin{pmatrix} S_{11} & S_{12} \\ S_{21} & S_{22} \end{pmatrix}$, Y is represented as accurately as possible by r PCs, where r is the number of PCs and the PCs are linear combinations of a submatrix Y_1, i.e. $Z = Y_1 A$ ($1 \leq r \leq q$). In order to derive $A = (a_1, \ldots, a_r)$, the following criteria can be used:

(Criterion 1) The prediction efficiency for Y is maximized using a linear predictor in terms of Z.

(Criterion 2) The RV-coefficient between Y and Z is maximized. The RV-coefficient is computed as

$$RV(Y, Z) = \mathrm{tr}(\tilde{Y}\tilde{Y}^\top \tilde{Z}\tilde{Z}^\top)/\{\mathrm{tr}(\tilde{Y}\tilde{Y}^\top)\mathrm{tr}(\tilde{Z}\tilde{Z}^\top)\}^{1/2}$$

where $\tilde{Y}$ and $\tilde{Z}$ are centered matrices of Y and Z, respectively.

The maximization criteria for the above (Criterion 1) and (Criterion 2) are given by the proportion P

$$P = \sum_{j=1}^{r} \lambda_j / \operatorname{tr}(S), \tag{14.1}$$

and the RV-coefficient

$$RV = \left\{ \sum_{j=1}^{r} \lambda_j^2 / \operatorname{tr}(S^2) \right\}^{1/2}, \tag{14.2}$$

respectively, where λ_j is the j-th eigenvalue, in order of magnitude, of the eigenvalue problem (EVP)

$$[(S_{11}^2 + S_{12}S_{21}) - \lambda S_{11}]a = 0. \tag{14.3}$$

When the number of variables in Y_1 is q, Y_1 should be assigned by a subset of q variables (Y_2 by a subset of $p - q$ remaining variables) which provides the largest value of P in (14.1) for (Criterion 1) or the largest value of RV in (14.2) for (Criterion 2), and the solution is obtained as a matrix A, the columns of which consist of the eigenvectors associated with the largest r eigenvalues of EVP (14.3).

Obviously, these criteria can be used to select a reasonable subset of size q, that is, "variable selection using criteria in M.PCA" is to find a subset of size q by searching for that which has the largest value of the above criterion P or RV among all possible subsets of size q.

14.4   Selection Procedures

Although the best method by which to find a subset of variables of size q provides the optimum value for a specified criterion among all possible $_pC_q$ combinations of variables, this method is usually impractical due to the high computational cost of computing criterion values for all possible subsets. Therefore, as practical strategies, Tanaka and Mori (1997) introduced the two-stage *Backward elimination* procedure, and later Mori (1997) proposed three procedures, *Forward selection*, *Backward-forward stepwise selection* and *Forward-backward stepwise selection*, in which only one variable is removed or added sequentially. These procedures allow automatic selection of any number of variables.

Let V be the criterion value P or RV obtained by assigning q variables to Y_1.

Backward elimination

Stage A. Initial fixed-variable stage

A-1 Assign q variables to subset Y_1, usually $q := p$.

A-2 Solve the EVP (14.3).

A-3 Look carefully at the eigenvalues, determine the number r of PCs to be used.

A-4 Specify kernel variables which should always be involved in Y_1, if necessary. The number of kernel variables is less than q.

Stage B. Variable selection stage (Backward)

B-1 Remove one variable from among q variables in Y_1, make a temporary subset of size $q - 1$, and compute V based on the subset. Repeat this for each variable in Y_1, then obtain q values of V. Find the best subset of size $q - 1$ which provides the largest V among these q values and remove the corresponding variable from the present Y_1. Put $q := q - 1$.

B-2 If V or q is larger (or smaller) than the preassigned values, go to B-1. Otherwise stop.

Forward selection

Stage A. Initial fixed-variable stage

A-1 $\sim$ 3 Same as A-1 to 3 in Backward elimination.

A-4 Redefine q as the number of kernel variables (here, $q \geq r$). If you have kernel variables, assign them to Y_1. If not, put $q := r$, find the best subset of q variables which provides the largest V among all possible subsets of size q and assign it to Y_1.

Stage B. Variable selection stage (Forward)

Basically the opposites of Stage B in Backward elimination

Backward-forward stepwise selection

Stage A. Initial fixed-variable stage

A-1 $\sim$ 4 Same as A-1 to 4 in Backward elimination.

Stage B. Variable selection stage (Backward-forward)

B-1 Put $i := 1$.

B-2 Remove one variable from among q variables in Y_1, make a temporary subset of size $q - 1$, and compute V based on the subset. Repeat this for each variable in Y_1, then obtain q values of V. Find the best subset of size $q-1$ which provides the largest V (denoted by V_i) among these q values and remove the corresponding variable from the present Y_1. Set $q := q - 1$.

B-3 If V or q is larger (or smaller) than preassigned values, go to B-4. Otherwise stop.

B-4 Remove one variable from among q variables in Y_1, make a temporary subset of size $q - 1$, and compute V based on the subset. Repeat this for each variable in Y_1, then obtain q values of V. Find the best subset of size $q-1$ which provides the largest V (denoted by V_{i+1}) among these q values and remove the corresponding variable from the present Y_1. Set $q := q - 1$.

B-5 Add one variable from among $p - q$ variables in Y_2 to Y_1, make a temporary subset of size $q+1$ and compute V based on the subset. Repeat this for each variable, except for the variable removed from Y_1 and moved to Y_2 in B-4, then obtain $p - q - 1$ Vs. Find the best subset of size $q + 1$ which provides the largest V (denoted by V_{temp}) among $p - q - 1$ Vs.

B-6 If $V_i < V_{temp}$, add the variable found in B-5 to Y_1, set $V_i := V_{temp}$, $q := q + 1$ and $i := i - 1$, and go to B-5. Otherwise set $i := i + 1$ and go to B-3.

Forward-backward stepwise selection

Stage A. Initial fixed-variable stage

    A-1 to **4** Same as A-1 to 4 in Forward selection.

Stage B. Variable selection stage (Forward-backward)

    Basically the opposites of Stage B in Backward-forward stepwise selection

Mori, Tarumi and Tanaka (1998) showed that criteria based on the subsets of variables selected by the above procedures differ only slightly from those based on the best subset of variables among all possible combinations in the case of variable selection using criteria in M.PCA. Mori, Tarumi and Tanaka (1998) also reported that stepwise-type selections (Backward-forward and Forward-backward) can select better subsets than single-type selections (Backward and Forward) and that forward-type selections (Forward and Forward-backward) tend to select better subsets than backward-type selections (Backward and Backward-forward).

14.5   Quantlet

The command

```
mpca (x{ ,r})
```

performs variable selection using criteria in M.PCA

Before calling the quantlet mpca, load quantlib metrics by typing:

```
library("metrics")
```

in the input line. This quantlib includes main quantlets such as mpca which select subsets of variables automatically and sub quantlets which are used in main quantlets: geigensm (solves the generalized EVP), divide (divides a matrix Y into two submatrices Y_1 and Y_2), delcol (deletes specified columns from the original matrix and generates a new matrix) and other necessary modules for selection.

The quantlet mpca has a required argument, a data set X, and an optional argument, r – number of PCs. If the number of PCs of the data is unknown, type the quantlet only using the first argument, e.g. mpca(data). If known, type the quantlet with both arguments, e.g. mpca(data, 2) and then the specification of the second parameter (the number of PCs) will be skipped.

When the mpca starts, four parameters are required for selection: a matrix type (covariance or correlation), the number r of PCs ($1 \leq r < p$), a criterion (the proportion P or the RV-coefficient) and a selection procedure (Backward, Forward, Backward-forward, Forward-backward or All-possible at q). We optionally implemented the All-possible selection procedure at a particular number q of variables to obtain the best subset of that size. Note that computation may take a long time.

After computation based on the specified parameters, two outputs are displayed: a list which indicates the criterion values and variable numbers to be assigned to Y_1 and Y_2 for every number q of selected variables ($r \leq q \leq p$) and a graph which illustrates the change of the criterion value. See the practical actions in the next section.

Note that this quantlet has no function to specify initial variables and the number of variables at the first stage. This quantlet simply selects a reasonable subset of variables automatically as q changes from p to r (or from r to p). In addition, mpca performs All-possible selection at the first stage of Forward and Forward-backward procedures to find the initial subset of size r.

14.6   Examples

14.6.1   Artificial Data

Here, we apply variable selection using M.PCA criteria to an artificial data set which consists of 87 individuals and 20 variables. Suppose the file name of the artificial data set is artif and the data set is saved in the folder in which XploRe is installed. Although this data set was generated artificially, the data set was modified in a clinical test (87 observations on 25 qualitative variables) to make the data meaningful.

Q XCSvaspca01.xpl

Based on the specified parameters variable selection is performed. Here, we apply variable selection with the following parameters: correlation matrix, two PCs, the proportion P criterion and Backward procedure. After calculation, the process of removing variables is displayed in the output window: the criterion value and variable numbers of Y_1 and Y_2 separated by "|" for every number q of selected variables $(q = p, p - 1, \ldots, r = 20, 19, \ldots, 2)$.

Table 14.1: Variable Selection in Principal Component Analysis using selection criteria in Modified PCA, Correlation matrix, Proportion P, Backward, r: 2

q	Criterion Y_1—Y_2 Value	1	2	3	4	5	6	7	8	9	10	11	12	13	14	15	16	17	18	19	20
20	0.74307	1	2	3	4	5	6	7	8	9	10	11	12	13	14	15	16	17	18	19	20|
19	0.74262	1	2	3	4	5	6	7	8	9	10	11	12	13	14	15	17	18	19	20|	16
18	0.74212	1	2	3	4	5	6	7	9	10	11	12	13	14	15	17	18	19	20|	8	16
17	0.74160	1	2	3	4	5	6	7	10	11	12	13	14	15	17	18	19	20|	8	9	16
16	0.74105	1	2	4	5	6	7	10	11	12	13	14	15	17	18	19	20|	3	8	9	16
15	0.74026	1	2	4	5	7	10	11	12	13	14	15	17	18	19	20|	3	6	8	9	16
14	0.73931	1	2	4	5	7	10	11	13	14	15	17	18	19	20|	3	6	8	9	12	16
13	0.73826	1	2	4	5	7	10	11	13	14	15	17	18	20|	3	6	8	9	12	16	19
12	0.73650	1	2	4	5	7	11	13	14	15	17	18	20|	3	6	8	9	10	12	16	19
11	0.73467	1	2	4	5	7	11	13	15	17	18	20|	3	6	8	9	10	12	14	16	19
10	0.73276	1	2	5	7	11	13	15	17	18	20|	3	4	6	8	9	10	12	14	16	19
9	0.73010	1	2	5	7	13	14	17	18	20|	3	4	6	8	9	10	11	12	15	16	19
8	0.72736	1	2	7	13	14	17	18	20|	3	4	5	6	8	9	10	11	12	15	16	19
7	0.72372	1	2	7	13	14	17	18|	3	4	5	6	8	9	10	11	12	15	16	19	20
6	0.71891	1	2	7	13	14	17|	3	4	5	6	8	9	10	11	12	15	16	18	19	20
5	0.71329	1	2	13	14	17|	3	4	5	6	7	8	9	10	11	12	15	16	18	19	20
4	0.70133	7	13	14	17|	1	2	3	4	5	6	8	9	10	11	12	15	16	18	19	20
3	0.68264	13	14	17|	1	2	3	4	5	6	7	8	9	10	11	12	15	16	18	19	20
2	0.65580	13	17|	1	2	3	4	5	6	7	8	9	10	11	12	14	15	16	18	19	20

r: number of principal components, q: number of selected variables,
Y_1: subset of variables to be selected, and Y_2: subset of variables to be deleted

The graph of criterion values is also displayed (Figure 14.2). You can observe the change in the criterion visually using this graph.

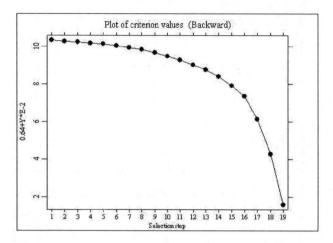

Figure 14.2: Index plot of the proportion Ps as q changes from 20 to 2. (Artificial data, $r=2$, correlation matrix, the proportion P and Backward)

These outputs show that the proportion P changes slightly until the number of variables is six (at step 15). The range of the proportion P's is only 0.02416 ($= 0.74307 - 0.71891$). This means that 14 of the 20 variables are almost redundant for composing PCs to be used to reproduce the original variables. Furthermore, if a subset of size 11 or more is selected, the difference between the proportion based on the selected subset and that based on all of the variables is less than 0.01.

Looking at the results, a subset of any number of variables displayed as Y1 can be selected in the output list.

Here, we show another result obtained by applying Forward-backward stepwise selection to the same data set. The index plot of the criterion value is illustrated in Figure 14.3 and selected variables are

Table 14.2: Variable Selection in Principal Component Analysis using selection criteria in Modified PCA
Correlation matrix, Proportion P, Forward-backward, r: 2

q	Criterion Value	$Y_1 - Y_2$																			
		1	2	3	4	5	6	7	8	9	10	11	12	13	14	15	16	17	18	19	20
2	0.65658	4	16|	1	2	3	5	6	7	8	9	10	11	12	13	14	15	17	18	19	20
3	0.68161	4	11	15|	1	2	3	5	6	7	8	9	10	12	13	14	16	17	18	19	20
4	0.69858	4	11	13	15|	1	2	3	5	6	7	8	9	10	12	14	16	17	18	19	20
5	0.71210	3	10	11	15	20|	1	2	4	5	6	7	8	9	12	13	14	16	17	18	19
6	0.72047	3	5	10	11	15	20|	1	2	4	6	7	8	9	12	13	14	16	17	18	19
7	0.72514	3	5	9	10	11	15	20|	1	2	4	6	7	8	12	13	14	16	17	18	19
8	0.72944	1	3	4	5	9	10	11	20|	2	6	7	8	12	13	14	15	16	17	18	19
9	0.73298	1	3	4	5	6	9	10	11	20|	2	7	8	12	13	14	15	16	17	18	19
10	0.73480	1	3	4	5	6	7	9	10	11	20|	2	8	12	13	14	15	16	17	18	19
11	0.73660	1	3	4	5	6	7	8	9	10	11	20|	2	12	13	14	15	16	17	18	19
12	0.73766	1	3	4	5	6	7	8	9	10	11	19	20|	2	12	13	14	15	16	17	18
13	0.73886	1	3	4	5	6	7	8	9	10	11	15	19	20|	2	12	13	14	16	17	18
14	0.73995	1	3	4	5	6	7	8	9	10	11	13	15	19	20|	2	12	14	16	17	18
15	0.74087	1	3	4	5	6	7	8	9	10	11	13	15	18	19	20|	2	12	14	16	17
16	0.74131	1	3	4	5	6	7	8	9	10	11	12	13	15	18	19	20|	2	14	16	17
17	0.74179	1	3	4	5	6	7	8	9	10	11	12	13	14	15	18	19	20|	2	16	17
18	0.74223	1	3	4	5	6	7	8	9	10	11	12	13	14	15	16	18	19	20|	2	17
19	0.74262	1	2	3	4	5	6	7	8	9	10	11	12	13	14	15	17	18	19	20|	16
20	0.74307	1	2	3	4	5	6	7	8	9	10	11	12	13	14	15	16	17	18	19	20|

r: number of principal components, q: number of selected variables
Y_1: subset of variables to be selected, Y_2: subset of variables to be deleted

r : number of principal components, q : number of selected variables Y_1: subset of variables to be selected, Y_2: subset of variables to be deleted

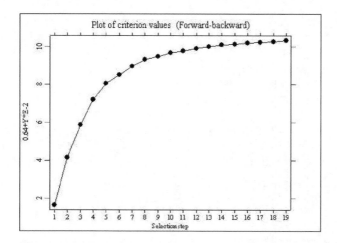

Figure 14.3: Index plot of the proportion Ps as q changes from 2 to 20. (Artificial data, $r=2$, correlation matrix, the proportion P and Forward-backward)

The outputs are displayed in selected order (in reverse order of backward-type selection). Although stepwise-type selection takes longer than single-type selection, stepwise-type selection can provide more reasonable results. In fact, when the number of variables is six, for example, the selected subset {3, 5, 10, 11, 15, 20} is the same result as that obtained by All-possible selection (see the result of All-possible selection described below).

If you choose All-possible at a specified q in the fourth selection box, one additional box opens to specify the number of variables to be investigated. Then, the best subset of the specified size q is displayed in the output window:

Table 14.3: Variable Selection in Principal Component Analysis using selection criteria in Modified PCA
Correlation matrix, Proportion P, All-possible at a specified q, r: 2

q	Criterion Value	Y_1						—	Y_2													
6	0.72047	3	5	10	11	15	20		1	2	4	6	7	8	9	12	13	14	16	17	18	19

r: the number of principal components, q: the number of selected variables
Y_1: a subset of variables to be selected, Y_2: a subset of variables to be deleted

If mpca is called using the second argument, for example, mpca(artif, 2), solving the prior EVP and the second selection to specify the number of PCs are skipped.

14.6.2 Application Data

As the second numerical example, we analyze a data set of alate adelges (winged aphids), which was analyzed originally by Jeffers (1967) using ordinary PCA and later by various authors, including Jolliffe (1973) and Krzanowski (1987a, 1987b), using PCA with variable selection functions. We applied our variable selection method to the data set given in Krzanowski (1987a). The data set consists of 40 individuals and 19 variables. Eigenvalues and their cumulative proportions of the data are 13.8379 (72.83%), 2.3635 (85.27%), 0.7480 (89.21%), ..., therefore we use two PCs as in previous studies. Since Jeffers (1967) found four clusters by observing the plot of PCs obtained by ordinary PCA based on the correlation matrix of whole variables, we choose the RV-coefficient as a selection criterion to detect a subset providing the close configuration of PCs to the original configuration. Here, we apply Forward-backward stepwise selection based on the correlation matrix to the data.

The results of (Y_1, Y_2) for every q are obtained as the following output and their RV-coefficients changes as shown in Figure 14.4.

Table 14.4: Variable Selection in Principal Component Analysis
using selection criteria in Modified PCA
Correlation matrix, RV-coefficient, Forward-backward, r: 2

q	Criterion Value	Y_1 — Y_2																	
2	0.97069	5	13|	1	18	17	16	15	14	12	11	10	9	8	7	6	4	3	2	19
3	0.98413	5	13	18|	17	16	15	14	12	11	10	9	8	7	6	4	3	2	1	19
4	0.98721	5	7	13	18|	17	16	15	14	12	11	10	9	8	6	4	3	2	1	19
5	0.99066	3	7	13	16	18|	17	15	14	12	11	10	9	8	6	4	3	2	1	19
6	0.99198	3	7	13	16	15	18|	17	14	12	11	10	9	8	6	4	3	2	1	19
7	0.99311	3	7	13	15	14	18	17|	16	12	11	10	9	8	6	4	3	2	1	19
8	0.99371	3	4	7	13	15	16	17	18|	14	12	11	10	9	8	6	5	2	1	19
9	0.99435	3	4	5	13	15	16	17	18	2|	14	12	11	10	9	8	7	6	1	19
10	0.99496	3	4	5	13	15	16	17	18	1	2|	14	12	11	10	9	8	7	6	19
11	0.99540	1	5	6	2	8	9	10	18	17	16	15	13|	14	12	11	7	4	3	19
12	0.99593	1	4	5	6	2	8	9	10	18	17	16	15	13|	14	12	11	7	3	19
13	0.99634	1	4	5	6	7	8	9	10	11	18	17	16	15	13|	14	12	3	2	19
14	0.99671	1	4	5	6	7	8	9	10	11	13	18	17	16	15|	14	12	3	2	19
15	0.99693	1	3	4	6	7	8	9	10	11	13	12	18	17	16	15|	14	7	2	19
16	0.99704	1	2	3	6	8	11	7	8	9	12	13	16	17	18	14|	7	14	15	19
17	0.99712	1	2	3	6	8	9	7	7	11	13	12	14	16	17	18	19|	7	14	15
18	0.99723	1	2	3	6	7	8	19|	12	10	11	12	16	15	17	16	18	7	19	13
19	0.99726	1	2	3	6	7	8	9	11	12	11	12	13	14	15	16	17	18	19|	—

r: number of principal components, q: number of selected variables
Y_1: subset of variables to be selected, Y_2: subset of variables to be deleted

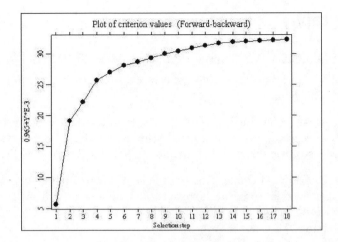

Figure 14.4: Index plot of the RV-coefficients as q changes from 2 to 19. (Alate data, $r=2$, correlation matrix, the RV-coefficient and Forward-backward)

The results illustrate that the RV-coefficient changes slightly when the number of variables is over five (at step 4). In particular, the sequential difference is less than 0.0007 when the number of variables is over 7 (step 6).

Here, we draw a scatter plot of PC scores based on the seven selected variables {3, 7, 13, 15, 16, 17, 18} and compare this plot with that based on the 19 original variables.

Q XCSvaspca02.xpl

Using these arguments in the quantlet `geigensm` to solve the generalized EVP (14.3), we obtain the sorted eigenvalues `mevp.values` and the associated eigenvectors `mevp.vectors`. Thus, the modified PC scores `mpc` are obtained after scale adjustment. The last block draws two scatter plots of the first two PC scores. These are shown in Figure 14.1 in Section 14.1 (The figures can be rotated and the first three PCs can be observed as the three-dimensional display by mouse operation. Note, however, that the modified PCs were calculated as the number of PCs is two).

As the plots illustrate, little difference exists between the two configurations, i.e. the use of only seven among 19 variables is sufficient to obtain PCs that provide almost the same information as the original PCs.

Bibliography

Bonifas, I., Escoufier, Y., Gonzalez, P.L. et Sabatier, R. (1984).
Choix de variables en analyse en composantes principales, *Rev. Statist. Appl.*, **23**: 5-15.

Falguerolles, A. De et Jmel, S. (1993). Un critere de choix de variables en analyse en composantes principales fonde sur des modeles graphiques gaussiens particuliers, *Rev. Canadienne Statist.*, **21**(3): 239-256.

Iizuka, M., Mori, Y., Tarumi, T. and Tanaka, Y. (2002a). Implementation of variable selection program for principal component analysis to WWW, *Proceedings of the Institute of Statistical Mathematics*, **49**(2): 277-292 (in Japanese).

Iizuka, M., Mori, Y., Tarumi, T. and Tanaka, Y. (2002b). Statistical software VASMM for variable selection in multivariate methods, In: W. Härdle and B. Rönz (eds.) *COMPSTAT2002 Proceedings in Computational Statistics*, Springer-Verlag, pp. 563-568.

Iizuka, M., Mori, Y., Tarumi, T. and Tanaka, Y. (2003). Computer intensive trials to determine the number of variables in PCA, *Journal of the Japanese Society of Computational Statistics*, **14**(2) (Special Issue of ICNCB) (to appear).

Jeffers, J. N. R. (1967). Two case studies in the application of principal component analysis, *Applied Statistics*, **16**: 225–236.

Jolliffe, I. T. (1972). Discarding variables in a principal component analysis I - Artificial data -, *Applied Statistics*, **21**: 160-173.

Jolliffe, I. T. (1973). Discarding variables in a principal component analysis II - Real data -, *Applied Statistics*, **22**: 21-31.

Krzanowski, W. J. (1987a). Selection of variables to preserve multivariate data structure, using principal components, *Applied Statistics*, **36**: 22-33.

Krzanowski, W. J. (1987b). Cross-validation in principal component analysis, *Biometrics*, **43**: 575-584.

McCabe, G. P. (1984). Principal variables, *Technometrics*, **26**: 137-44.

Mori,Y. (1997). Statistical software VASPCA - Variable selection in PCA, *Bulletin of Okayama University of Science,* **33**(A): 329-340.

Mori, Y. (1998). Principal component analysis based on a subset of variables - Numerical investigation using RV-coefficient criterion, *Bulletin of Okayama University of Science*, **34**(A): 383-396 (in Japanese).

Mori, Y. and Iizuka, M. (2000). Study of variable selection methods in data analysis and its interactive system, *Proceedings of ISM Symposium - Recent Advances in Statistical Research and Data Analysis*: 109-114.

Mori, Y., Iizuka, M. Tarumi, T. and Tanaka, Y. (1999). Variable selection in "Principal Component Analysis Based on a Subset of Variables", *Bulletin of the International Statistical Institute (52nd Session Contributed Papers Book2)*: 333-334.

Mori, Y., Iizuka, M. Tarumi, T. and Tanaka, Y. (2000a). Statistical software "VASPCA" for variable selection in principal component analysis, In: W. Jansen and J.G. Bethlehem (eds.) *COMPSTAT2000 Proceedings in Computational Statistics (Short Communications)*, pp. 73-74.

Mori, Y., Iizuka, M., Tarumi, T. and Tanaka, Y. (2000b). Study of variable selection criteria in data analysis, *Proceedings of the 10th Japan and Korea joint Conference of Statistics*: 547-554.

Mori, Y., Tarumi, T. and Tanaka, Y. (1994). Variable selection with RV-coefficient in principal component analysis, In: R. Dutter and W. Grossman (eds.), *COMPSTAT1994 Proceedings in Computational Statistics (Short Communications)*, pp. 169-170.

Mori, Y., Tanaka, T. and Tarumi, T. (1997). Principal component analysis based on a subset of qualitative variables, In: C. Hayashi et al. (eds.), *Proceedings of IFCS-96: Data Science, Classification and Related Methods*, Springer-Verlag, pp. 547-554.

Mori, Y., Tarumi, T. and Tanaka, Y. (1998). Principal Component analysis based on a subset of variables - Numerical investigation on variable selection procedures, *Bulletin of the Computational Statistics of Japan*, **11**(1): 1-12 (in Japanese).

Rao, C. R. (1964). The use and interpretation of principal component analysis in applied research, *Sankhya*, **A26**: 329-358.

Robert, P. and Escoufier, Y. (1976). A unifying tool for linear multivariate statistical methods: the RV-coefficient, *Appl. Statist.*, **25**: 257-65.

Tanaka, Y. and Mori, Y. (1997). Principal component analysis based on a subset of variables: Variable selection and sensitivity analysis, *American Journal of Mathematics and Management Sciences*, **17**(1&2): 61-89.

15 Spatial Statistics

Pavel Čížek, Wolfgang Härdle and Jürgen Symanzik

15.1 Introduction

This chapter deals with the analysis of spatial data. Such data can be the structure of biological cells, the distribution of plants and animals in a geographic region, the occurrence of diseases in a county or state, economic data in different administrative districts, climate data such as temperature or precipitation over geographic regions, and the distribution of galaxies in space. Spatial data often are not independent. Temperature and precipitation measurements at two locations that are 10 km apart will be more similar than such measurements at two locations that are 1000 km or even 100 km apart. Infectious diseases often occur in spatial clusters. One region of a country may encounter hundreds of cases while another region may encounter only very few cases. Thus, spatial data analysis/spatial statistics deals with the quantitative study of phenomena that are located in some two- or higher-dimensional space.

There are three main types of spatial data: spatial point patterns (we speak of spatial point processes when we refer to the underlying stochastic processes that result in observable point patterns), geostatistical data (also called spatially continuous data), and lattice data (also called area data). If there is an additional temporal component, we speak of spatio-temporal data.

Throughout this chapter, we will be dealing with a two-dimensional area of interest, called D. We assume that we have n sample locations $\mathbf{x}_i$ that are usually located in D, but some may occasionally be located outside of D. We make n observations $Z(\mathbf{x}_i)$ at these locations and want to describe the underlying spatial process $Z(\mathbf{x})$.

For spatial point patterns, the point locations in D are random and their number n is unknown in advance. We are primarily interested in the observed locations $\mathbf{x}_i \in D$ that represent particular point events, such as the occurrence of a disease, a species habitat, or the location of trees. A typical question for spatial point patterns is whether the observed locations are clustered, randomly distributed, or regularly distributed. In this case, we simply assume that $Z(\mathbf{x}_i) = 1$ for all $\mathbf{x}_i \in D$, i.e., there is no other data being recorded than the spatial locations of the n point events. Sometimes, additional variables such as the time of the occurrence of an event or physical measurements such as height, diameter, and crown-defoliation of a tree are measured. Then, $Z(\mathbf{x}_i)$ represents a random variable (or a random vector) at location $\mathbf{x}_i \in D$. Details on spatial point patterns can be found, for example, in Diggle (2003).

For geostatistical data, D is a fixed subset of the two-dimensional space. We observe $Z(\mathbf{x}_i)$ that represents a random variable (or a random vector) at location $\mathbf{x}_i \in D$. We are usually not interested in the locations $\mathbf{x}_i$ at which the sample measurements were taken. In fact, we assume the locations have been randomly chosen or are predetermined by towns or measurement stations. Of interest are only the univariate or multivariate measurements $Z(\mathbf{x}_i)$, such as amount of precipitation or number and concentration of different air pollutants measured at a particular measurement station. Because the number of locations n where actual measurements were taken is sparse, we usually want to estimate the values for the variable(s) of interest at locations where no actual measurements were taken. The term spatially continuous data relates to the fact that measurements at least theoretically can be taken at any location $\mathbf{x}_i \in D$. However, time and cost constraints usually only allow measurements to be taken at a limited number of locations. Details on geostatistical data can be found, for example, in Isaaks and Srivastava (1989) and Wackernagel (1998).

For lattice data, D is a fixed subset of the two-dimensional space that consists of countably many sub-areas of regular or irregular shape. We observe $Z(\mathbf{x}_i)$ that represents a random variable (or a random vector) at sub-area $\mathbf{x}_i \in D$. Lattice data represents spatial data that has been aggregated to areal units. Instead of knowing the exact locations where a disease occurred, or the exact residence addresses and income of all employees, we may only know the total number of occurrences (or the incidence rate) of a disease for different health service areas, or the average annual income of employees in different countries of the European Community. Statistical variables associated with areas often do not vary continuously over space. For example, the tax rate on goods might be 6% in one state and 8% in the next state. Often (but not always), the given spatial areas are considered to be the only spatial locations at which the variables of interest can be measured. We typically want to describe and model the observed spatial pattern and determine possible explanations for this pattern, for example, which other factors might be associated with higher disease rates in many of the urban health service areas.

In addition to the specific references cited above, the reader is referred to Bailey and Gatrell (1995), Ripley (1981), or Cressie (1993) for comprehensive overviews dealing with all three main types of spatial data and beyond. This chapter closely follows Chapter 14 in Venables and Ripley (1999) and, therefore, the notation used in Ripley (1981). The XploRe quantlets used in this chapter have been adapted from the S-Plus and underlying C code that accompanies Venables and Ripley (1999), with kind permission from Brian D. Ripley. The XploRe quantlets support techniques for spatial point patterns and geostatistical data. In the electronic version of this chapter, the **Q** symbol underneath each figure provides a direct link to the XploRe code that was used to create the figure. At this point, the XploRe quantlib spatial does not support any techniques for lattice data.

In Section 15.2, we discuss techniques for the analysis of geostatistical data. In Section 15.3, we discuss techniques for the analysis of spatial point processes. We finish with a short discussion in Section 15.4.

15.2   Analysis of Geostatistical Data

In this section, we discuss techniques for the analysis of geostatistical data, in particular spatial interpolation, smoothing, kriging, correlograms, and variograms. We assume that we have n fixed sampling locations $\mathbf{x}_i \in D$ and observe $Z(\mathbf{x}_i)$. Our goal is to predict the spatial process $Z(\mathbf{x})$ for any $\mathbf{x} \in D$ or, rather, the mean value $E(Z(\mathbf{x}))$ for this spatial process for any $\mathbf{x} \in D$. A simple, but often unrealistic, assumption is that $\{Z(\mathbf{x}) \mid \mathbf{x} \in D\}$ are independent and the distributions of $Z(\mathbf{x})$ only differ in the mean but otherwise are identical. More realistically, we should assume some degree of spatial correlation and therefore incorporate spatial dependence into our model. This leads to first order effects and second order effects. First order effects relate to variation in the mean value of a process in space, i.e., a global (or large scale) trend. Second order effects relate to the spatial correlation structure, i.e., these are local (or small scale) effects.

Our examples in this section are based on the `topo` dataset, introduced in Davis (1973), Table 6.4, and further discussed in Ripley (1981, p. 58–72). This dataset consists of $n = 52$ spatial locations with measurements of topographic elevation, measured in feet above sea level. The area D is an approximate square with side lengths of about 305 feet. The coordinates have been labelled in 50 feet units, such that the actual spatial locations $\mathbf{x}_i$ fall into the area $(0.2, 6.3) \times (0.1, 6.2)$, where the first represent East-West coordinates and the second represent North-South coordinates. For convenience, the origin $(0, 0)$ is assumed to be located in the Southwest corner of the area D. In all of our calculations and plots, we assume that the area of interest actually is the square area $(0, 6.5) \times (0, 6.5)$. The examples in this section show how to do computations and produce graphics similar to those in Sections 14.1 and 14.2 in Venables and Ripley (1999), using XploRe.

15.2.1   Trend Surfaces

A trend surface analysis is a simple approach to model the global first order effect in the mean value of a spatially continuous process. First, we assume that $\{Z(\mathbf{x}) \mid \mathbf{x} \in D\}$ are independent. Let us further express the spatial coordinates as $\mathbf{x} = (x, y)$. Often, the expected value $E(Z(\mathbf{x})) = f(\mathbf{x})$ of a spatial process is expressed as a trend surface, i.e., a polynomial regression surface of the form

$$f(\mathbf{x}) = \sum_{0 \leq r+s \leq p} a_{rs} x^r y^s,$$

where the parameter p is called the order (or the degree) of the trend surface. For example, a quadratic trend surface is of the form

$$f(\mathbf{x}) = a_{00} + a_{10}x + a_{01}y + a_{20}x^2 + a_{11}xy + a_{02}y^2$$

and has $P = 6$ coefficients. In general, a least squares (LS) trend surface of degree p has $P = (p+1)(p+2)/2$ coefficients that are chosen to minimize

$$\sum_{i=1}^{n}(Z(\mathbf{x}_i) - f(\mathbf{x}_i))^2,$$

where $\mathbf{x}_i \in D, i = 1, \ldots, n$, are the locations at which the n sample measurements were taken.

Figure 15.1 shows trend surfaces of degree 2, 3, 4, and 6 fitted to the `topo.dat` dataset. The 52 spatial locations are overlaid as small red crosses on the trend surfaces. This figure looks similar to Figure 14.1 in Venables and Ripley (1999). When fitting a trend surface of degree $p = 6$, $P = 28$ coefficients have to be estimated from only 52 spatial locations. As a consequence, problems with the visual appearance of the trend surface of degree 6 can be noticed due to extrapolation near the edges.

Another problem with fitting trend surfaces is that often the spatial locations are not regularly spaced. Instead, the spatial locations are often more dense where the surface is high (e.g., for air pollution, we want to determine the spatial locations where the pollution level might be critical for human health

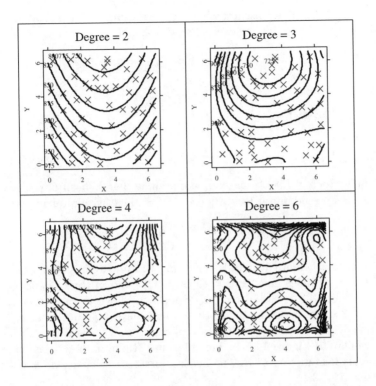

Figure 15.1: Least squares trend surfaces of degree 2, 3, 4, and 6 for the
topo.dat dataset.

Q XCSspa01.xpl

and thus we take additional measurements in regions with elevated pollution
levels). It becomes necessary to consider the spatial correlation of the errors
as well. Venables and Ripley (1999) suggested the model

$$Z(\mathbf{x}) = \mathbf{f}(\mathbf{x})^\top \boldsymbol{\beta} + \varepsilon(\mathbf{x}),$$

where $\mathbf{f}(\mathbf{x}) = (f_1(\mathbf{x}), \ldots, f_P(\mathbf{x}))^\top$ is a parametrized trend term as above, $\boldsymbol{\beta} =$
$(\beta_1, \ldots, \beta_P)^\top$ is a parameter vector, and $\varepsilon(\mathbf{x})$ is a zero-mean spatial stochastic
process of errors. In our previous example of a quadratic trend surface, we
have $\mathbf{f}(\mathbf{x}) = (1, x, y, x^2, xy, y^2)^\top$ and $\boldsymbol{\beta} = (a_{00}, a_{10}, a_{01}, a_{20}, a_{11}, a_{02})^\top$. It is
further assumed that $\varepsilon(\mathbf{x})$ possesses second moments and has the covariance
function

$$C(\mathbf{x}, \mathbf{y}) = Cov(\varepsilon(\mathbf{x}), \varepsilon(\mathbf{y})),$$

where $\mathbf{x}, \mathbf{y} \in D$. If we assume that we obtain measurements at n spatial locations $\mathbf{x}_1, \ldots, \mathbf{x}_n \in D$, we can define the model

$$\mathbf{Z} = \mathbf{F}\boldsymbol{\beta} + \boldsymbol{\varepsilon},$$

where

$$\mathbf{Z} = \begin{bmatrix} Z(\mathbf{x}_1) \\ \vdots \\ Z(\mathbf{x}_n) \end{bmatrix}, \quad \mathbf{F} = \begin{bmatrix} \mathbf{f}(\mathbf{x}_1)^\top \\ \vdots \\ \mathbf{f}(\mathbf{x}_n)^\top \end{bmatrix}, \quad \text{and} \quad \boldsymbol{\varepsilon} = \begin{bmatrix} \varepsilon(\mathbf{x}_1) \\ \vdots \\ \varepsilon(\mathbf{x}_n) \end{bmatrix}.$$

If we further define $K = [C(\mathbf{x}_i, \mathbf{x}_j)]$ and assume that K has full rank, we can estimate $\boldsymbol{\beta}$ by generalized least squares (GLS), i.e., by minimizing

$$(\mathbf{Z} - \mathbf{F}\boldsymbol{\beta})^\top K^{-1} (\mathbf{Z} - \mathbf{F}\boldsymbol{\beta}).$$

Additional mathematical details regarding the underlying calculations can be found in Venables and Ripley (1999, p. 436) and in Ripley (1981, p. 47). The resulting GLS trend surface of degree 2 is shown in the upper right of Figure 15.2 and it is contrasted to the ordinary least squares trend surface of the same degree in the upper left (a replicate from Figure 15.1). This figure looks similar to Figure 14.5 in Venables and Ripley (1999). The choice of the covariance function C that is needed for these calculations is discussed in Section 15.2.3.

15.2.2 Kriging

Kriging is a technique developed in the early 1960s by Matheron and his school in the mining industry. The term kriging is named after the South African mining engineer D. G. Krige. When we speak of kriging, we basically mean an optimal prediction of unobserved values of the spatial process

$$Z(\mathbf{x}) = \mathbf{f}(\mathbf{x})^\top \boldsymbol{\beta} + \varepsilon(\mathbf{x}),$$

as introduced before.

Several forms of kriging exist. In its most general form, called universal kriging, the process $Z(\mathbf{x})$ is fitted by generalized least squares, predicting the value of the functional term as well as the value of the error term at location $\mathbf{x} \in D$ and taking their sum. In contrast to the generalized least squares approach discussed in Section 15.2.1, it is no longer assumed that $\varepsilon(\mathbf{x})$ is a zero-mean process of errors.

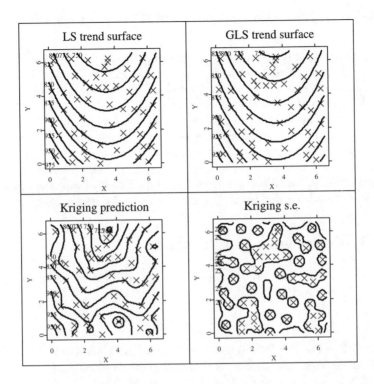

Figure 15.2: Least squares trend surface (upper left), generalized least
squares trend surface (upper right), kriging surface (lower left),
and kriging standard errors (lower right) for the topo.dat
dataset.

Q XCSspa02.xpl

A simplification of universal kriging is (ordinary) kriging where the trend
surface is assumed to be of degree 0, i.e., the process $Z(\mathbf{x})$ has constant mean
$E(Z(\mathbf{x})) = \mu$ for all $\mathbf{x} \in D$, with $\mu \in \mathbb{R}$ unknown. To meet this condition,
the process $Z(\mathbf{x})$ often is first detrended as described in Section 15.2.1 and
the spatial residuals are used for the next analysis steps.

A further simplification of ordinary kriging is simple kriging where it is assumed that $\mu \in \mathbb{R}$ is known in advance and thus does not have to be estimated
from the data. Other forms of kriging, such as robust kriging, disjunctive
kriging, block kriging, and co-kriging have been discussed in the literature.

Details can be found in Bailey and Gatrell (1995) or Cressie (1993) for example.

The computational steps for universal kriging and the calculation of the error variances have been discussed in Venables and Ripley (1999, p. 439), with additional mathematical details provided in Ripley (1981, p. 47–50). Universal kriging predictions (based on a trend surface of degree 2) and kriging standard errors are displayed in the lower left and lower right of Figure 15.2. There are considerable differences in the appearances of the kriging surface and the previously introduced least squares trend surface (upper left) and the generalized least squares trend surface (upper right). This figure looks similar to Figure 14.5 in Venables and Ripley (1999). The choice of the covariance function C that is needed for these calculations is discussed in Section 15.2.3.

15.2.3   Correlogram and Variogram

In the previous sections, we have made the often unrealistic assumption that the covariance function

$$C(\mathbf{x}, \mathbf{y}) = Cov(\varepsilon(\mathbf{x}), \varepsilon(\mathbf{y}))$$

is known. However, if C is unknown, we have to make additional assumptions for the underlying spatial process that will allow us to estimate C.

One common assumption for second order effects is that the spatial process $\{Z(\mathbf{x}) \mid \mathbf{x} \in D\}$ exhibits stationarity (also called homogeneity). This means that the statistical properties of $Z(\mathbf{x})$ are independent of the absolute locations in D, i.e., $E(Z(\mathbf{x})) = \mu$ and $Var(Z(\mathbf{x})) = \sigma^2$ are constant in D. This also implies that $Cov(Z(\mathbf{x}), Z(\mathbf{y}))$ for $\mathbf{x} \neq \mathbf{y}$ depends only on the relative locations (i.e., distance and direction) of $\mathbf{x}$ and $\mathbf{y}$, but it does not depend on their absolute locations in D. Thus, for any $\mathbf{x}, \mathbf{y} \in D$ with $\mathbf{x} + \mathbf{r} = \mathbf{y}$, it holds that $Cov(Z(\mathbf{x}), Z(\mathbf{y})) = C(\mathbf{r})$.

Moreover, we call the spatial process $\{Z(\mathbf{x}) \mid \mathbf{x} \in D\}$ isotropic if it is stationary and $Cov(Z(\mathbf{x}), Z(\mathbf{y}))$ depends only on the distance r between $\mathbf{x}$ and $\mathbf{y}$, but it does not depend on the direction in which they are separated. If mean, variance, or covariance differ over D, the spatial process exhibits non-stationarity (also called heterogeneity).

A somewhat weaker assumption than stationarity (or even isotropy) is intrinsic stationarity where we assume that $E(Z(\mathbf{x} + \mathbf{r}) - Z(\mathbf{x})) = 0$ and $Var(Z(\mathbf{x} + \mathbf{r}) - Z(\mathbf{x})) = 2\gamma(\mathbf{r})$ for any separation vector $\mathbf{r}$. Thus, we have constant variance in the differences between values at locations that are separated by a given distance and direction $\mathbf{r}$. The quantity $2\gamma(\mathbf{r})$ is called the variogram while the quantity $\gamma(\mathbf{r})$ is called the semi-variogram. Often, the prefix "semi" is omitted and we speak of a variogram although we mean a semi-variogram. The factor 2 has the effect that $\gamma(\mathbf{r}) = \sigma^2$ (and not $2\sigma^2$) for large separation vectors $\mathbf{r}$, i.e., $\lim\limits_{||\mathbf{r}|| \to \infty} \gamma(\mathbf{r}) = \sigma^2$.

If we assume isotropy, the covariance function

$$Cov(Z(\mathbf{x}), Z(\mathbf{y})) = c(d(\mathbf{x}, \mathbf{y})) = c(r)$$

becomes a function c that entirely depends on the Euclidean distance $r = ||\mathbf{r}|| = d(\mathbf{x}, \mathbf{y})$ between $\mathbf{x}$ and $\mathbf{y}$. Common choices for theoretical covariance functions c are discussed further below.

Given that $c(0) > 0$, we define

$$\rho(r) = \frac{c(r)}{c(0)} = \frac{c(r)}{\sigma^2}$$

and call this function the correlogram (also known as autocorrelation function) at distance r. It should be noted that

$$\sigma^2 = Var(Z(\mathbf{x})) = Cov(Z(\mathbf{x}), Z(\mathbf{x})) = c(d(\mathbf{x}, \mathbf{x})) = c(0).$$

Apparently, it must hold that $\rho(0) = 1$. However, there is no reason why $\lim\limits_{r \to 0+} \rho(r)$ could not be less than one for very small distances r. If this is the case, we speak of a nugget effect that represents a microscale variation of the spatial process. A possible explanation of such an effect are measurement errors, i.e., if multiple measurements at location $\mathbf{x}$ were made, they would all be slightly different. Extensions of theoretical covariance functions that include a nugget effect can be found in the previously cited literature. We will include a nugget effect in some of our examples later in this section, though, and ask the reader to carefully check what happens for very small distances r.

One other relationship between semi-variogram γ and covariance function C (for stationary processes) should be noted. It holds that

$$
\begin{aligned}
\gamma(\mathbf{r}) &= \frac{1}{2} Var(Z(\mathbf{x} + \mathbf{r}) - Z(\mathbf{x})) \\
&= \frac{1}{2} \{ Var(Z(\mathbf{x} + \mathbf{r})) + Var(Z(\mathbf{x})) - 2C(Z(\mathbf{x} + \mathbf{r}), Z(\mathbf{x})) \} \\
&= \sigma^2 - C(\mathbf{r}).
\end{aligned}
$$

While this holds for the theoretical relationship, it should be noted that this does not hold in general for the empirical functions, i.e., commonly we have $\hat{\gamma}(\mathbf{r}) \neq \hat{C}(0) - \hat{C}(\mathbf{r})$, where $\hat{\gamma}$ and $\hat{C}$ relate to the estimates of γ and C.

Before we consider theoretical covariance functions, we take a closer look at empirical correlograms and empirical variograms for isotropic processes. For both of these, we first divide the range of the data into m bins $[a_i, b_i)$ that are usually equally wide. For an empirical correlogram, for each bin i, we then determine the covariance $\hat{c}$ for those pairs of sample locations $\mathbf{x}, \mathbf{y} \in D$ where $d(\mathbf{x}, \mathbf{y}) \in [a_i, b_i)$. We finally divide by the overall variance to obtain $\hat{\rho}$ for bin i. Similarly, for an empirical variogram, for each bin i, we determine the average squared difference between $Z(\mathbf{x})$ and $Z(\mathbf{y})$ for those pairs of sample locations $\mathbf{x}, \mathbf{y} \in D$ where $d(\mathbf{x}, \mathbf{y}) \in [a_i, b_i)$. More formally,

$$\hat{c}(r_i) = \frac{1}{n(r_i)} \sum_{d(\mathbf{x}_i, \mathbf{x}_j) \in [a_i, b_i)} (Z(\mathbf{x}_i) - \overline{x})(Z(\mathbf{x}_j) - \overline{x}),$$

where $\overline{x} = 1/n \sum_{i=1}^{n} Z(\mathbf{x}_i)$ is the mean of all observed sample values and $n(r_i)$ is the number of the pairs of locations $\mathbf{x}_i, \mathbf{x}_j \in D$ that have a separation distance that falls into the interval $[a_i, b_i)$. r_i for which $\hat{c}$ is calculated is usually chosen as the mean of all separation distances that fall into bin i (although variations in the literature also choose $r_i = (a_i + b_i)/2$, i.e., the midpoint of the interval $[a_i, b_i)$). Similarly,

$$2\hat{\gamma}(r_i) = \frac{1}{n(r_i)} \sum_{d(\mathbf{x}_i, \mathbf{x}_j) \in [a_i, b_i)} (Z(\mathbf{x}_i) - Z(\mathbf{x}_j))^2.$$

A common way to suppress unreliable estimates of $\hat{\rho}$ and $\hat{\gamma}$ is to use the calculated results only for bins i that contain at least six pairs of sample locations.

An empirical correlogram and an empirical variogram for the residuals of the topo.dat dataset, based on a least squares quadratic trend surface as described in Section 15.2.1, are shown in Figure 15.3. This figure looks similar to Figure 14.6 in Venables and Ripley (1999).

General requirements for theoretical covariance functions for general spatial processes are symmetry and non-negative definiteness. For stationary processes, or even isotropic processes, exponential, Gaussian, and spherical families of covariance functions meet the general requirements and are frequently fitted to the data. An exponential covariance function has the form

$$c(r) = \sigma^2 \exp\left(-\frac{r}{d}\right).$$

An exponential covariance function has been overlaid on the correlogram

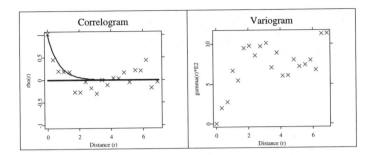

Figure 15.3: Empirical correlogram (left) and empirical variogram (right) for
the residuals of the `topo.dat` dataset after fitting a least squares
quadratic trend surface.

Q XCSspa03.xpl

(left) in Figure 15.3. A Gaussian covariance function has the form

$$c(r) = \sigma^2 \exp\left(-\frac{r^2}{d^2}\right).$$

A spherical covariance function in two dimensions has the form

$$c(r) = \sigma^2 \left\{ 1 - \frac{2}{\pi}\left(\frac{r}{d}\sqrt{1 - \frac{r^2}{d^2}} + \sin^{-1}\frac{r}{d}\right)\right\} \boldsymbol{I}_{(r \in [0,d])}$$

and a spherical covariance function in three dimensions (but also valid as a
covariance function in two dimensions) has the form

$$c(r) = \sigma^2 \left(1 - \frac{3r}{2d} + \frac{r^3}{2d^3}\right) \boldsymbol{I}_{(r \in [0,d])},$$

where $\boldsymbol{I}_{(r \in [0,d])}$ is the indicator function that takes value 1 if $r \in [0,d]$ and
0 otherwise. Within XploRe, the first version of these spherical covariance
functions is used in case the optional parameter "D" in the XploRe quantlet
call is omitted or takes the value 2, whereas the second version is used for all
other values of "D".

In the formulas above, the fixed distance $d = d(\mathbf{x}, \mathbf{y})$ is called the range
and basically represents the lag distance beyond which $Z(\mathbf{x})$ and $Z(\mathbf{y})$ are
uncorrelated. In this context, σ^2 is called the sill and represents the variance
of the process $Z(\mathbf{x})$ as defined above.

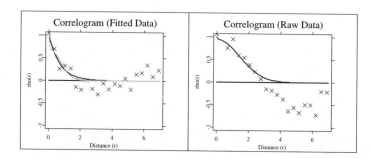

Figure 15.4: Empirical correlograms for the `topo.dat` dataset, based on
residuals from a quadratic trend surface (left) and the raw data
(right). An exponential covariance function (solid blue line) and
a Gaussian covariance function (dashed cyan line) have been fitted to the empirical correlogram of the residuals (left) while a
Gaussian covariance function has been fitted to the empirical
correlogram of the raw data (right).

Q XCSspa04.xpl

Figure 15.4 shows two empirical correlograms with overlaid covariance functions. In the left plot, we look at an empirical correlogram for the residuals
from a quadratic trend surface. An exponential covariance function [1] (solid
blue line) and a Gaussian covariance function with some nugget effect [2]
(dashed cyan line) have been overlaid. In the right plot, we look at an empirical correlogram for the raw data. A Gaussian covariance function [3] with
a small nugget effect and wide range has been overlaid. This figure looks
similar to Figure 14.7 in Venables and Ripley (1999).

The effect on the kriging surface and kriging standard errors when using
[1] as the covariance function has already been shown in Figure 15.2 in the
bottom row. In Figure 15.5, we see the effect on the kriging surface and
kriging standard errors when using covariance function [2] in the top row and
when using covariance function [3] in the bottom row. While all three kriging
surfaces look similar in the center of our region of interest D, we can notice
considerable differences on the edges of D. However, considerable differences
can be noticed in the structure of the kriging standard errors in the center of
D, depending on which of the three covariance functions has been selected.
Figure 15.5 looks similar to Figure 14.8 in Venables and Ripley (1999).

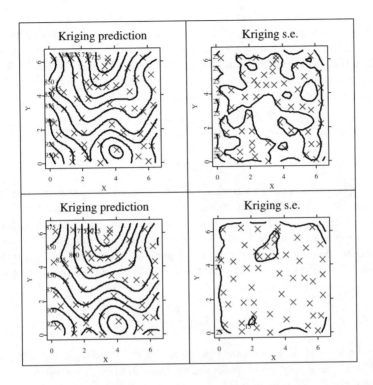

Figure 15.5: Kriging predictions (left) and kriging standard errors (right) for the residuals of the `topo.dat` dataset using covariance function [2] (top) and for the raw data without fitting a trend surface using covariance function [3] (bottom).

Q XCSspa05.xpl

15.3 Spatial Point Process Analysis

In this section, we discuss techniques for the analysis of spatial point patterns. A spatial point pattern is a set of randomly observed locations $\mathbf{x}_i$ that are more or less irregularly distributed in the area of interest D. One of the questions we are interested in when analyzing a spatial point pattern is whether the observed locations $\mathbf{x}_i$ are completely randomly distributed in D or whether there exists some spatial pattern, e.g., clustering or regularity.

Our examples in this section are based on the `pines` dataset, introduced in Strand (1972) and further discussed in Ripley (1981, p. 172–175). This dataset consists of $n = 71$ spatial locations, representing pine saplings in a 10×10-meter square. The spatial locations of the pines are shown in the upper left plot of Figure 15.6. The examples in this section show how to do computations and produce graphics similar to those in Section 14.3 in Venables and Ripley (1999), using XploRe.

One way to describe a spatial point process is to describe the number of events that are occurring in arbitrary sub-areas D_i of D, i.e.,

$$\{Z(D_i) \mid D_i \subseteq D\},$$

where $Z(D_i)$ is a random variable that represents the number of events in sub-area D_i. Obviously, this means that $E(Z(D_i))$ and any higher-order moments depend on the size(s) of the sub-areas that are involved, which is of little practical use. Instead, we characterize spatial point patterns based on the limiting behavior of these quantities per unit area. First order properties are described as intensity $\lambda(\mathbf{x})$ that represents the mean number of events per unit area at point $\mathbf{x}$, i.e.,

$$\lambda(\mathbf{x}) = \lim_{dx \to 0} \frac{E(Z(\mathbf{dx}))}{dx},$$

where $\mathbf{dx}$ is a small area around point $\mathbf{x}$ and $dx = ||\mathbf{dx}||$ is the size of area $\mathbf{dx}$. For a stationary point process, we have $\lambda(\mathbf{x}) = \lambda$ for all $\mathbf{x} \in D$, i.e., the intensity is constant over D. An obvious estimate of λ then is $\hat{\lambda} = n/A$, where n is the number of observed points in D and $A = ||D||$ is the size of area D.

A point process that is used to model a completely random appearance of the point pattern in D is the homogeneous Poisson process. Given such a process, we speak of complete spatial randomness (CSR). For the process $\{Z(D_i) \mid D_i \subseteq D\}$, it holds that $Z(D_i)$ and $Z(D_j)$ are independent for any choices of $D_i, D_j \in D$. The probability distribution of $Z(D_i)$ is a Poisson distribution with mean value λA_i where $A_i = ||D_i||$ is the size of area D_i. The corresponding probability density function (pdf) of $Z(D_i)$ is

$$f_{Z(D_i)}(z) = \frac{(\lambda A_i)^z}{z!} e^{-\lambda A_i},$$

where λ represents the constant intensity over D. CSR usually represents the null hypotheses when we want to assess whether an observed point pattern shows clustering or regularity instead.

The second moment of a point process can be specified via the K function, where $\lambda K(r)$ is the expected number of points within distance r of any of the

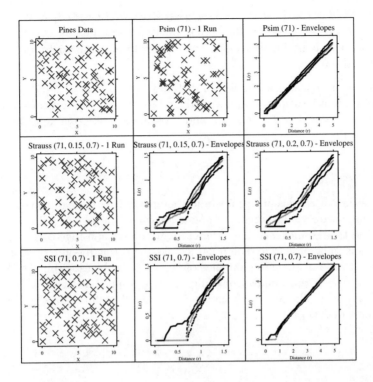

Figure 15.6: Observed point pattern for the `pines.dat` dataset (upper left),
and comparisons with a CSR process (upper middle and upper
right), two Strauss processes (middle row), and a SSI process
(bottom row). In the plots titled "Envelopes", the dark (blue)
lines represent the lower and upper simulation envelopes and
the light (cyan) line the average of the simulations runs of the
specified point process. The solid black line shows the observed
$\hat{L}(r)$ for the `pines.dat` dataset.

Q XCSspa06.xpl

points of the observed point pattern. For the homogeneous Poisson process,
it can be shown that $K(r) = \pi r^2$. If we obtain values that are significantly
greater than this value at a distance r_0 or significantly less than this value at a
distance r_0, this would be an indicator of clustering or regularity, respectively,
at this distance.

Instead of working with $K(r)$, one often switches to $L(r) = \sqrt{K(r)/\pi}$ (or $\tilde{L}(r) = \sqrt{K(r)/\pi} - r$). For the homogeneous Poisson process, $L(r)$ therefore would be a straight line with slope 1 that goes through the origin (or $\tilde{L}(r) = 0$ for all distances r).

Let us define r_{ij} as the Euclidean distance between the ith and j^{th} of the observed point locations $\mathbf{x}_i$ and $\mathbf{x}_j$ and let $\boldsymbol{I}_{(r_{ij} \in [0,r])}$ be the indicator function that takes value 1 if $0 \leq r_{ij} \leq r$ and 0 otherwise. A possible estimator of $K(r)$ then is

$$\hat{K}(r) = \frac{A}{n^2} \sum_{i,j;i \neq j} \boldsymbol{I}_{(r_{ij} \in [0,r])}.$$

This estimator reveals one problem for points that are close to the edge of D. The summation excludes pairs of points for which the second point is outside of D and thus is unobservable. Therefore, we need some edge-correction. Let us consider a circle centered on point $\mathbf{x}_i$, passing through point $\mathbf{x}_j$. Let w_{ij} be the proportion of the circumference of the circle that lies within D, i.e., this represents the conditional probability that a point is observed in D, given that it is within distance r_{ij} from the ith point. Therefore, an edge-corrected estimator of $K(r)$ is

$$\hat{K}(r) = \frac{A}{n^2} \sum_{i,j;i \neq j} \frac{\boldsymbol{I}_{(r_{ij} \in [0,r])}}{w_{ij}}.$$

An edge-corrected estimator of $L(r)$ can be obtained as $\hat{L}(r) = \sqrt{\hat{K}(r)/\pi}$ (or $\hat{\tilde{L}}(r) = \sqrt{\hat{K}(r)/\pi} - r$).

A graphical assessment for CSR is to plot $\hat{L}(r)$ (or $\hat{\tilde{L}}(r)$) versus r. Any major departure from a straight line at distance r_0 then indicates clustering (if above the straight line) or regularity (if below the straight line), respectively. Apparently, an empirical plot based on observed point locations will rarely produce a straight line, even if the observed pattern originates from a homogeneous Poisson process. Therefore, we work with simulation envelopes of the assumed process.

To produce simulation envelopes, we simulate the assumed point process s times, say 100 times, in our examples. At each distance r, the minimum, average, and maximum, i.e., $l(r) = \min_{i=1,\dots,s} \hat{L}_i(r)$, $a(r) = \operatorname*{avg}_{i=1,\dots,s} \hat{L}_i(r)$, and $u(r) = \max_{i=1,\dots,s} \hat{L}_i(r)$ are calculated, where $\hat{L}_i(r)$ is the estimate of $L(r)$ in the ith simulation run. We call $l(r)$ and $u(r)$ the lower and upper simulation envelopes of the simulated process. If we treat $\hat{L}(r)$ as a random variable, then we can approximate that

$$P(\hat{L}(r) > u(r)) = P(\hat{L}(r) < l(r)) = \frac{1}{s+1}.$$

Thus, for $s = 100$ independent simulation runs, we obtain a two-sided test at the approximate 2% significance level that rejects the null hypothesis of CSR if the observed $\hat{L}(r)$ falls above the upper or below the lower simulation envelope at some distance r.

We first make $s = 100$ independent simulation runs of a Poisson process with $n = 71$ observations that inhibit the same spatial domain as the original data. We draw the result of the first simulation run in the upper center plot in Figure 15.6. It is expected that for a Poisson process, we visually get the impression that points are clustered in some sub-areas of D while other sub-areas of D only contain few points.

The upper right plot in Figure 15.6 shows the lower and upper simulation envelopes as well as the average of the $s = 100$ simulation runs. The observed $\hat{L}(r)$ for the `pines.dat` dataset (the solid black line) falls below the lower simulation envelope for distances $r \in [0.7, 1.2]$ approximately. This means, our observed process is significantly different from a homogeneous Poisson process. Instead, we have some regularity for distances from around 0.7 to 1.2 meters.

Common departures from CSR towards clustering processes, such as heterogeneous Poisson processes, Cox processes, and Poisson cluster processes, can be found in the previously cited literature on spatial point patterns. Here, we take a closer look at two processes that are used as models for regularity, i.e., Strauss processes and sequential spatial inhibition processes.

Many regular point patterns can be described by simple inhibition rules. For example, the cell centers of animal cells cannot be located closer than the diameter of the cells, or two plants in close proximity are less likely to survive and grow to maximum height (although this is not impossible) than plants that are further apart. A general class of spatial point patterns that describes such processes are Markov point processes. A subclass of such processes are pairwise interaction point processes with Strauss processes as special cases.

In a Strauss process, points in D that are less than some distance $R > 0$ apart are called neighbors. The joint density function for n point locations $\mathbf{x}_1, \ldots, \mathbf{x}_n \in D$ which contains m distinct pairs of neighbors is specified as

$$f(\mathbf{x}_1, \ldots, \mathbf{x}_n) = ab^n c^m,$$

where $a > 0$ is a normalizing constant, $b > 0$ reflects the intensity of the process, and c with $0 \leq c \leq 1$ describes the interactions between neighbors. Special cases for c are $c = 1$ which gives a homogeneous Poisson process with intensity b and $c = 0$ which results in a simple inhibition process that contains no events at a distance less than or equal to R. All other cases with $0 < c < 1$ represent some form of regularity. The smaller c and the larger m, the less likely it becomes that another point occurs in proximity to these n points.

In the plots in the middle row of Figure 15.6, we consider two Strauss processes as possible alternatives to CSR. The middle left plot shows one simulation run of a Strauss process with $R = 0.7$ (i.e., the distance at which regularity starts based on the CSR simulation envelopes) and $c = 0.15$. In the middle center plot, we show the lower and upper simulation envelopes as well as the average of the $s = 100$ simulation runs of a Strauss process with these parameters. In the middle right plot, we show the lower and upper simulation envelopes as well as the average of the $s = 100$ simulation runs of another Strauss process with $R = 0.7$ and $c = 0.2$. In both plots, the observed $\hat{L}(r)$ for the pines.dat dataset (the solid black line) falls within the lower and upper simulation envelopes of these Strauss processes. Thus, both of these Strauss processes are possible models for the observed point pattern.

Just for illustrative purposes, we also look at $s = 100$ simulation runs of Matern's sequential spatial inhibition (SSI) process in the bottom row of Figure 15.6. The bottom left plot shows one simulation run of a SSI process that prohibits any two points to occur at a distance less than $R = 0.7$. In the bottom center plot and bottom right plot, we show the lower and upper simulation envelopes as well as the average of the $s = 100$ simulation runs of an SSI process with this parameter. While the observed $\hat{L}(r)$ for the pines.dat dataset (the solid black line) falls within the lower and upper simulation envelopes of this SSI process for larger values of r, say $r > 2$, shown in the bottom right plot, the observed $\hat{L}(r)$ falls clearly above the upper simulation envelope of this SSI process. This means that a process that requires a minimum distance of $R = 0.7$ between any two points is not a valid model for the observed point pattern. Pine saplings are less likely (than what we would expect under CSR) to occur in proximity of $R = 0.7$ meters or less, but it is not impossible for them to occur in such a close proximity.

15.4 Discussion

In this chapter, we have discussed some basic methods for the analysis of spatial data, in particular for the analysis of geostatistical data and for spatial point patterns. Each of the figures has been produced in XploRe, using quantlets from the XploRe quantlib spatial. A quick glance at the literature introduced in Section 15.1 reveals that the methods discussed here represent only a small fraction of the methods commonly used for spatial data. However, many additional methods can be directly implemented in XploRe as they only require linear algebra and matrix operations. Additional point processes can be simulated by following simple rules. In fact, Symanzik et al. (1998) provided examples of additional user-written spatial functions in XploRe for the analysis of spatial data. Thus, this chapter hopefully has provided some insights how to conduct an analysis of spatial data within XploRe.

15.5 Acknowledgements

Symanzik's work was partially supported by the Deutsche Forschungsgemeinschaft, Sonderforschungsbereich 373 "Quantifikation und Simulation ökonomischer Prozesse", Humboldt-Universität zu Berlin, Germany. Thanks are due to Anton Andriyashin, William B. Morphet, and Qian Zhao for their helpful comments on a late draft of this chapter.

Bibliography

Bailey, T. C. and Gatrell, A. C. (1995). *Interactive Spatial Data Analysis*, Longman/Wiley, Burnt Mill, UK/New York, NY.

Cressie, N. A. C. (1993). *Statistics for Spatial Data (Revised Edition)*, Wiley, New York, NY.

Davis, J. C. (1973). *Statistics and Data Analysis in Geology*, Wiley, New York, NY.

Diggle, P. J. (2003). *Statistical Analysis of Spatial Point Patterns (Second Edition)*, Arnold/Oxford University Press, London/New York, NY.

Isaaks, E. H. and Srivastava, R. M. (1989). *An Introduction to Applied Geostatistics*, Oxford University Press, New York, NY.

Ripley, B. D. (1981). *Spatial Statistics*, Wiley, New York, NY.

Strand, L. (1972). A Model for Stand Growth, *IUFRO Third Conference Advisory Group of Forest Statisticians*, Institut National de la Recherche Agronomique (INRA), Paris, 207–216.

Symanzik, J., Kötter, T., Schmelzer, S., Klinke, S., Cook, D. and Swayne, D. F. (1998). Spatial Data Analysis in the Dynamically Linked Arc-View/XGobi/XploRe Environment, *Computing Science and Statistics*, 29(1):561–569.

Venables, W. N. and Ripley, B. D. (1999). *Modern Applied Statistics with S-Plus (Third Edition)*, Springer, New York, NY.

Wackernagel, H. (1998). *Multivariate Geostatistics (Second, Completely Revised Edition)*, Springer, Berlin.

16 Functional Data Analysis

Michal Benko

In many different fields of applied statistics the object of interest is depending on some continuous parameter, i.e. continuous time. Typical examples in biostatistics are growth curves or temperature measurements. Although for technical reasons, we are able to measure temperature just in discrete intervals – it is clear that temperature is a continuous process. Temperature during one year is a function with argument "time". By collecting one-year-temperature functions for several years or for different weather stations we obtain bunch (sample) of functions – *functional data set*. The questions arising by the statistical analysis of functional data are basically identical to the standard statistical analysis of univariate or multivariate objects. From the theoretical point, design of a stochastic model for functional data and statistical analysis of the functional data set can be taken often one-to-one from the conventional multivariate analysis. In fact the first method how to deal with the functional data is to discretize them and perform a standard multivariate analysis on the resulting random vectors. The aim of this chapter is to introduce the functional data analysis (FDA), discuss the practical usage and implementation of the FDA methods.

This chapter is organized as follows: Section 16.1 defines the basic mathematical and statistical framework for the FDA, Section 16.2 introduces the most popular implementation of functional data analysis – the functional basis expansion. In Section 16.4 we present the basic theory of the functional principal components, smoothed functional principal components and a practical application on the temperature data set of the Canadian Weather-stations.

16.1 Introduction

In the traditional multivariate framework the random objects are modeled through a T-dimensional random vector X. More formally a random vector is a measurable function $X : (\Omega, \mathcal{A}, P) \to (\mathbb{R}^T, \mathcal{B}^T)$, that maps a probability space $(\Omega, \mathcal{A}, P)$ on the real measurable space $(\mathbb{R}^T, \mathcal{B}^T)$, where $\mathcal{B}^T$ are the

Borel sets on $\mathbb{R}^T$. Observing N realizations of X we analyze the random vector X using the data set

$$\mathcal{X}_M \stackrel{\text{def}}{=} \{x_{i1}, x_{i2} \ldots x_{iT}, i = 1, \ldots, N\}.$$

In the functional data framework, objects are typically modeled as realizations of a stochastic process $X(t)$, $t \in J$, where J is a bounded interval in $\mathbb{R}$. Thus, the set of functions

$$\mathcal{X}_f \stackrel{\text{def}}{=} \{x_i(t), \; i = 1, 2, \ldots N, \; t \in J\}$$

represents the data set. More formally, the random function X in the functional data framework is modelled as a measurable function mapping $(\Omega, \mathcal{A}, \mathcal{P})$ into $(\mathcal{H}, \mathcal{B}_{\mathcal{H}})$, where $\mathcal{B}_{\mathcal{H}}$ is a Borel field on the functional Hilbert space $\mathcal{H}$.

We will mainly work with functional Hilbert space $L^2(J)$ with standard L^2 scalar product defined by

$$\langle f, g \rangle \stackrel{\text{def}}{=} \int_J f(t)g(t)dt, \text{ for } \forall f, g \in L^2(J). \tag{16.1}$$

The corresponding $L^2(J)$ norm is determined by the scalar product (16.1) by $\|f\| \stackrel{\text{def}}{=} \langle f, f \rangle^{1/2}$.

Moreover assume the existence of the mean, variance, covariance and functions of X, and denote these by $EX(t)$, $Var_X(t)$, $Cov_X(s,t)$ and $Corr_X(s,t)$ respectively:

$$Var_X(t) \stackrel{\text{def}}{=} E\{X(t) - EX(t)\}^2, \; t \in J,$$
$$Cov_X(s,t) \stackrel{\text{def}}{=} E\{X(s) - EX(s)\}\{X(t) - EX(t)\}, \; s, t \in J,$$
$$Corr_X(s,t) \stackrel{\text{def}}{=} \frac{Cov_X(s,t)}{\sqrt{Var_X(s) \, Var_X(t)}}.$$

Note that the $Corr_X(s,t)$ is defined under the assumption $Var_X(s)$, $Var_X(t) > 0$.

For the functional sample $x_i(t)$, $i = 1, \ldots N$ we can define the estimators of

$EX(t)$, $Var_X(t)$, $Cov_X(s,t)$ and $Corr_X(s,t)$ in a straightforward way:

$$\bar{x}(t) \;=\; \tfrac{1}{N} \sum_{i=1}^{N} x_i(t),$$

$$\widehat{Var}_X(t) \;=\; \tfrac{1}{N-1} \sum_{i=1}^{N} \{x_i(t) - \bar{x}(t)\}^2,$$

$$\widehat{Cov}_X(s,t) \;=\; \tfrac{1}{N-1} \sum_{i=1}^{N} \{x_i(s) - \bar{x}(s)\}\{x_i(t) - \bar{x}(t)\}.$$

$$\widehat{Corr}_X(s,t) \;=\; \frac{\widehat{Cov}_X(s,t)}{\sqrt{\widehat{Var}_X(s)\,\widehat{Var}_X(t)}}.$$

Dauxois, Pousse and Romain (1982) show that

$$\|Cov_X(s,t) - \widehat{Cov}_X(s,t)\| \to 0, \text{ with probability one.}$$

16.2   Functional Basis Expansion

In the previous section, we have presented the problem of statistical analysis of random functions. As we will see, from a theoretical point of view, the multivariate statistical concepts can be often introduced into the functional data analysis easily. However, in practice we are interested in the implementation of these techniques in fast computer algorithms, where a certain finite-dimensional representation of the analyzed functions is needed.

A popular way of FDA-implementation is to use a truncated functional basis expansion. More precisely, let us denote a functional basis on the interval J by $\{\theta_1, \theta_2, \dots, \}$ and assume that the functions x_i are approximated "well" by the first L basis functions θ_l, $l = 1, 2, \dots L$

$$x_i(t) = \sum_{l=1}^{L} c_{il}\theta_l(t) = \mathbf{c}_i^\top \boldsymbol{\theta}(t), \tag{16.2}$$

where $\boldsymbol{\theta} = (\theta_1, \dots, \theta_L)^\top$ and $\mathbf{c}_i = (c_{i1}, \dots, c_{iL})^\top$. The first equal sign in (16.2) is not formally adequate – in practice we are just approximating the x_i. However, in order to keep the notation simple we will neglect this difference between the real $x_i(t)$ and its approximation.

In practice, the analysis of the functional objects will be implemented through the coefficient matrix

$$\mathbf{C} = \{c_{il},\; i = 1, \dots, N,\; l = 1, \dots, L\},$$

e.g. the mean, variance, covariance and correlation functions can be approximated by:

$$
\begin{aligned}
\bar{x}(t) &= \bar{\mathbf{c}}^\top \boldsymbol{\theta}(t), \\
\widehat{Var}_X(t) &= \boldsymbol{\theta}(t)^\top Cov(\mathbf{C})\boldsymbol{\theta}(t), \\
\widehat{Cov}_X(s,t) &= \boldsymbol{\theta}(s)^\top Cov(\mathbf{C})\boldsymbol{\theta}(t), \\
\widehat{Corr}_X(s,t) &= \frac{\widehat{Cov}_X(s,t)}{\left\{\widehat{Var}_X(t)\,\widehat{Var}_X(s)\right\}^{1/2}}
\end{aligned}
$$

where $\bar{\mathbf{c}}_l \overset{def}{=} \frac{1}{N} \sum_{i=1}^{N} c_{il},\ l = 1, \ldots, L,\ Cov(\mathbf{C}) \overset{def}{=} \frac{1}{N-1} \sum_{i=1}^{N} (\mathbf{c}_i - \bar{\mathbf{c}})(\mathbf{c}_i - \bar{\mathbf{c}})^\top.$
The scalar product of two functions corresponds to:

$$
\langle x_i, x_j \rangle \overset{def}{=} \int_J x_i(t)x_j(t)dt = \mathbf{c}_i^\top \mathbf{W} \mathbf{c}_j,
$$

where

$$
\mathbf{W} \overset{def}{=} \int_J \boldsymbol{\theta}(t)\boldsymbol{\theta}(t)^\top dt. \tag{16.3}
$$

There are three prominent examples of functional bases: Fourier, Polynomial and B-Spline basis.

16.2.1 Fourier Basis

A well known basis for periodic functions on the interval J is the Fourier basis, defined on J by

$$
\theta_l(t) = \left\{
\begin{array}{ll}
1, & l = 0 \\
\sin(r\omega t), & l = 2r - 1 \\
\cos(r\omega t), & l = 2r
\end{array}
\right.
$$

where ω is so called frequency, determines the period and the length of the interval $|J| = 2\pi/\omega$. The Fourier basis defined above can easily be transformed to an orthonormal basis, hence the scalar-product matrix in (16.3) is simply the identity matrix. The popularity of this basis is based partially on the possibility of fast coefficient calculation by the Fast Fourier Transformation (FFT) Algorithm. In XploRe one can use the quantlet **Fourierevalgd** for general case or the quantlet **fft** that performs the FFT Algorithm for the equidistant design.

16.2.2 Polynomial Basis

The polynomial basis, appropriate for non-periodic functions is defined by

$$\theta_l(t) = (t - w)^k, k = 0, 1, \ldots, L - 1$$

where w is a shift parameter. The polynomial (or monomial) functions are easy to calculate for example by a simple recursion. However, the higher order polynomials become too fluctuating especially in the boundaries of J. In XploRe one can use the quantlet `polyevalgd`.

16.2.3 B-Spline Basis

A very popular functional basis for non-periodic data is the B-Spline basis. This basis is defined by the sequence of knots on the interval J and is roughly speaking a basis for piecewise polynomial functions of order K smoothly connected in the knots. More formally, the basis functions are

$$\theta_l(t) = B_{l,K}(t), l = 1, \ldots, m + k - 2 \tag{16.4}$$

where $B_{l,K}$ is l-th B-Spline of order K, for the non-decreasing sequence of knots $\{\tau_i\}_{i=1}^m$ defined by following recursion scheme:

$$B_{i,1}(t) = \begin{cases} 1, & \text{for } t \in [\tau_i, \tau_{i+1}] \\ 0, & \text{otherwise} \end{cases}$$

$$B_{i,k}(t) = \frac{t - \tau_i}{\tau_{i+k-1} - \tau_i} B_{i,k-1}(t) + \frac{\tau_{i+k} - t}{\tau_{i+k} - \tau_{i+1}} B_{i+1,k-1}(t)$$

for $i = 1, \ldots, m + k$, $k = 0, \ldots, K$. The number of the basis function will uniquely be defined by the B-spline order and the number of knots. The advantage of the B-spline basis is its flexibility, relatively easy evaluation of the basis functions and their derivatives. In XploRe one can use the quantlet `Bsplineevalgd`.

The detailed discussion of the implementation of the B-spline basis expansion in XploRe can be found in Ulbricht (2004).

16.2.4 Data Set as Basis

Let us briefly discuss an interesting special case – the use of the functions $x_i(t), i = 1, \ldots, N$ themselves as the basis. This directly implies that the coefficient matrix $\mathbf{C}$ is the identity matrix. Information about the data set $\mathcal{X}_f$ is "stored" in the matrix $\mathbf{W}$.

As we will show in next sections this case has an direct application in practice, despite its pathological first-sight impression.

16.3 Approximation and Coefficient Estimation

In practice, we observe the function values

$$\mathcal{X} = \{x_i(t_{i1}), x_i(t_{i2}), \ldots, x_i(t_{iT_i}), \ i = 1, \ldots, N\}$$

only on a discrete grid $\{t_{i1}, t_{i2}, \ldots, t_{iT_i}\} \in J$, where T_i are the numbers of design points for the i-th observation. In this case we may approximate the function $x_i(t)$ by functions $\theta_l(t), l = 1, \ldots L$ by minimizing some loss function, e.g. sum of squares. This approach is known as the least squares approximation. In case of using the data set as basis we need to approximate integrals $\int x_l(t)x_k(t)dt$ by some numerical integration techniques.

A slightly different setup occurs if we assume that the data set is contaminated by some additive noise. A standard statistical approach is to assume that the data set consist of $\mathcal{X}_\varepsilon \overset{\text{def}}{=} \{Y_{ij}, j = 1, \ldots, T_i, \ i = 1, \ldots, N\}$, where

$$Y_{ij} = x_i(t_{ij}) + \varepsilon_{ij} \tag{16.5}$$

and ε_{ij} is the realization of a random variable with zero mean and variance function $\sigma_i^2(t)$, i.e. we are faced with the N regression problems. The estimated coefficient matrix $\mathbf{C}$ can be obtained by minimizing an appropriate loss function. The method of regularization by the roughness penalty can be applied. Defining the roughness penalty as the norm of an operator on the (Hilbert) space $\mathcal{H}$, $R \overset{\text{def}}{=} \| \mathcal{L} \|^2$, $\mathcal{L} \in \mathcal{H}^*$ we will minimize:

$$\sum_{j=1}^{T_i} \left\{ Y_{ij} - \mathbf{c_i}^\top \boldsymbol{\theta}(t_{ij}) \right\}^2 + \alpha \parallel \mathcal{L}(\mathbf{c_i}^\top \boldsymbol{\theta}) \parallel^2 \tag{16.6}$$

where α is a parameter controlling the degree of penalization. Clearly $\alpha = 0$ yields the least square regression. A popular example of the roughness penalty is $\mathcal{L} = \mathcal{D}^2$ where we penalize nonlinearity of the estimated function $\mathbf{c_i}^\top \boldsymbol{\theta}$. A more general approach assumes $\mathcal{L}$ is a linear differential operator, i.e. $\mathcal{L} = a_1 \mathcal{D}^1 + a_2 \mathcal{D}^2 + \ldots + a_P \mathcal{D}^P$. The proper choice of the operator should have background in some additional information about the underlying function. Assume for example that $x_i \in \mathcal{V}, \mathcal{V} \subset \mathcal{H}$, then we should try to find an operator $\mathcal{L}$ so that $\text{Ker}(\mathcal{L}) = \mathcal{V}$. Doing so we will penalize the coefficients that yield functions $\hat{x}_i = \mathbf{c_i}^\top \boldsymbol{\theta} \notin \mathcal{V}$.

Clearly, we can write $\mathcal{L}(\mathbf{c_i}^\top \boldsymbol{\theta}) = \mathbf{c_i}^\top \mathcal{L}(\boldsymbol{\theta})$, hence for implementation we only need to be able to calculate the function $\mathcal{L}(\theta_l)$.

Note that in the standard FDA setup, one assumes that the functions x_i are observed without additional error. This assumption is often violated in practice. Again in order to keep notation simple we will neglect the difference between the estimated and real coefficients. We can do so if we assume that the additional noise is of smaller order in compare to the variation of the functions x_i. However, from a statistical point of view we should keep this difference in mind.

One important question of practitioners is how many functions should be used in the basis expansion. Although, as stated by Ramsay and Silverman (1997), even a subjective selection of the smoothing parameter leads usually to the reasonable choice, from a statistical point of view the automated (data driven selection) is needed. In the simplest case of e.g. Fourier basis without using additional regularization we need to set just the L. This can be done easily by Cross-Validation, Generalized Cross Validation or other similar criteria described in Härdle (1990) among others. Much more complicated is the case of B-splines – in practice we need to choose the knots sequence in addition to the number of functions. In some special applications the choice of knot points is naturally given by the underlying problem. One practical rule of thumb can be a good starting point: set at least 3 knots in the neighborhood of the "interesting" point of the function, e.g. around expected extreme-point or another change in the function.

An alternative approach may be applied in case we have additional information about the function of interest transformed into the roughness penalty $\| \mathcal{L} \|$.

The algorithm is as follows:

1. Use a "nested" model for the data set, i.e. use $L \approx$ number of observations. Using this basis directly would lead to a highly volatile estimator with a small (zero) bias.

2. Transform additional information about the function into the kernel of some appropriate linear differential operator.

3. Use the roughness penalty approach and estimate "smoothed" coefficients vector $\mathbf{c}_i$.

For the cubic B-splines basis, the first step corresponds to setting the knots into each design point. If we set $\mathcal{L} = \mathcal{D}^2$, we in fact penalize nonlinear functions, and obtain a special case of the very popular nonparametric technique – smoothing splines. In the third step of the algorithm we might easily set the smoothing parameter by Cross-Validation (CV) or Generalized Cross-Validation (GCV), for details see Hastie, et al (2002). This method is fully data driven for a given operator $\mathcal{L}$.

16.3.1   Software Implementation

Software implementation This paragraph gives just brief insight into the philosophy of the FDA-implementation, deeper discussion can be found in Ulbricht (2004) and Benko (2004). The implementation presented here is designed for Statistical environment XploRe, similar packages for R and Matlab can be found in Ramsay (2003).

We implemented in XploRe general functional basis as a list object `basisfd` with following elements:

> `fbname` – string, the name of the functional basis, supported are: `Fourier, Polynomial, Bspline`, that are mentioned above
>
> `range` – vector of two elements, range of interval J
>
> `param` – abstract set of elements, functional basis specific parameters that uniquely determine the functional basis `fbname`
>
> `W` – optional parameter, the scalar product matrix $\mathbf{W}$
>
> `penmat` – optional parameter, the penalty matrix

A functional object `fd` is similarly a list containing:

> `basisfd` – object of type functional basis
>
> `coef` – array of coefficients

These two objects can be created by following two quantlets: `createfdbasis` (fbname, range, param) that creates the fdbasis object, on the interval [`range[1]`,`range[2]`] using parameters `param` and `data2fd` (y, argvals, basisfd, Lfd, W, lambda) that converts an array y of function values, or penalized regression with `Lfd` and `lambda` observed on an array `argvals` of argument values into a functional data object. The statistical functions operating on these objects will be presented in the following text on the simple Temperature data set. In addition one can use XploRe help system (APSS) for further reference.

16.3.2   Temperature Example

In this section we want to analyze a data set containing 35 weather stations in Canada, listed in the Table 16.3.2.

Table 16.1: Names of the Canadian weather stations

Arvida	Bagottvi	Calgary	Charlott	Churchil	Dawson
Edmonton	Frederic	Halifax	Inuvik	Iqaluit	Kamloops
London	Montreal	Ottawa	Princeal	Princege	Princeru
Quebec	Regina	Resolute	Scheffer	Sherbroo	Stjohns
Sydney	Thepas	Thunderb	Toronto	Uraniumc	Vancouvr
Victoria	Whitehor	Winnipeg	Yarmouth	Yellowkn	

This data set is taken from Ramsay and Silverman (1997), the data with the description can be found in the online database MD*Base. We choose this example as a "guinea pig" data set that illustrates the defined concepts and the use of the implemented quantlets and gives the possibilities of comparison.

Due to the cyclical behavior of the temperature during years it is usual in comparable studies to assume the temperature functions to be periodic. Thus we may employ the Fourier basis functions.

Figure 16.1 shows estimated temperature functions using 31 Fourier functions.

For our Temperature data set we obtained the following functions that correspond to the basic statics in multivariate framework:

Looking at the functions in the Figures 16.2 and 16.4 we observe the mean function with a bump in the summer, which is not surprising – temperatures are higher in summer than in winter. Another fact may be, however, not so expected: in the winter we can observe higher variance than in the summer. This fact can possibly be explained by the higher impact of the geographical differences on the winter temperature than on the summer temperature. Looking at the correlation function, plotted in the Figure 16.4 we can see that the autumn temperatures seems to be higher correlated with the spring temperatures than winter and summer temperatures.

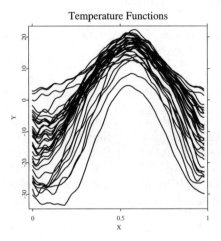

Figure 16.1: Example of functional data, temperatures measured by Canadian weather stations listed in the Table 16.3.2.

XCSfdaTempf.xpl

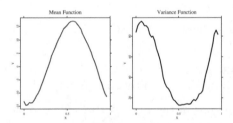

Figure 16.2: Mean and variance function (temperature).

XCSfdaMeanVar.xpl

16.4   Functional Principal Components

Principal Components Analysis (PCA) yields dimension reduction in the multivariate framework. The idea is to find the normalized weight vectors $\gamma_m \in \mathbb{R}^T$ for which the linear transformations of a T-dimensional random

Covariance Surface

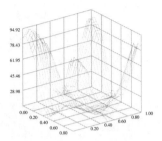

Figure 16.3: Covariance function (temperature). The plotted surface is the linear interpolation of grid on $[0, 1]$ and step $1/30$.

Q XCSfdaCov.xpl

vector **x**:

$$\beta_m = \gamma_m^\top(\mathbf{x} - E\mathbf{x}) = \langle \gamma_m, \mathbf{x} - E\mathbf{x} \rangle, \ m = 1, \dots, T, \qquad (16.7)$$

have maximal variance subject to:

$$\gamma_l^\top \gamma_m = \langle \gamma_l, \gamma_m \rangle = \boldsymbol{I}(l = m) \text{ for } l \leq m.$$

The problem is solved by the means of the Jordan spectral decomposition of the covariance matrix, Härdle and Simar (2003), p. 63.

In Functional Principal Components Analysis (FPCA) the dimension reduction can be achieved via the same route: Find orthonormal weight functions $\gamma_1, \gamma_2, \dots$, such that the variance of the linear transformation is maximal.

The weight functions satisfy:

$$||\gamma_m||^2 = \int \gamma_m(t)^2 dt = 1,$$

$$\langle \gamma_l, \gamma_m \rangle = \int \gamma_l(t)\gamma_m(t)dt = 0, \ l \neq m.$$

Corr. Surface

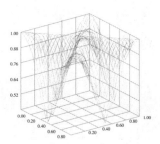

Figure 16.4: Correlation function (temperature). The plotted surface is the
linear interpolation of grid on $[0,1]$ and step $1/30$.

XCSfdaCorr.xpl

The linear combination is:

$$\beta_m = \langle \gamma_m, X - \mathbf{E}X \rangle = \int \gamma_m(t)\{X(t) - \mathbf{E}X(t)\}dt, \qquad (16.8)$$

and the desired weight functions solve:

$$\underset{\langle \gamma_l, \gamma_m \rangle = \mathbf{I}(l=m), l \leq m}{\arg \max} Var \langle \gamma_m, X \rangle, \qquad (16.9)$$

or equivalently:

$$\underset{\langle \gamma_l, \gamma_m \rangle = \mathbf{I}(l=m), l \leq m}{\arg \max} \int \int \gamma_m(s) \, Cov(s,t)\gamma_m(t)dsdt.$$

The solution is obtained by solving the Fredholm functional eigenequation

$$\int Cov(s,t)\gamma(t)dt = \lambda\gamma(s). \qquad (16.10)$$

The eigenfunctions $\gamma_1, \gamma_2, \ldots$, sorted with respect to the corresponding eigenvalues $\lambda_1 \geq \lambda_2 \geq \ldots$ solve the FPCA problem (16.9). The following link

between eigenvalues and eigenfunctions holds:

$$\lambda_m = Var(\beta_m) \quad = \quad Var\left[\int \gamma_m(t)\{X(t) - \mathrm{E}X(t)\}dt\right] =$$

$$= \int\int \gamma_m(s)\ Cov(s,t)\gamma_m(t)dsdt.$$

In the sampling problem, the unknown covariance function $Cov(s,t)$ needs to be replaced by the sample covariance function $\widehat{Cov}(s,t)$. Dauxois, Pousse and Romain (1982) show that the eigenfunctions and eigenvalues are consistent estimators for λ_m and γ_m and derive some asymptotic results for these estimators.

16.4.1 Implementation

In this section we will present three possibilities of implementation of the functional PCA. We will start with a simple discretization technique. In the second step we will focus more on the implementation by the basis expansion, including the application on the temperature data set.

Discretization

One possibility of calculating the functional PCA is simply to perform the multivariate PCA on a dense grid $\{t_1,\ldots,t_T\}$, obtain the eigenvectors $(\widehat{\gamma}_j(t_i),\ i = 1,\ldots,T)^\top$ for $j = 1,\ldots,r$ and estimate the coefficients of eigenvectors $b_1,\ldots,b_r$. The implementation is very simple since the routines of the multivariate PCA or matrix spectral analysis are needed. However, in the next section we will present a implementation method that corresponds more to the functional nature of the underlying problem. Secondly, the estimated eigenfunctions are not necessarily orthonormal in the functional sense, due to the dependence of the integrals on the length of the interval and of the vector scalar product of the discretized functions on the number of discretization points T . Thus an additional correction is needed. A simple way is to orthonormalize the coefficient with respect to the matrix $\mathbf{W}$ using Gramm-Schmidt procedure.

Basis Expansion

Suppose that the weight function γ has the expansion

$$\gamma = \sum_{l=1}^{L} \mathbf{b}_l \theta_l = \boldsymbol{\theta}^\top \mathbf{b}.$$

Using this notation we can rewrite the left hand side of eigenequation (16.10):

$$\begin{aligned} \int Cov(s,t)\gamma(t)dt &= \int \boldsymbol{\theta}(s)^\top Cov(\mathbf{C})\boldsymbol{\theta}(t)\boldsymbol{\theta}(t)^\top \mathbf{b}\,dt \\ &= \boldsymbol{\theta}^\top Cov(\mathbf{C})\mathbf{W}\mathbf{b}, \end{aligned}$$

so that:

$$Cov(\mathbf{C})\mathbf{W}\mathbf{b} = \lambda \mathbf{b}.$$

The functional scalar product $\langle \gamma_l, \gamma_k \rangle$ corresponds to $\mathbf{b}_l^\top \mathbf{W} \mathbf{b}_k$ in the truncated basis framework, in the sense that if two functions γ_l and γ_k are orthogonal, the corresponding coefficient vectors $\mathbf{b}_l, \mathbf{b}_k$ satisfy $\mathbf{b}_l^\top \mathbf{W} \mathbf{b}_k = 0$. Matrix $\mathbf{W}$ is symmetric by definition, thus, defining $\mathbf{u} = \mathbf{W}^{1/2}\mathbf{b}$, one needs to solve finally a symmetric eigenvalue problem:

$$\mathbf{W}^{1/2} Cov(\mathbf{C})\mathbf{W}^{1/2}\mathbf{u} = \lambda \mathbf{u},$$

and to compute the inverse transformation $\mathbf{b} = \mathbf{W}^{-1/2}\mathbf{u}$. For the orthonormal functional basis (i.e. also for Fourier basis) $\mathbf{W} = \mathbf{I}$, i.e. the problem of FPCA is reduced to the multivariate PCA performed on the matrix $\mathbf{C}$.

Algorithm

1. calculate $\mathbf{C}$ and $\mathbf{W}$

2. using Cholesky decomposition calculate $\mathbf{W}^{1/2}$

3. use symmetric matrix eigenvalue routine and obtain eigenvalues and eigenvectors ($\mathbf{u}$) of $\mathbf{W}^{1/2} Cov(\mathbf{C})\mathbf{W}^{1/2}$

4. calculate $\mathbf{b} = \mathbf{W}^{-1/2}\mathbf{u}$

Notice: The estimated coefficient of eigenfunctions are orthonormal with respect to the scalar product $\mathbf{b}_i^\top \mathbf{W} \mathbf{b}_j$, however, numerical errors can cause small deviances.

16.4.2 Data Set as Basis

As announced in the previous section, if we use the data set $\mathcal{X}_f$ as the basis we need to estimate the matrix $\mathbf{W}$ rather than the coefficient matrix $\mathbf{C}$. We will show how to use this concept in the functional principal components analysis.

Estimation procedure is based on the Karhunen-Loèvy decomposition – we use eigenfunctions as factor functions in the model of following type:

$$x_i = \bar{x} + \sum_{j=1}^{K} \beta_{ij} \gamma_j, \tag{16.11}$$

recall, $\bar{x}$ is the sample mean, $\bar{x} = 1/N \sum_{i=1}^{N} x_i$. The K is the number of nonzero eigenvalues of the (empirical) covariance operator.

$$\mathcal{C}_N(\xi) = \frac{1}{N} \sum_{i=1}^{N} \langle x_i - \bar{x}, \xi \rangle (x_i - \bar{x}) \tag{16.12}$$

This is the sample version of the covariance operator used in (16.10), compare also with definition of $\widehat{\mathrm{Cov}}_X$. Let us denote the eigenvalues, eigenvectors of $\mathcal{C}_N$ by $\lambda_1^{\mathcal{C}_N}, \lambda_2^{\mathcal{C}_N} \ldots, \gamma_1^{\mathcal{C}_N}, \gamma_2^{\mathcal{C}_N} \ldots$, and the principal scores $\beta_{ir}^{\mathcal{C}_N} \stackrel{\text{def}}{=} \langle \gamma_r^{\mathcal{C}_N}, x_i - \bar{x} \rangle$.

Using this notation model (16.11) is based on the known fact, that the first L eigenfunctions of the empirical covariance operator, ordered by the corresponding eigenvalues, construct the "best empirical basis" in the integrated square error sense, i.e. the residual integrated square error:

$$\rho(m_1, \ldots, m_L) = \sum_{i=1}^{N} \| x_i - \bar{x} - \sum_{j=1}^{L} \beta_{ij} m_j(t) \|^2 \tag{16.13}$$

is minimized with respect to all L orthogonal functions $m_j \in L^2$, $j = 1, \ldots, L$ by setting $m_j(t) \equiv \gamma_j^{\mathcal{C}_N}(t), t \in J$. In the estimation procedure, we follow the idea of Kneip and Utikal (2001), introduced for the case where $x_i(t)$ is a density function. Instead of estimating the eigenfunction $\gamma_j^{\mathcal{C}_N}$ by discretization or functional basis expansion of x_i we focus on the spectral analysis of matrix

$$M_{lk} = \langle x_l - \bar{x}, x_k - \bar{x} \rangle. \tag{16.14}$$

This procedure is motivated by the following two facts: firstly all nonzero eigenvalues of the empirical covariance operator $\mathcal{C}_N$ and the eigenvalues of the matrix M denoted by $\lambda_1^M, \lambda_2^M, \ldots$ are related as follows: $\lambda_r^M = N.\lambda_r^{\mathcal{C}_N}$.

Secondly, for the eigenvectors of M denoted by $p_1, p_2, \ldots$ and principal scores $\beta_{jr}^{\mathcal{C}_N}$ holds:

$$\beta_{jr}^{\mathcal{C}_N} = \sqrt{\lambda_r^M} p_{jr} \tag{16.15}$$

and

$$\gamma_r^{\mathcal{C}_N} = \left(\sqrt{\lambda_r^M}\right)^{-1} \sum_{i=1}^{N} p_{ir} (x_i - \bar{x}) = \left(\sqrt{\lambda_r^M}\right)^{-1} \sum_{i=1}^{N} p_{ir} x_i = \frac{\sum_{i=1}^{N} x_i \beta_{ir}^{\mathcal{C}_N}}{\sum_{i=1}^{N} (\beta_{ir}^{\mathcal{C}_N})^2}. \tag{16.16}$$

The estimation procedure follows now in two steps. First we estimate the M by an appropriate estimator $\widehat{M}$ and in the second step we use (16.16) to obtain the estimators $\hat{\beta}_{ir}, \hat{\gamma}_r$ of principal scores and eigenfunctions $\beta_{ir}^{\mathcal{C}_N}, \gamma_r^{\mathcal{C}_N}$.

There are several aspects of this technique that need to be mentioned. First we need to mention that we virtually separate the spectral analysis and move it into the (feature) space of scalar products. On the other hand in the general case of unequal designs the estimation of the scalar products can be complicated. The deeper discussion, for the special case of the density functions can be found in above mentioned Kneip and Utikal (2001), discussion of using this idea in the regression case can be found in Benko and Kneip (2005).

Temperature Example

For our temperature example we obtained the weight functions (eigenfunctions) displayed in the Figure 16.5, using the same setup as in the previous section (31 Fourier functions), with the following variance proportions (eigenvalues):

Table 16.2: Eigenvalues of functional PCA

variance proportions	cum. variance proportions
0.88671	0.88671
0.084837	0.971547
0.019451	0.990998
0.0052221	0.9962201

The first eigenfunction (black curve) explains 89% of variation. The second eigenfunction (blue curve) explains 8% of variation, the third eigenfunction

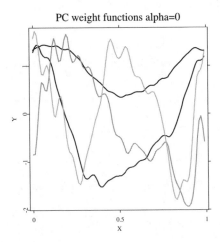

Figure 16.5: Weight functions for temperature data set.

XCSfdaTempPCA.xpl

(green curve) 2% of variation and the fourth function (cyan curve) 0.5% of variation.

However, the eigenfunctions are rough (non-smooth). This roughness is caused by sampling variance or by the observation noise and flexibility of used functional basis. In the Section 16.5 we will discuss the method of smoothing the eigenfunctions in order to get more stable and better interpretable results.

16.5 Smoothed Principal Components Analysis

As we see in the Figure 16.5, the resulting eigenfunctions are often very rough. Smoothing them could result in morex stable and better interpretable results. Here we apply a popular approach known as the roughness penalty. The downside of this technique is that we loose orthogonality in the L^2 sense.

Assume that the underlying eigenfunctions have a continuous and square-integrable second derivative. Recall that $\mathcal{D}\gamma = \gamma'(t)$ is the differential operator and define the roughness penalty by $\Psi(\gamma) = ||\mathcal{D}^2\gamma||^2$. Moreover, suppose that γ_m has square-integrable derivatives up to degree four and that the second and the third derivative satisfy one of the following conditions:

1. $\mathcal{D}^2\gamma$, $\mathcal{D}^3\gamma$ are zero at the ends of the interval J

2. the periodicity boundary conditions of $\gamma, \mathcal{D}\gamma$, $\mathcal{D}^2\gamma$ and $\mathcal{D}^3\gamma$ on J.

Then we can rewrite the roughness penalty in the following way:

$$
\begin{aligned}
||\mathcal{D}^2\gamma||^2 &= \int \mathcal{D}^2\gamma(s)\mathcal{D}^2\gamma(s)ds \\
&= \mathcal{D}\gamma(u)\mathcal{D}^2\gamma(u) - \\
&\quad - \mathcal{D}\gamma(d)\mathcal{D}^2\gamma(d) - \int \mathcal{D}\gamma(s)\mathcal{D}^3\gamma(s)ds & (16.17) \\
&= \gamma(u)\mathcal{D}^3\gamma(u) - \gamma(d)\mathcal{D}^3\gamma(d) - \int \gamma(s)\mathcal{D}^4\gamma(s)ds & (16.18) \\
&= \langle\gamma, \mathcal{D}^4\gamma\rangle, & (16.19)
\end{aligned}
$$

where d and u are the boundaries of the interval J and the first two elements in (16.17) and (16.18) are both zero under both conditions mentioned above.

Given a principal component function γ, with norm $||\gamma||^2 = 1$, we can penalize the sample variance of the principal component by dividing it by $1 + \alpha\langle\gamma, \mathcal{D}^4\gamma\rangle$:

$$
PCAPV = \frac{\int\int \gamma(s)\widehat{Cov}(s,t)\gamma(t)dsdt}{\int \gamma(t)(\mathcal{I} + \alpha\mathcal{D}^4)\gamma(t)dt}, \tag{16.20}
$$

where $\mathcal{I}$ denotes the identity operator. The maximum of the penalized sample variance of the principal component (PCAPV) is an eigenfunction γ corresponding to the largest eigenvalue of the generalized eigenequation:

$$
\int \widehat{Cov}(s,t)\gamma(t)dt = \lambda(\mathcal{I} + \alpha\mathcal{D}^4)\gamma(s). \tag{16.21}
$$

As already mentioned above, the resulting weight functions are no longer orthonormal in the L^2 sense. Since the weight functions are used as smoothed estimators of principal components functions, we need to rescale them to satisfy $||\gamma_l||^2 = 1$. The weight functions γ_l can be interpreted as orthogonal in modified scalar product of the Sobolev type

$$
(f,g) \stackrel{\text{def}}{=} \langle f,g\rangle + \alpha\langle\mathcal{D}^2 f, \mathcal{D}^2 g\rangle.
$$

A more extended theoretical discussion can be found in Silverman (1991).

16.5.1   Implementation Using Basis Expansion

Define $\mathbf{K}$ to be a matrix whose elements are $\langle D^2\theta_j, D^2\theta_k \rangle$. Then the generalized eigenequation (16.21) can be transformed to:

$$\mathbf{W}\,Cov(\mathbf{C})\mathbf{W}\mathbf{u} = \lambda(\mathbf{W} + \alpha\mathbf{K})\mathbf{u}. \tag{16.22}$$

Finding matrix L for that holds: $\mathbf{L}\mathbf{L}^\top = \mathbf{W} + \alpha\mathbf{K}$ and defining $\mathbf{S} = \mathbf{L}^{-1}$ we can rewrite (16.22) into:

$$\{\mathbf{S}\mathbf{W}\,Cov(\mathbf{C})\mathbf{W}\mathbf{S}^\top\}(\mathbf{L}^\top\mathbf{u}) = \lambda\mathbf{L}^\top\mathbf{u}.$$

Algorithm

1. calculate $\mathbf{C}$ and $\mathbf{W}$

2. using Cholesky decomposition calculate $\mathbf{L}$ and their inverse $\mathbf{L}^{-1}$

3. use symmetrical matrix eigenvalue-eigenvector routine and obtain eigenvalues and eigenvectors $(\mathbf{u})$ of $\mathbf{S}\mathbf{W}\,Cov(\mathbf{C})\mathbf{W}\mathbf{S}^\top$

4. calculate $\mathbf{b} = \mathbf{L}^{-1}\mathbf{u}$

5. renormalize $\mathbf{b}$ with respect to matrix $\mathbf{W}$, so that $\mathbf{b}^\top\mathbf{W}\mathbf{b} = 1$

If we are looking at the first K eigenfunctions as the best empirical basis for the functional observations $\mathcal{X}_f$, we may also re-orthonormalize coefficients $\mathbf{b}_j$ with respect to matrix $\mathbf{W}$, using Gramm-Schmidt procedure.

In this section we have presented the case with roughness penalty $\| \mathcal{D}^2\gamma \|$ similarly we could consider a more general case with rougness penalty $\| \mathcal{L}\gamma \|$.

16.5.2   Temperature Example

Performing the idea of Smoothed Functional PCA (SPCA) on the temperature data set, we obtained with the same setup as in previous sections (31 Fourier functions and $\alpha = 10^{-6}$) the weight functions plotted in Figure 16.6. We can observe that the high frequency variance is smoothed out and the interpretation of the eigenfunctions is more obvious.

The first eigenfunction (black curve) can be explained as a weighted level of the temperature over the year with a high weighting of the winter temperatures, this eigenfunction explains 89% of variation. The second eigenfunction

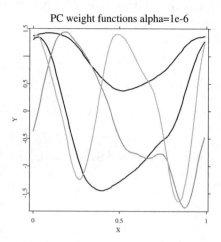

Figure 16.6: Weight functions for temperature data set, using $\alpha = 10^{-6}$ and L=31

Q XCSfdaTempSPCA.xpl

Table 16.3: Eigenvalues of penalized functional PCA

variance proportions	cum. variance proportions
0.88986	0.88986
0.08461	0.97447
0.018512	0.992982
0.0048335	0.9978155

(blue curve) has different signs for winter and summer and explains 8% of variation. The third eigenfunction (green curve) changes the sign in a similar way for autumn and spring and explains 2% of variation and the fourth function (cyan curve) could be explained as changes of seasons and explains 0.5% of variation.

Another possibility of interpreting the result is the plot of the estimated principal scores, sample analogue of β_m:

$$\widehat{\beta}_{im} \stackrel{\text{def}}{=} \langle \widehat{\gamma}_m, x_i - \bar{x} \rangle = \mathbf{b}_m^\top \mathbf{W}(\mathbf{c}_i - \bar{\mathbf{c}})$$

The estimated principal scores are plotted in the Figure 16.7, the abbre-

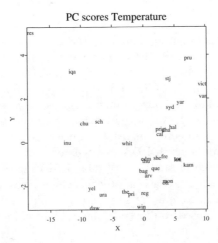

Figure 16.7: Principal scores for temperature data set

XCSfdaTempPCAsc.xpl

viations of the names, listed in Table 16.5.2 have been used (compare with Table 16.3.2).

Table 16.4: Abbreviations of the names of the Canadian weather stations

arv	bag	cal	cha	chu	daw
edm	fre	hal	inu	iqa	kam
lon	mon	ott	pri	prig	pru
que	reg	res	sch	she	stj
syd	the	thu	tor	ura	van
vict	whit	win	yar	yel	

A simple observation is that **res** is a kind of outlier, with high loading of second component. The **res** stands for Resolute, using similar arguments as in Ramsay and Silverman (1997). Resolute is known for having a very cold winter relative (PC1) to the other weather stations but only a small difference between summer and winter temperatures (PC 2). This corresponds to our interpretation of the first two eigenfunctions.

Conclusions

To summarize, the functional data analysis technique described in this chapter takes the functional nature of the observed variable in to account. This approach becomes frequently used especially in biostatistics, chemometrics, enables to use the smoothness of the underlying objects (functions) and "overcomes" the problem of dimensions, in functional sense one observation is just one-dimensional object. The main motivation of this chapter is not to give a extensive overview of theoretical results, rather to give a practical guide to basic descriptive methods in FDA we focus on basic statistics and functional principal components analysis. We mainly discuss the implementation of these techniques functional basis approach. The macros (quantlets) are designed for the statistical computing environment XploRe. A typical example from the biostatistic is used to illustrate the FDA technique.

Bibliography

Benko, M. (2004). Functional Principal Components Analysis, Implementation and Applications, *Master thesis, Statistics*, Humboldt Universität zu Berlin.

Benko, M. and Kneip, A. (2005). Common functional component modelling *Proceedings of 55th Session of the International Statistical Institute*, Sydney 2005.

Dauxois, J., Pousse, A. and Romain, Y. (1982). Asymptotic Theory for the Principal Component Analysis of a Vector Random Function: Some Applications to Statistical Inference, *Journal of Multivariate Analysis 12*: 136-154.

Hastie, T., Tibshirani, R. and Friedman, J., (2002). *The Elements of Statistical Learning*, Springer.

Härdle, W. (1990). *Applied Nonparametric Regression*, Cambridge University Press.

Härdle, W., Müller, M., and Klinke, S. (2001). *XploRe Learning Guide*, Springer, Berlin.

Härdle, W. and Simar, L. (2003). *Applied Multivariate Statistical Analysis*, Springer-Verlag Berlin Heidelberg.

Kneip, A. and Utikal, K. (2001). Inference for Density Families Using Functional Principal Components Analysis, *Journal of the American Statistical Association 96*: 519-531.

Ramsay, J. (2003). *Matlab, R and S-Plus Functions for Functional Data Analysis*, McGill University,
ftp://ego.psych.mcgill.ca/pub/FDAfuns

Ramsay, J. and Silverman, B. (1997). *Functional Data Analysis*, Springer, New York.

Rice, J. and Silverman, B. (1991). Estimating the Mean and Covariance Structure Nonparametrically when the Data are Curves, *Journal of Royal Statistical Society, Ser. B 53*: 233-243.

Silverman, B. (1996). Smoothed Functional Principal Components Analysis by Choice of Norm, *Annals of Statistics 24*: 1-24.

Ulbricht, J. (2004). Representing smooth functions, *Master Arbeit, Statistics*, Humboldt Universität zu Berlin.

XploRe Inner Group. (2005). XploRe, Auto Pilot Support System, *MD*Tech*, Berlin.

17 Analysis of Failure Time with Microearthquakes Applications

Graciela Estévez-Pérez and Alejandro Quintela del Rio

17.1 Introduction

The problem of searching for stochastic models to describe the sequence of occurrence times of earthquakes from some geographic region is of great interest in sysmology sciences. In effect, a detailed analysis of such process might reveal new aspects of the pattern of occurrence of earthquakes, and suggest important ideas about the mechanism of earthquakes.

The development of detailed stochastic models to describe the list of origin times or equivalently that of time intervals between consecutive earthquakes is quite recent. Vere-Jones (1970) surveys some of the stochastic models (clustering models and stochastic models for aftershock sequences) proposed in the literature and describes their behavior in several data sets. Other more recent models include the Trigger models (Lomnitz and Nava, 1983), the Epidemic-Type Aftershock Sequence (ETAS) model (Ogata, 1988), or refinements of Hawkes (1971) self-exciting point process model, which describes spatial-temporal patterns in a catalog.

However, standard models applied to seismic data do not always fit the data well. In part, this is because parametric models are usually only well suited for a sequence of seismic events that have similar causes. Moreover, parametric models can be insensitive to poorly-fitting events, which often are at least as interesting as well-fitting ones, (Ogata, 1989).

In this work we use nonparametric methods for analyzing seismic data. They involve several different approaches to nonparametric estimation of the hazard and intensity functions of point processes that evolve with time. This enables us to split up and analyze the occurrence of temporal processes of earthquakes within a region without constraining them to having predetermined properties. We argue that nonparametric methods for the analysis of earthquake data are valuable supplements to more conventional parametric approaches, especially as tools for exploratory data analysis.

The objective of our analysis is to show two statistical tools (hazard and intensity functions) which could help to describe the whole cycle of seismic activity in a region without imposing predetermined conditions on this activity. That is, our analysis is based on the information provided by the data and on the universally accepted assumption of temporal grouping of earthquakes. The hazard function is used to confirm this grouping and characterizes the occurrence process of main shocks. On the other hand, the aftershock sequences (clusters) have been studied by means of the intensity function.

Obviously, in this chapter we only deal in detail with one of the several applications of the hazard function on the study of failure times, that is, the seismology. However, the methodology presented below is available in many others biological problems that emerge in reliability studies, survival analysis, ambient studies, etc.

The work is organized as follows: In Section 17.2 we introduce the nonparametric estimator of hazard function. Section 17.3 describes the occurrence process of earthquakes in terms of its evolution in time, and contains the analysis of seismic activity of the Galician region (Spain) - during a specially active time period - using the nonparametric methods mentioned before. Section 17.4 concludes the chapter.

This research has been supported by the PGIDT01PXI10504PR (Xunta de Galicia) and BFM2002-00265 (Ministerio de Ciencia y Teconologia) grants.

17.2   Kernel Estimation of Hazard Function

Let X be a nonnegative real random variable with absolutely continuous distribution function $F(\cdot)$, and probability density function $f(\cdot)$. The hazard function is defined by

$$r(x) = \frac{f(x)}{1 - F(x)} = \frac{f(x)}{\bar{F}(x)},$$

when $\bar{F}(x) > 0$, that is, $r(\cdot)$ is defined in the set $\{x \in \mathbb{R}/\bar{F}(x) > 0\}$. Nonparametric estimation of hazard function started with Watson and Leadbetter (1964a) and Watson and Leadbetter (1964b) who introduced the kernel estimator, and from that time on, a lot of papers on this topic have come out in the nonparametric literature. Most of the previous literature on non-parametric smoothing of hazard function was based on the assumption of independence on the sample variables. However, in several fields of applications the independence assumption is far from being realistic. This is for instance the case of microearthquake studies, see for details Rice and Rosenblatt (1976) and Estévez, Lorenzo and Quintela (2002). Previous papers on dependent hazard estimation involve Sarda and Vieu (1989), Vieu (1991) or Estévez and Quintela (1999) in which several asymptotic properties for kernel hazard estimation are proved.

Here we consider a random sample $X_1, ..., X_n$, each X_i having the same distribution as X, which proceeding from a strictly stationary sequence of strong mixing variables (Rosenblatt, 1956). This dependence structure, which is satisfied by a large class of time series (autoregressive processes and autoregressive moving average time series models), is one of the least restrictive among the numerous asymptotic independence conditions usually considered. One among the conventional nonparametric estimators of $r(\cdot)$ is the kernel estimator defined by

$$r_h(x) = \frac{f_h(x)}{1 - F_h(x)} \tag{17.1}$$

A similar estimator uses the empirical distribution function in the denominator,

$$r_n(x) = \frac{f_h(x)}{1 - F_n(x)} \tag{17.2}$$

In this expression $f_h(x) = \frac{1}{nh}\sum_{i=1}^{n} K\left(\frac{x - X_i}{h}\right)$ is the known Parzen-Rosenblatt estimator of $f(\cdot)$ and $F_h(\cdot)$ is the kernel estimator of $F(\cdot)$, defined by

$$F_h(x) = \frac{1}{n}\sum_{i=1}^{n} H\left(\frac{x - X_i}{h}\right) = \int_{-\infty}^{x} f_h(t)dt,$$

with $K(\cdot)$ a kernel function, $H(x) = \int_{-\infty}^{x} K(u)du$, and $h = h(n) \in \mathbb{R}^+$ is the smoothing parameter, or bandwidth.

In Xplore, we use the following quantlets (`hazard` library):

```
rh = XCSkernelhazard(x,h,v)
```

estimates a hazard function using the ratio of the nonparametric density estimation and 1 minus the nonparametric kernel distribution estimation;

```
rn = XCSkernelempirichazard(x,h,v)
```

estimates a hazard function using the ratio of the nonparametric density estimation and 1 minus the empirical distribution estimation;

```
Fh = XCSkerneldistribution(x,h,v)
```

nonparametric kernel distribution estimator;

```
Fn = XCSempiricaldistribution(x,v)
```

empirical distribution function estimator;

```
H = XCSepadistribution(x)
```

integral of the Epanechnikov kernel applied to the estimation points in distribution function estimation.

Q XCSkernelhazard.xpl

Q XCSkernelempirichazard.xpl
Q XCSkerneldistribution.xpl
Q XCSempiricaldistribution.xpl
Q XCSepadistribution.xpl

In a L_2 framework, to assess the global performance of $r_h(\cdot)$ as estimator of $r(\cdot)$, we will consider the following quadratic measures of accuracy:

Integrated Squared Error (ISE)

$$ISE(h) = \int (r_h(x) - r(x))^2 w(x) f(x) \, dx,$$

and the Mean Integrated Squared Error $(MISE^*)$

$$MISE^*(h) = E \int \left[(r_h(x) - r(x)) \frac{1 - F_h(x)}{1 - F(x)} \right]^2 w(x) f(x) \, dx,$$

where $w(\cdot)$ is a nonnegative weight function introduced to allow reduction of boundary effects. It is well-known that such measures are asymptotically equivalent (Vieu, 1991) and that their convergence rates are the same as in density estimation (Estévez, 2002).

The main practical problem associated with applying the estimator $r_h(\cdot)$ is the choice of h. A first method that we can consider, having into account that we are working in a dependent data framework, is the "leave-$(2l_n + 1)$-out" version of the cross-validation procedure. That is, we select the bandwidth h_{cv} that minimizes

$$CV_{l_n}(h) = \int r_h^2(x)\, w(x)\, dx - \frac{2}{n} \sum_{i=1}^{n} \frac{f_h^{-i}(X_i)}{\left(1 - F_h^{-i}(X_i)\right)\left(1 - F_n(X_i)\right)} w(X_i),$$

where

$$f_h^{-i}(x) = (h n_{l_n})^{-1} \sum_{|j-i|>l_n} K\left(\frac{x - X_j}{h}\right)$$

and

$$F_h^{-i}(x) = n_{l_n}^{-1} \sum_{|j-i|>l_n} H\left(\frac{x - X_j}{h}\right)$$

are the kernel estimators of the density and distribution function, respectively, when we use in the estimation all the data except the closest points (in time) from X_i. Here $F_n(x)$ is the classical empirical distribution function and l_n is a positive integer such that n_{l_n} satisfies $n n_{l_n} = \#\{(i,j)\,/\,|i - j| > l_n\}$. With this definition, an attempt is made to classify the data as a function of their temporal proximity, and l_n indicates when two data can be handle as if they were independent. For $l_n = 0$, we have the classical cross-validation rule when independence is assumed, which is asymptotically optimal (Youndjé, Sarda and Vieu, 1996).

Similar criteria, based on cross-validation techniques, have already been discussed in other settings related with hazard estimation, see e.g. Sarda and Vieu (1989), Sarda and Vieu (1991) or Patil (1993a), Patil (1993b). In the paper of Estévez and Quintela (1999) it is shown that the "leave-$(2l_n + 1)$-out" version of cross-validation bandwidth is asymptotically optimal for strong-mixing or α-mixing data (Rosenblatt, 1956), in the sense that

$$\frac{MISE^*(h_{cv})}{MISE^*(h_0)} \to 1 \ a.s., \tag{17.3}$$

or

$$\frac{h_{cv}}{h_0} \to 1 \ a.s., \tag{17.4}$$

where h_0 is the minimizer of $MISE^*(h)$. Note that by the Theorem 4.1 of Vieu (1991), the previous expressions also remain valid when changing $MISE^*$ in ISE, that is, if $\widehat{h}_0$ is the minimizer of $ISE(h)$ then

$$\frac{ISE(h_{cv})}{ISE(\widehat{h}_0)} \to 1 \ a.s., \tag{17.5}$$

and

$$\frac{h_{cv}}{\widehat{h}_0} \to 1 \ a.s.. \tag{17.6}$$

While asymptotic optimality is very encouraging, an important question is to know the convergence rates in (17.3) and (17.4) ((17.5) and (17.6), respectively). Hence, Estévez, Quintela and Vieu (2002) present the following results, which describe the relative amount by which h_{cv} fails to minimize the $MISE^*$ and ISE, respectively:

$$\left| \frac{MISE^* \ (h_{cv}) - MISE^* \ (h_0)}{MISE^* \ (h_0)} \right| = \mathcal{O}_p \left(n^{-(1/2-r/p)/(2k+1)} \right), \tag{17.7}$$

and

$$\left| \frac{ISE \ (h_{cv}) - ISE \ \left(\widehat{h}_0\right)}{ISE \ \left(\widehat{h}_0\right)} \right| = \mathcal{O}_p \left(n^{-(1/2-r/p)/(2k+1)} \right),$$

provided r is a positive integer ($r < p/2$), p is some integer $p > 3$ controlling the dependence amount, and k is the order of kernel function.

As a result of (17.7) it is easy to establish the following rates, which quantifies the relative distance between h_{cv} or $\widehat{h}_0$ towards the optimal bandwidth, h_0:

$$\left| \frac{h_{cv} - h_0}{h_0} \right| = \mathcal{O}_p \left(n^{-(1/2-r/p)/(2k+1)} \right) \tag{17.8}$$

and

$$\left| \frac{\widehat{h}_0 - h_0}{h_0} \right| = \mathcal{O}_p \left(n^{-(1/2-r/p)/(2k+1)} \right). \tag{17.9}$$

Note that the relative difference between h_{cv} and h_0 seems, at first glance, to be fairly slow (17.8). However, we should not be too worried because it is of the same order as the difference between $\widehat{h}_0$ and h_0 (17.9). This means that the automatically selected bandwidth h_{cv} is as close (at least asymptotically) to the referential bandwidth h_0 as $\widehat{h}_0$ (which is another reasonable candidate to be a referential bandwidth) does.

On the other hand, if we observe with care the proof of these theorems, we conclude that these rates are basically determined by the rates estimating $f\,(\cdot)$. Hence, the rates of convergence under independence conditions ($p = \infty$) are the same as in density estimation, that is, $\mathcal{O}_p\left(n^{-1/2(2k+1)}\right)$ (Hall and Marron, 1987).

In spite of the above quality properties, it's well known that if the observations are dependent, cross-validation procedure will produce an undersmoothed bandwidth. This has been observed in several functional estimation contexts, and also confirmed in hazard estimation by the computational studies of Estévez and Quintela (1999).

The observation of the rates of convergence given previously suggests us to introduce the following version of cross-validation: we propose to penalize the cross-validation bandwidth h_{cv} in such a way that the new bandwidth h^p_{cv} still has the same convergence rate as h_{cv}. So, we take

$$h^p_{cv} = h_{cv} + \lambda_n, \tag{17.10}$$

with

$$\lambda_n = \mathcal{O}\left(n^{-(3/2-r/p)/(2k+1)}\right), \tag{17.11}$$

and it is possible to establish the following results, which are obvious corollaries of (17.7) and (17.8):

With the conditions and notations of (17.7), and if, in addition, (17.11) is satisfied,

$$\left|\frac{MISE^*\left(h^p_{cv}\right) - MISE^*\left(h_0\right)}{MISE^*\left(h_0\right)}\right| = \mathcal{O}_p\left(n^{-(1/2-r/p)/(2k+1)}\right). \tag{17.12}$$

In addition, under the conditions of (17.8),

$$\left|\frac{h^p_{cv} - h_0}{h_0}\right| = \mathcal{O}_p\left(n^{-(1/2-r/p)/(2k+1)}\right). \tag{17.13}$$

Hence, these results guarantee us that the penalized cross-validated bandwidth is still asymptotically optimal.

A complete simulation study has allowed to derive an empirical formula for the penalized cross-validated bandwidth and proves that such bandwidth works better than ordinary cross-validation (Estévez, Quintela and Vieu, 2002).

17.3   An Application to Real Data

17.3.1   The Occurrence Process of Earthquakes

Earthquakes can be represented by point events in a five-dimensional $(\Psi_i, \lambda_i, d_i, \ t_i, M_i)$ space-time-energy continuum, where Ψ_i and λ_i are the latitude and longitude of the epicenter, d_i the depth of the focus, t_i the origin time and M_i the magnitude. The starting point of consideration is the one-dimensional series of occurrence times $\{t_i\}$. To give a precise meaning to this time series, its space, time and magnitude boundaries must be specified. Obviously, these boundaries will be chosen according to the objectives of the study: to characterize different seismic areas in the same time period, to analyze several seismic series in a particular region, etc.

Space specifications define the volume from which the population of earthquakes, represented by the time series $\{t_i\}$, is taken. This may be done in practice by specifying an area A and a lower limit in depth H. Since detectability is limited, a lower limit of magnitude M_0 must also be specified. This limit is a function of the station distribution and sensitivity, and defines the lowest magnitude for which all events from anywhere in the bounded region can be detected.

Once a bounded set of time occurrence is established, a series can be constructed with the time intervals between consecutive earthquakes $\{\Delta t_i\}$, such that for $\Delta t_i = t_i - t_{i-1}$. The distribution of the values of these intervals is of great interest to specify the time structure of the seismicity of a region.

The simplest statistical model to fit a series of occurrence times of earthquakes is the Poisson process, under which the time intervals between consecutive events are exponentially distributed. This model presupposes independence of the events, so that the occurrence of one earthquake is not influenced by that of previous ones, which is very far away from reality. In effect, several authors, Vere-Jones (1970), Udias and Rice (1975), have found, for different populations of earthquakes, that the Poisson fit to the time series of microearthquakes is very poor, especially for active periods. The deviation from the model is principally due to the existence of a much larger number of small intervals than expected. The reason for such a large number of small intervals is that the earthquakes happen forming clusters, that is, one main shock is followed and/or preceded by a stream of smaller shocks, called aftershocks and/or precursors, see for details Lomnitz and Hax (1967) and Vere-Jones and Davies (1966), produced in the same general focal region.

Therefore, some authors   (Vere-Jones, 1970) have defined the occurrence process of earthquakes in terms of two components: (i) a process of cluster centers; and (ii) a subsidiary process defining the configuration of the members within a cluster. The final process is taken as the superposition of all the clusters. Several possible models for these processes can be found in the literature, for example the Compound Poisson Processes (Vere-Jones and Davies, 1966), Trigger Models (Lomnitz and Nava, 1983) or Epidemic-type Models (Ogata, 1988 and references therein). All these models assume structural conditions on the occurrence of earthquakes, as for example, that the process of cluster centers is stationary and follows a Poisson distribution. This hypothesis is not very likely either for particular cases. A drawback of these approaches is that they depend very much on the models, and so are subject to the instability and goodness of fit problems noted in Section 17.1.

As we mentioned in Section 17.1, nonparametric methods for analyzing the distribution of time intervals between consecutive earthquakes - occurred in Galicia- will be considered, obtaining another attempt to describe temporal behavior of an earthquake series in a geographic region.

17.3.2 Galicia Earthquakes Data

Seismic activity increased substantially in Galicia (Spanish region) during the 1990's, creating some times a significantly social alarm. The data analyzed correspond to the 978 earthquakes occurring from January 15, 1987 to May 3, 2000. Their epicenters, scattered throughout Galicia, show small spatial groupings at high risk areas named Sarria, Monforte and Celanova.

For this region Figures 17.1 and 17.2 show the sequence of time intervals between consecutive shocks $\{\Delta t_i\}_{i=1}^{978}$ and their magnitudes. These graphs indicate a quiet period until September 1995 and three temporal groupings in December 1995, May 1997 and May-June 1998, which are related with the strongest earthquakes.

The hazard function estimation (Figure 17.3), which has been built using the Epanechnikov kernel in r_h (17.1), presents a common shape in a seismology framework: it decreases suddenly in the first hours and then it fluctuates around a small risk. This shape confirms the well known fact that earthquakes form clusters. We use the example program XCSkernelhazard to make this figure (the bandwidth calculated by cross-validation with an Epanechnikov kernel in the quantlet denbwsel). XCSkernelhazard is the example that allows us to estimate the hazard function to our data.

Observation: In this work, we also have programmed three quantlets more, named   XCSempiricalfunction,   XCSkerneldistribfunction   and

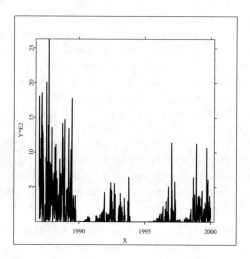

Figure 17.1: Secuence graph of time intervals between consecutive earthquakes $\{\Delta t_i\}_{i=1}^{977}$.

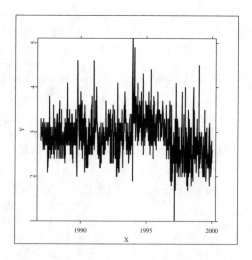

Figure 17.2: Sequence graph of magnitudes.

XCSkernelhazard2. The two first are examples of empirical and kernel distribution function of a normal random sample, respectively, and the third

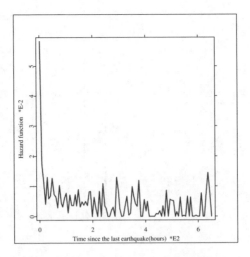

Figure 17.3: Hazard estimation of time intervals between consecutive shocks.

⌕ XCSkernelhazard.xpl

quantlet shows the kernel hazard estimations using 17.1 and 17.2.

⌕ XCSempiricalfunction.xpl

⌕ XCSkerneldistribfunction.xpl
⌕ XCSkernelhazard2.xpl

Therefore, 206 clusters with "cluster length" less than 144 hours have been formed (a cluster is defined as a set of earthquakes originating from a relatively small volume, and separated in time by intervals smaller than a fixed duration -"cluster length"-. The cluster center is a shock representative of the cluster -the first shock, for instance-. Then, the occurrence process of earthquakes is taken as the superposition of all the clusters.). The sequence of sizes and magnitudes of cluster centers (Figures 17.4 and 17.5) show three important clusters, the first one beginning with a big shock (4.7 on the Richter scale). Figures 17.4, 17.5 and 17.2 also suggest that the strongest earthquakes are related to small clusters, that is, such events are not followed or preceded by many earthquakes.

The behavior of the clusters will be studied using the process of origin times $\{t_i\}$ and its intensity function. This function gives, for each time t, $\lambda(t)$ the average number of earthquakes per unit of time, t hours after the main

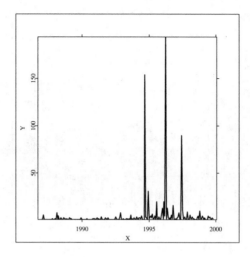

Figure 17.4: Sequence graph of cluster sizes (a total of 206).

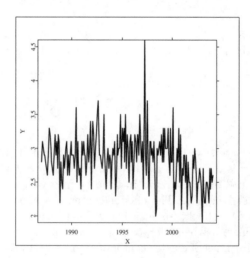

Figure 17.5: Sequence graph of magnitudes of cluster centers.

shock (cluster center). This function clearly shows the evolution of the cluster with time, and therefore, it is suitable for comparing the seismic activity of several geographic regions. In this work, we propose to estimate the intensity function by means of a kernel estimator, which is defined as:

$$\widehat{\lambda}(t) = \frac{1}{h} \sum_{i=1}^{n} K\left(\frac{t-t_i}{h}\right), \ \forall t \in \mathbb{R}^+$$

(Wand and Jones (1995), Choi and Hall (1999) and their references), where $K(\cdot)$ is the kernel function and h the bandwidth.

This function is easy to use in XploRe, only seeing that this is the density estimate multiplied by n.

The first cluster is composed of 147 shocks, whose epicenters are contained in a small area close to Sarria (Lugo). The intensity estimation (Figure 17.6) indicates that: (i) the cluster begins with a high number of shocks (the first of magnitude 4.6), (ii) there is another grouping of events coinciding with another earthquake of magnitude 4.6, and (iii) the intensity function is low in the remainder of the range. XCSintensityfunction allows us to calculate the intensity function with bandwidth h (you can select it as in the hazard case).

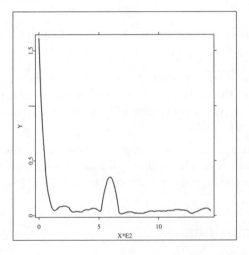

Figure 17.6: Intensity estimation for first cluster (December 1995).

Q XCSintensityfunction.xpl

The second cluster consists of 190 earthquakes, whose epicenters are also near Sarria (Lugo). The shape of the intensity function (Figure 17.7) reflects the behavior of the cluster members: a small group of precursors warns that important shocks are to arrive (one of magnitude 5.1 and another of 4.9) and then there is a sequence of aftershocks.

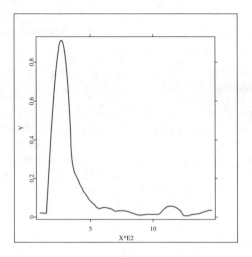

Figure 17.7: Intensity estimation for second cluster (May 1997).

Finally, the third cluster involves 79 events, with epicenters in Celanova (Orense). This is the weakest cluster (few shocks of low magnitude). Its estimated intensity function (Figure 17.8) shows fluctuations around quite small values the whole time.

A more detail study of the seismic activity of Galicia together with an similar analysis of another Spanish region – Granada, traditionally area of great seismic activity – can be seen in Estévez, Lorenzo and Quintela (2002).

17.4 Conclusions

In this work we show how the hazard and intensity functions represent another way of describing the temporal structure of seismic activity in a geographic region. Kernel estimation of hazard function has confirmed what Vere-Jones (1970), Udias and Rice (1975) and many others have noted: earthquakes have the tendency to group. The occurrence process of these groups has also been studied by means of the hazard function and each important cluster has been described using the intensity function.

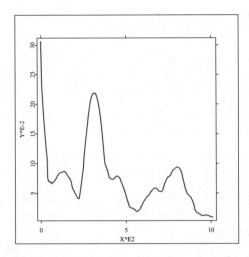

Figure 17.8: Intensity estimation for third cluster (June 1998).

As we argued, a major advantage of nonparametric methods is that they do not require formulation of structural models, which are often well suited only for data that have closely related seismic causes. Another novelty is that we take into account the possible dependence of the data to estimate the distribution of time intervals between earthquakes, which has not been considered in most statistics studies on seismicity.

Bibliography

Choi, E. and Hall, P. (1999). Nonparametric approach to analysis of space-time data on earthquake occurrences. *Journal of the Computational and Graphical Statistics*, **8**, 733-748.

Estévez, G. (2002). On convergence rates for quadratic errors in kernel hazard estimation. *Statistics & Probability Letters*, **57**, 231-241.

Estévez, G., Lorenzo, H. and Quintela, A. (2002). Nonparametric analysis of the time structure of seismicity in a geographic region. *Annals of Geophysics*, **45**, 497-511.

Estévez, G. and Quintela, A. (1999). Nonparametric estimation of the hazard function under dependence conditions. *Communications in Statistics: Theory and Methods*, **10**, 2297-2331.

Estévez, G., Quintela, A., and Vieu, P. (2002). Convergence rate for cross-validatory bandwidth in kernel hazard estimation from dependent samples. *Journal of Statistical Planning and Inference*, **104**, 1-30.

Hall, P. y Marron, J. (1987). On the amount of noise inherent in bandwidth selection for kernel density estimator. *Annals of Statistics*, **15**, 163-181.

Hawkes, A.G. (1971). Point spectra of some mutually exciting point processes. *Journal of the Royal Statistical Society, Series B*, **33**, 438-443.

Lomnitz, C. and Hax, A. (1967). *Clustering in aftershock sequences in The Earth Beneath the Continents*. Geophysical Monograph 10. American Geophysical Union.

Lomnitz, C. and Nava, F.A. (1983). The predictive value of seismic gaps. *Bulletin of the Seismological Society of America*, **73**, 1815-1824.

Ogata, Y. (1988). Statistical models for earthquakes occurrences and residual analysis for point processes. *J. Amer. Stat. Assoc.*, **83**, 9-27.

Ogata, Y. (1989). Statistical model for standard seismicity and detection of anomalies by residual analysis. *Tectonophysics*, **169**, 159-174.

Patil, P.N. (1993). Bandwidth choice for nonparametric hazard rate estimation. *Journal of Statistical Planning and Inference*, **35**, 15-30.

Patil, P.N. (1993). On the least squares cross-validation bandwidth in hazard rate estimation. *Annals of Statistics*, **21**, 1792-1810.

Rice, J. and Rosenblatt, M. (1976). Estimation of the log survival function and hazard function. *Sankhya*, **36**, 60-78.

Rosenblatt, M. (1956). A central limit theorems and a strong mixing condition. *Proceedings of the National Academy of Sciences of the United States of America*, **42**, 43-47.

Sarda, P. and Vieu, P. (1989). Empirical distribution function for mixing random variables. Application in nonparametric hazard estimation. *Statistics*, **20**, 559-571.

Sarda, P. and Vieu, P. (1991). Smoothing parameter selection in hazard estimation. *Statistics & Probability Letters*, **11**, 429-434.

Udias, A. and Rice, J. (1975). Statistical analysis of microearthquakes activity near San Andres Geophysical Observatory, Hollister, California. *Bulletin of the Seismological Society of America*, **65**, 809-828.

Vere-Jones, D. (1970). Stochastic models for earthquake occurrence. *Journal of the Royal Statistical Society, Series B*, **32**, 1-62.

Vere-Jones, D. and Davies, R.B. (1966). A statistical survey of earthquakes in the main seismic region of New Zealand. Part 2. Time Series Analyses. *Journal of Geology and Geophysics*, **3**, 251-284.

Vieu, P. (1991). Quadratic errors for nonparametric estimates under dependence. *Journal of Multivariate Analysis*, **39**, 324-347.

Wand, M.P. and Jones, M.C. (1995). *Kernel Smoothing*. Chapman and Hall. New York.

Watson, G.S. and Leadbetter, M.R. (1964a). Hazard analysis I. *Biometrika*, **51**, 175-184.

Watson, G.S. and Leadbetter, M.R. (1964b). Hazard analysis II. *Sankhya*, **26**, 101-116.

Youndjé, É., Sarda, P. and Vieu, P. (1996). Optimal smooth hazard estimates. *TEST*, **5**, 379-394.

18 Polychotomous Regression: Application to Landcover Prediction

Frédéric Ferraty, Martin Paegelow and Pascal Sarda

18.1 Introduction

An important field of investigation in Geography is the modelization of the evolution of land cover in view of analyzing the dynamics of this evolution and then to build predictive maps. This analysis is now possible with the increasing performance of the apparatus of measure: sattelite image, aerial photographs, ... Whereas lot of statistical methods are now available for geographical spatial data and implemented in numerous softwares, very few methods have been improved in the context of spatio-temporal data. However there is a need to develop tools for helping environmental management (for instance in view of preventing risks) and national and regional development.

In this paper, we propose to use a polychotomous regression model to modelize and to predict land cover of a given area: we show how to adapt this model in order to take into account the spatial correlation and the temporal evolution of the vegetation indexes. The land cover (map) is presented in the form of pixels, and for each pixel a value (a color) representing a kind of vegetation (from a given nomenclatura): we have several maps for different dates in the past. As a matter of fact the model allows us to predict the value of vegetation for a pixel knowing the values of this pixel and of the pixels in its neigbourhood in the past.

We study data from an area in the Pyrénées mountains (south of France). These data are quite interesting for our purpose since the mediterranean mountains knows from the end of the first half of the 19th century spectacular changes in the land covers. These changes come from the decline of the old agricultural system and the drift from the land.

The paper is organized as follows. In Section 18.2, we describe more precisely the data. The polychotomous regression model for land cover prediction is presented in Section 18.3. We show how to use this model for our problem and define the estimator in 18.4. Application of this model to the data is given in sections 18.5 and 18.6. Among others, we discuss how to choose the different parameters of the model (shape of the neighbourhood of a pixel, value for the smoothing parameter of the model).

18.2   Presentation of the Data

18.2.1   The Area: the Garrotxes

The "Garrotxes" is an area in the south of France (Pyrénées mountains). More exactly, it is localized in the department (administrative area) of Pyrénées Orientales: see Figure 18.1 below. The type of agriculture was essentially agropastoral traditional. Then, this area has known lot of changes in the landcover from the 19th century. Whereas agriculture has almost disapeared due to the city migration, the pastoral activity knows an increasing from the eighties. It is important for the near future to manage this pastoral activity by means of different actions on the landcover. For this, the knowledge of the evolution of the landcover is essential.

18.2.2   The Data Set

The data set consists in a sequence of maps of landcover for the years 1980, 1990 and 2000. The area we have studied is divided into 40401 pixels (201×201) which is a part of the Garrotxes: each pixel is a square with side of about 18 meters. For each pixel we have

- the type of vegetation with 8 types coded from 1 to 8:

    1 : "Coniferous forests",

    2 : "Deciduous forests",

    3 : "Scrubs",

    4 : "Broom lands",

    5 : "Grass pastures",

    6 : "Grasslands",

    7 : "Agriculture",

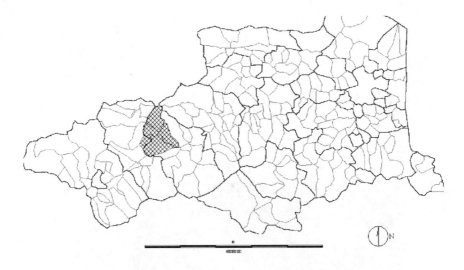

Figure 18.1: Localization of the Garrotxes in the department of Pyrénées
Orientales.

        8 : "Urban"

- several environmental variables:

  - elevation,

  - slope,

  - aspect,

  - distance of roads and villages,

  - type of forest management (administrative or not),

  - type of area (pastoral or not).

For each pixel, the environmental variables remain unchanged during the
period of observation. Figure 18.2 below shows the land cover of the aera for
the year 1980.

18.3   The Multilogit Regression Model

It is quite usual to modelize a regression problem where the response is categorical by a *multiple logistic regression model* also known as *polychotomous*

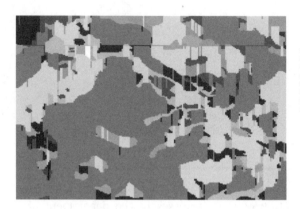

Figure 18.2: Land cover for the part of Garrotxes area in 1980.

regression model. We refer to Hosmer, Lemeshow (1989) for a description of this model and to Kooperberg, Bose, Stone (1987) for a smooth version of this model. In our context we aim at predicting the type of vegetation for a pixel at date t by the types of vegetation of this pixel and of neighbouring pixels at date $t-1$: thus the model takes into account both spatial and temporal aspects. Moreover we will include in the set of explanatory variables environmental variables which does not depend on time. Let us note that we have chosen a time dependence of order 1 since it allows to produce a model not too complex with a reasonable number of parameters to estimate (with respect to the number of observations). Note also that the size and the shape of the neighborhood will be essential (see below for a discussion on this topic).

We give now a more formal description of the polychotomous regression model for our problem. For each pixel i, $i = 1, \ldots, N$, let us note by $X_i(t)$ the type of vegetation at time t. We then define for pixel i a neighborhood, that is a set of pixels J_i. Our aim is to predict the value $X_i(t)$ knowing the value of $X_j(t-1)$, $j \in J_i$, and the value of environmental variables for pixel i denoted by $Y_i = (Y_i^1, \ldots, Y_i^K)$ (independent of t). Denoting by $D_i(t-1) = \{X_j(t-1), j \in J_i\}$ and by V the number of different vegetation types (8 in our case), we will predict $X_i(t)$ by an estimation of the quantity

$$\arg \max_{v=1,\ldots,V} P\left(X_i(t) = v | D_i(t-1), Y_i\right).$$

At first let us write

$$P\left(X_i(t) = v | D_i(t-1), Y_i\right) = \frac{\exp \theta \left(v | D_i(t-1), Y_i\right)}{\sum_{v=1}^{V} \exp \theta \left(v' | D_i(t-1), Y_i\right)},$$

where

$$\theta\left(v | D_i(t-1), Y_i\right) = \log \frac{P\left(X_i(t) = v | D_i(t-1), Y_i\right)}{P\left(X_i(t) = V | D_i(t-1), Y_i\right)}.$$

Now, the polychotomous regression model consists in writting $\theta(v | D_i(t-1), Y_i)$ as

$$\theta(v | D_i(t-1), Y_i) = \alpha_v + \sum_{x \in D_i(t-1)} \sum_{l=1}^{V} \beta_{vl} I(x=l) + \sum_{k=1}^{K} \gamma_{vj} Y_i^k,$$

where $\delta = (\alpha_1, \ldots, \alpha_{V-1}, \beta_{1,1}, \ldots, \beta_{1,V} \beta_{2,1}, \ldots, \beta_{2,V}, \ldots, \beta_{V-1,1}, \ldots, \beta_{V-1,V}, \gamma_{1,1}, \ldots, \gamma_{1,K}, \ldots, \gamma_{V-1,1}, \ldots, \gamma_{V-1,K})$ is the vector of parameters of the model. Note that since $\theta(V | D_i(t-1), Y_i) = 0$, we have $\alpha_V = 0$, $\beta_{V,l} = 0$ for all $l = 1, \ldots, V$ and $\gamma_{V,k} = 0$ for all $k = 1, \ldots, K$.

18.4 Penalized Log-likelihood Estimation

We estimate the vectors of parameters by means of a penalized log-likelihood maximization. The log-likelihood function is given by

$$l(\delta) = \log \left(\prod_{i=1}^{N} P\left(Z_i(t) | D_i(t-1), Y_i, \delta\right) \right).$$

Kooperberg, Bose, Stone (1987) have shown that introducing a penalization term in the log-likelihhod function may have some computational benefits: it allows numerical stability and guarantees the existence of a finite maximum. Following their idea, we then define the penalized log-likelihood function as

$$l_\epsilon(\delta) = l(\delta) - \epsilon \sum_{i=1}^{N} \sum_{v=1}^{V} u_{iv}^2,$$

where for $v = 1, \ldots, V$

$$u_{iv} = \theta(v|D_i(t-1), Y_i, \delta) - \frac{1}{V} \sum_{v'=1}^{V} \theta(v'|D_i(t-1), Y_i, \delta),$$

and ϵ is the penalization parameter. For reasonable small values of ϵ, the penalty term would not affect the value of the estimators.

For numerical maximization of the penalized log-likelihood function we use a Newton-Raphson algorithm.

18.5   Polychotomous Regression in Action

As pointed out above the estimators of the parameters of the model will depend on the size and on the shape of the neighborhood for pixels and on the value of the penalization parameter ϵ. For the shape of the neighborhood we choose to keep it as a square centered on the pixel. We have then to choose the (odd) number of pixels for the side of the square and the value of ϵ. The choice has been achieved through two steps namely an *estimation step* and a *validation step* described below.

- The *estimation step* is based on the maps from the years 1980 and 1990: it consists in calculating the estimator $\widehat{\delta}$ of δ for several values of the size of the neighborhood and of the penalization parameter ϵ. The computation of δ is achieved by the maximization of the penalized log-likelihood function defined at the previous Section.

- For the *validation step*, we use the map for the year 2000 and compare it with the predicted map for this year using the estimator computed previously in the following way. Once the estimator $\widehat{\delta}$ has been computed, we estimate the probability of transition replacing the parameter by its estimator. We then obtain the quantities

$$\widehat{P}(X_i(t+1) = v|D_i(t), Y_i), \quad v = 1, \ldots, V.$$

At time $t + 1$ (in this case $t + 1 = 2000$), we affect the most probable type of vegetation at pixel i, that is the value v which maximizes

$$\left\{ \widehat{P}(X_i(t+1) = v|D_i(t), Y_i) \right\}_{v=1,\ldots,V}.$$

We then keep the values of the size of the neighborhood and of ϵ which produces a map with the best percentage of well-predicted pixels (for the year 2000).

Finally we use the values selected in the last step above to produce a map for the year 2010. Concerning the implementation of such a method, all programs are written with the R language (R, 2004); maps and R sources are available on request.

18.6   Results and Interpretation

To see the accuracy of our porcedure we compare the (real) map for the year 2000 with the predicted map for this year. Figure 18.3 shows this true map of land cover.

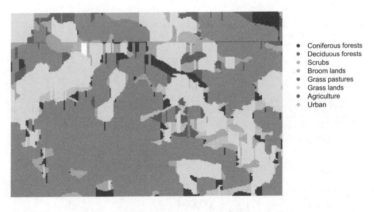

Figure 18.3: Land cover for the part of Garrotxes area in 2000

After having used the procedure as described in the previous Section, we have selected a squared neighborhood of size 3 pixels and a parameter ϵ equal to 0.1. With these values we produced an estimated map (for the year 2000) shown in Figure 18.4.

Table 18.1 below shows the percentage of different types of vegetation in the map of the year 2000 compared with the estimated perecentage. Table 18.1 shows that globally the predicted percentage are quite near of the real percentages.

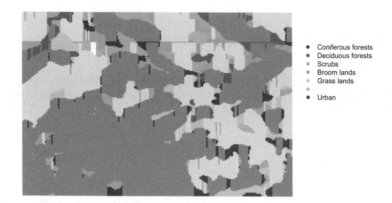

Figure 18.4: Estimated land cover for the part of Garrotxes area in 2000

Table 18.1: Percentage of different vegetation types in 2000

Land cover types	True percentage	Estimated percentage
Coniferous forests	44.5	49.6
Deciduous forests	17.4	10.1
Scrubs	19.1	11
Broom lands	4.7	12.3
Grass pastures	12.3	16
Grasslands	0.0001	0

However, we have to compare the position of the vegetation types to look at the accuracy of the procedure. We consider now the percentage of miss-classified pixels. The global percentage of missclassified pixels was 27.9%. This can be seen as a quite good percentage since only 3 dates are available. Also, the performance of such a procedure can be seen by comparing figures 18.3 and 18.4 which show similar global structures. However if we look at the details of missclassified pixels with respect to each type of vegetation we obtain the following Table 18.2 (we retain only the types of vegetation which cover at least 1 percent of the area).

Table 18.2: Percentage of missclassified pixels in 2000

Land cover types	True percentage	Percentage of missclassified pixels
Coniferous forests	44.5	7.1
Deciduous forests	17.4	44.8
Scrubs	19.1	65.5
Broom lands	4.7	28.1
Grasslands	12.3	18.5

Table 18.2 shows that the results are quite different for different types of vegetation: Coniferous forests, Broom lands and Grasslands are well predicted for the two firsts and quite well for the third. At the opposite, Deciduous forests and Scrubs are badly predicted (more than half of the pixels are not well predicted). This fact can be explain in two ways. At first, Deciduous forests and Scrubs are unstable in the sense that they are submitted to random effects that our model does not take into account. For instance, into the period of ten years separating two maps a fire can transform deciduous forest into scrubs. This can explain that scrubs is the more dynamic type of vegetation. Moreover, the classification of several types of vegetation is subject to some measure of error: as a matter of fact the frontier between deciduous forests and scrubs is not so easy to determine.

As a conclusion to our study, we have seen that the polychotomous procedure introduced to predict land cover maps has given in a certain sense some quite good results and also has shown some limitations. Stable and frequent vegetation types have been well predicted. In the opposite, results for vegetation types submitted to random changes are not so good. We see several ways to improve further studies for land cover prediction. On the geographical ground, it is important to have closer dates of measures which will lead to have a more precise idea of the dynamics. It is also important to think of defining a precise nomenclatura of vegetations. For the modelization aspects, the polychotomous regression could also be improved for instance by taking different shapes of neighborhood (rectangular, not centered in the pixel that we want to predict or with a size depending of this pixel). We can also think to integrate additional variables in order to modelize effects such as forest fires. Finally we can compare this procedure with other modelizations: this has been done in Paegelow, Villa, Cornez, Ferraty, Ferré, Sarda (2004) and in Villa, Paegelow, Cornez, Ferraty, Ferré, Sarda (2004) where a Geographic Information System and a neural netwok procedure have been investigated on the same data sets. The third approaches lead to quite similar reults (and similar rates of missclassified pixels). Also the same limitations have been highlighted.

Bibliography

Cardot, H., Faivre, R. and Goulard, M. (2003). Functional approaches for predicting land use with the temporal evolution of coarse resolution remote sensing data. *Journal of Applied Statistics*, **30**, 1201-1220.

Hosmer, D. and Lemeshow, S. (1989). *Applied Logistic Regression*. Wiley, New York.

Kooperberg, C., Bose, S. and Stone, C.J. (1987). *Partially Linear Models*. Springer-Physica-Verlag, Heidelberg.

Paegelow, M., Villa, N., Cornez, L., Ferraty, F., Ferré, L. and Sarda, P. (2004). Modélisations prospectives de données géoréférencées par approches croisées SIG et statistiques. Application à l'occupation du sol en milieu montagnard méditerranéen. *CyberGEO*, **295**, http://www.cybergeo.presse.fr.

R Development Core Team (2004). *R: A language and environment for statistical computing*. R Foundation for Statistical Computing, Vienna, Austria.

Villa, N., Paegelow, M., Cornez, L., Ferraty, F., Ferré, L. and Sarda, P. (2004). Various approaches to predicting land cover in Mediterranean mountain areas. Preprint

19 The Application of Fuzzy Clustering to Satellite Images Data

Hizir Sofyan, Muzailin Affan and Khaled Bawahidi

19.1 Introduction

Recent advances in the field of aerospace technology have led to the collection of huge amounts of satellite image data. Since the availability of data is abundant, it will be easier to study the environmental change in a specific area by monitoring the land use and land cover. Land use is one of the factors that influences environmental changes. Most of the land use changes are caused by human activities, such as deforestation for expanding agricultural land or for urban use. This will be major aspects of attention we relation to the city such as Ipoh in Malaysia with the reduction in the rain forest stand, air pollution, extremely rapid extension of its urban area and many other environmental changes (Günther, Radermacher, and Riekert, 1995).

Clustering can be used to obtain some initial information from satellite images. This method constructs groups in such a way that the profiles of objects in the same groups are relatively homogenous whereas the profiles of objects in different groups are relatively heterogeneous.

The main advantage of using the method is that interesting structures or clusters can be found directly from the images data without using any background knowledge. By conventional clustering methods, a class is either assigned to or not assigned to a defined group.

Fuzzy clustering which applies the concept of fuzzy sets to cluster analysis allocates members pertaining to a group at each pixel of the images data by use of a membership function which associates to each cluster ranging between 0 and 1.

The primary objective in this article is to use the technique of unsupervised fuzzy classification in monitoring the urban land use change using Ipoh city as the case study area. In this study, fuzzy clustering methods were implemented using the statistical software package XploRe and GIS (GRASS) and Remote Sensing (ERDAS) were used to classify multi-spectral Landsat TM images. The result of this investigation shows that the underlying structures and patterns from satellite image data can be classified more precisely than the conventional ones.

In the subsequent Section 2 and 3, we present reviews of remote sensing and fuzzy clustering method. Section 4 describes data and methods. Section 5 presents the results and discussions.

19.2   Remote Sensing

Remote sensing is a form of measuring physical characteristics of remote object without being in contact with them (Günther, Radermacher, and Riekert, 1995). In this case, the earth surface is used as the target of observation. The remote sensing system is a repeatedly consistent activity toward the earth surface which is supposed to monitor the earth system and its effect on the human activities. Here, the measurement is focused on images which is essentially a two dimensional spatial grid of spectral and spatial information.

Satellite image consists of several bands. These bands give information about the spectral reflection from the earth surface. Each band will have a different pixel value which depends on the measuring frequency. Each band has a value between $0 - 255$ representing the spectral distribution of these bands. In this paper we just concentrate on images as data without attention to the process of how the data have been physically absorbed. A more comprehensive overview of the evaluation of remote sensor data can be found at Günther, Hess, Mutz, Riekert, and Ruwwe (1993).

Traditionally, the thematically classification of an image follows the following stages (Schowengerdt, 1997):

- **Feature extraction**: Transformation of the multispectral image by a spatial or spectral transform to a feature image.

- **Classification**: Extraction of the pixels to be classified either by training the classifier to recognize certain classes through the supervised or unsupervised classification method and using statistical procedures to aggregate the pixels.

- **Labelling**: Labelling the output map by analysts, consisting of one label for each pixel.

More references about land use-land change classification hierarchy can be found at Anderson, Hardy, Roach, and Witmer (1976).

A case that emerges in relation to mapping the urban land-use class is to differentiate between classes which are closely related to each other such as "urban residential" or "light industrial" areas. Therefore, it will be necessary to see the more complex relationship among the physical measurement, multi-spectral image and destination map class. However, sometimes having known this all is not enough, we still need additional information which is referred to as ancillary information.

19.3   Fuzzy C-means Method

```
v = xcfcme(x, c, m, e, alpha)
```

This quantlet performs a fuzzy C-means cluster analysis.

One approach to fuzzy clustering is the fuzzy C-Means (Bezdek, 1981). Before Bezdek, Dunn (1973) had developed the fuzzy C-Means Algorithm. The idea of Dunn's algorithm is to extend the classical within groups sum of squared error objective function to a fuzzy version by minimizing this objective function. Bezdek generalized this fuzzy objective function by introducing the weighting exponent m, $1 \leq m < \infty$:

$$J_m(U, V) = \sum_{k=1}^{n} \sum_{i=1}^{c} (u_{ik})^m d^2(x_k, v_i), \qquad (19.1)$$

where U is a partition of X in c part, $V = v = (v_1, v_2, ..., v_c)$ are the cluster centers in $\mathbb{R}^p$, and A is any $(p \times p)$ symmetric positive definite matrix defined as the following:

$$d(x_k, v_i) = \sqrt{(x_k - v_i)^\top (x_k - v_i)} \qquad (19.2)$$

where $d(x_k, v_i)$ is an inner product induced norm on $\mathbb{R}^p$, u_{ik} is referred to as the grade of membership of x_k to the cluster i. This grade of membership satisfies the following constraints:

$$0 \leq u_{ik} \leq 1, \quad \text{for } 1 \leq i \leq c, 1 \leq k \leq n, \tag{19.3}$$

$$0 < \sum_{k=1}^{n} u_{ik} < n, \qquad \text{for } 1 \leq i \leq c, \tag{19.4}$$

$$\sum_{i=1}^{c} u_{ik} = 1, \qquad \text{for } 1 \leq k \leq n. \tag{19.5}$$

The fuzzy C-Means (FCM) uses an iterative optimization of the objective function, based on the weighted similarity measure between x_k and the cluster center v_i.

Steps of the fuzzy C-Means algorithm, according to Hellendorn and Driankov (1998) follow:

Algorithm

1. Given a data set $X = \{x_1, x_2, ..., x_n\}$, select the number of clusters $2 \leq c < N$, the maximum number of iterations T, the distance norm $d^2(x_k, v_i)$, the fuzziness parameter $m > 1$, and the termination condition $\varepsilon > 0$.

2. Give an initial value $U^{(0)}$.

3. For $t = 1, 2, ..., T$

   a) Calculate the c cluster centers $\{v_{i,t}\}, i = 1, ..., c$

   $$v_{i,t} = \frac{\sum_{k=1}^{n} u_{ik,t-1}^{m} x_k}{\sum_{k=1}^{n} u_{ik,t-1}^{m}} \tag{19.6}$$

   b) Update the membership matrix. Check the occurrence of singularities. Let $I = \{1, ..., c\}$,

   $$I_{k,t} = \{i | 1 \leq i \leq c, d_{ik,t} = \parallel x_k - v_{i,t} \parallel = 0\},$$

   and $\bar{I}_{k,t} = \{1, 2, ..., c\}/I_{k,t}$
   Then calculate the following

   $$u_{ik,t} = \sum_{j=1}^{c} \left(\frac{d_{ik,t}}{d_{jk,t}} \right)^{\frac{2}{m-1}}, \text{ if } \Upsilon_{k,t} = 0 \tag{19.7}$$

   Choose $a_{ik,t} = 1/\#(\Upsilon_{k,t}), \forall i \in \Upsilon; \#(\cdot)$ denotes the ordinal number.

4. If $E_t = \| U_{t-1} - U_t \| \leq \varepsilon$ then stop otherwise return to step 3.

This procedure converges to a local minimum or a saddle point of J_m. The FCM algorithm computes the partition matrix U and the clusters' prototypes in order to derive the fuzzy models from these matrices.

19.3.1 Data and Methods

The data set consists of 7 channels from a Landsat TM scene (256×256 pixels) around Ipoh city in Malaysia. The data were obtained from the School of Aerospace Engineering, Universiti Sains Malaysia, Malaysia. The image was georeferenced to Malaysian RSO projection, with RMS error less than 0.5 pixel.

The chosen area of study will therefore concentrate itself around the Ipoh city. Some reasons for this choice are that:

- This location lies in the Kinta valley, once a thriving for mining area, which is currently undergoing changes to its land-use.

- There is an availability of satellite digits data since 1991 such as Landsat and SPOT.

The site and its surroundings include the urban and suburban area where the major land cover comprises the mixture of building, vegetation, bare soil, and water. The land classes that appear in Figure 19.1 show a fairly complex mixture that obviously will create a big challenge to determine the right class.

The methodology that we will used are unsupervised classification (fuzzy clustering) and then compare this with the ISODATA unsupervised classification method. More information of ISODATA unsupervised classification algorithm can be found at Ball and Hall (1967).

Firstly, we manipulated the data with XploRe. The value of the spectrum frequency of the seven bands is to be extracted, where the total observations that we have $256 \times 256 \times 7 = 458752$ pixels. We then apply fuzzy clustering to all of the seven bands. As a default, we set the value of $m = 2$ and $c = 5$. The choice of $m = 2$ is due to its fast convergence compared to other numbers of m. Meanwhile the $c = 5$ what we have chosen is based on the research undertaken by Bawahidi, *et al.* (2003).

We conducted also with the similar data using ISODATA algorithm. This process done by ERDAS software, in which this algorithm already implemented in ERDAS.

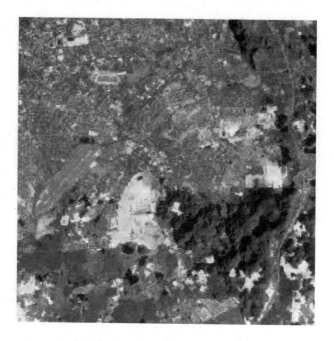

Figure 19.1: Image of Ipoh City

19.4   Results and Discussions

By analyzing the data, it is assumed that there is no more noise. Multi-resolution image is usually high correlated. Either when it is seen visually or numerically (Schowengerdt, 1997).

Figure 19.2 shows the test data and all 7 bands of Ipoh City. Bawahidi, *et al.* (2003) has carried out a classification using an unsupervised ISODATA classification method. This method classified the data into 15 classes. These classes were then clustered into 5 classes and named as: water, agriculture, grass, urban areas, barren and mining area.

However, it is known that classifying an urban area using Landsat TM data is not easy. Especially when it is done in a rural settlement surrounded with meadows, brush land, and agricultural fields. When the area is fallow, the brightness value obtained will be the same with that of the urban area itself. This will result in a false process of classification of the classes.

Next, we will see the performance algorithm of the suggested unsupervised

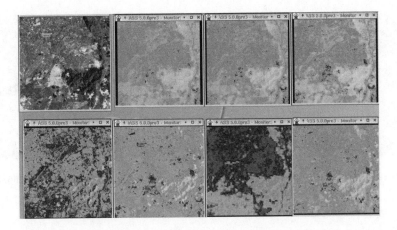

Figure 19.2: Scenes from test data and 7 band images of Ipoh City

classification (fuzzy clustering) and then compare this with the ISODATA classification methods.

We got the cluster results of the fuzzy clustering method from XploRe and transferred to GRASS for display purposes. We only choose the observation of pixels where the membership value is greater than 0.5. Pixels which have membership value smaller than 0.5, we leave it for further investigation. There are around 800 pixels which are not belong to certain cluster but to two or three cluster together.

We also got the cluster results of ISODATA from ERDAS and transferred to GRASS for display purposes. All of the two clustering results together with the test images are shown in Figure 19.3.

We also presented the accuracy assessment of both methods. These accuracy assessments were done by ERDAS Imagine. We choose the pixel to be compared randomly. From the Figure 19.3, it is shown clearly that an airport is lying on Grass Land. There is a relationship with the table of accuracy assessment, where for the Grass Land class, the accuracy is increased from 88% to 92%.

In general, it can be clearly seen that the latter method (fuzzy clustering) attains a greater level of accuracy than the first one (ISODATA). The overall accuracy is significantly increased from 85% to 91%.

We have presented fuzzy clustering method for remotely sensed imagery of Ipoh City will be proposed in this study. It seems to be clear from its accu-

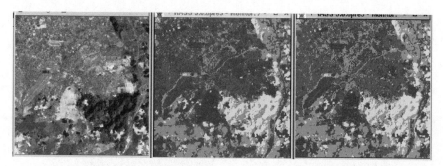

Figure 19.3: Scenes of test image, five clusters with the ISODATA method
and the Fuzzy method

Table 19.1: Accuracy assessment for the ISODATA clustering

Class name	W/S	F/A	U/B	G	B/M	Total	User's
Water/shadow	33	2	2	1	1	39	0.85
Forset/agriculture	1	108	8	5	2	124	0.87
Urban/built-up	2	6	67	7	3	85	0.79
Grass Land	2	2	4	77	3	88	0.88
Barren/Mining area	1	0	2	1	26	30	0.87
Total	39	118	83	91	35	366	
Producers' accuracies	0.85	0.92	0.81	0.85	0.74		
Overall Accuracy 85%							

racy that the fuzzy c-means method significantly outperforms the ISODATA
approach.

Table 19.2: Accuracy assessment for the fuzzy clustering

Class name	W/S	F/A	U/B	G	B/M	Total	User's
Water/shadow	55	2	0	1	1	59	0.93
Forset/agriculture	1	112	2	1	0	116	0.97
Urban/built-up	0	6	59	7	3	75	0.79
Grass Land	1	2	0	65	3	71	0.92
Barren/Mining area	0	0	2	2	41	45	0.91
Total	57	122	63	76	48	366	
Producers' accuracies	0.96	0.92	0.94	0.86	0.85		
Overall Accuracy 91%							

Bibliography

Anderson, J.R., Hardy, E.E., Roach, J.T., and Witmer, R.E. (1976). A Land
    Use and Land Cover Classification System for Use with Remote Sensor
    Data, *Washington D.C., U.S. Geological Survey*, No. Professional paper
    964.

Ball, G. and Hall, D. (1967). A clustering technique for summarizing multi-
    variate data, *Behavioral Science*, **12**:152:155.

Bawahidi, K., Affan, M., Md. Said, M. A. and Razali, R. (2003). *The appli-
    cation of remote sensing and GIS in monitoring Land-Use/Land Cover
    changes for a study area Ipoh*, Kuala Lumpur Conference.

Bezdek, J. C. (1981). *Pattern Recognition with Fuzzy Objective Function
    Algoritmss*, Plenum Press, New York.

Dunn, J. C. (1973). A Fuzzy Relative of the ISODATA Process and Its Use
    in Detecting Compact Well-Separated Clusters, *Journal of Cybernetics*
    3: 32–57.

Günther, O., Hess, G., Mutz, M., Riekert, W.-F., and Ruwwe, T. (1993).
    RESEDA : A Knowledge-Based Advisory System for Remote Sensing,
    Applied Intelligence, **3(4)**: 317–341.

Günther, O., Radermacher, F. J., and Riekert, W.-F. (1995). Environmental
    Monitoring: Models, Methods and Systems, *in* : Avouris, N. M. and
    Page, B. (eds.), *Environmental Informatics*, Kluwer Academic Publish-
    ers.

Hellendorn, H. and Driankov, D. (1998). Fuzzy: Model Identification,
    Springer Verlag, Heidelberg.

Ruspini, E. H. (1969). A New Approach to Clustering, *Information Control*
    15: 22–32.

Schowengerdt, R. A (1997). *Remote Sensing, Models and Methods for Image
    Processing*, Academic Press.

Index

XCSFuncKerReg, 255
Bsplineevalgd, 309
createfdbasis, 312
data2fd, 312
denbwsel, 337
fft, 308
Fourierevalgd, 308
hazdat, 216
hazreg, 216
haztest, 216
kaplanmeier, 208
panfix, 38
panrand, 38
plmhetexog, 98
plmhetmean, 100
plmhett, 99
plmk, 90–93, 95, 98–100
plmls, 96, 101
plmp, 92, 93, 95
polyevalgd, 309
stree, 169, 173–175
XCSbsplineini, 228
XCSbspline, 228
XCSdensestim, 75
XCSdensiterband, 75
XCSempiricalfunction, 337
XCSFuncKerDiscrim, 260, 261
XCSFuncKerReg, 255, 257
XCSHFestimci, 76
XCSHFestim, 76
XCSHFiterband, 76
XCSintensityfunction, 341
XCSkerneldistribfunction, 337
XCSkernelhazard2, 338
XCSkernelhazard, 337

XCSSemiMetricDer2, 251, 260
XCSSemiMetricDer, 251
XCSSemiMetricPCA, 252, 260
XCSsflmgcvmult, 229
XCSsflmgcv, 229
XCSsquantgcv, 234
XSCbspline, 252

Analysis of contingency tables, 105
    computing statistics for log-
        linear models, 113
    estimation of parameter vec-
        tor, 113
    fitting to log-linear models, 111
    generalized linear models, 109
    interference for log-linear mod-
        els using XploRe, 113
    log-linear models, 105
    log-linear models for three-way
        contigency tables, 107
    log-linear models for two-way
        contigency tables, 106
    model comparison and selec-
        tion, 114, 119
    testing independence, 115
artif data, 273

Bootstrap methods for testing in-
        teractions in GAMs, 147
    application to real data sets,
        156
    bootstrap approximation, 153
    bootstrap-based testing for in-
        teractions, 152
    direct test, 153

estimation of GAM with interactions, 150
likelihood ratio-based test, 153
neural basis for decision making, 156
risk of post-operative infection, 159
simulation study, 154

data sets
Early Lung Cancer Detection, 175
HFdata1, 76, 79
artif, 273
pines, 297
topo, 287
Discriminant analysis based on continuous and discrete variables, 3
application to the location model, 5
asymptotic distribution of Matusita distance, 10
comparison with the linear discriminant analysis, 24
example, 22
generalisation of the Mahalanobis distance, 4
Kullback–Leibler divergence, 5
location model, 22
methods and stopping rules for selecting variables, 13
rejection option, 15
simulations, 12

Early Lung Cancer Detection data, 175
estimation and nonparametric fits, 89

forward selection, 270
forward-backward stepwise selection, 271

Functional data analysis, 305
approximation and coefficient estimation, 310
B-Spline basis, 309
basis expansion, 318
data set as basis, 309, 319
discretization, 317
Fourier basis, 308
functional basis expansion, 307
functional principal components, 314
polynomial basis, 309
smoothed principal components analysis, 321
software implementation, 312
temperature example, 313, 320, 323
Fuzzy clustering for satellite images, 357
data and methods, 361
fuzzy C-means method, 359
remote sensing, 358

hazard library, 331
hazker library, 75
hazreg library, 169, 214
HFdata1 data, 76, 79

Identifying coexpressed genes, 125
clustering, 132
methodology and implementation, 127
weighting adjustment, 128
introduction, 63

Kernel estimates of hazard functions, 63
application, 75
bandwidth selection, 69
kernel estimate, 64
procedure, 74
shape of kernel, 68

Kernel method used for replicated micro-array experiments, 45
  data analysis, 52
  fully non-paprametric approach, 49
  implementation of the nonparametric method, 51
  mixture model approach, 48
  nonparametric approach results, 53
  normal mixture model results, 53
  reflection approach in kernel estimation, 50
  simulation study, 56
  statistical model and some existing methods, 46
  t-test, 47

Landcover prediction, 347
  multilogit regression model, 349
  penalized log-likelihood estimation, 351
  polychotomous regression in action, 352
  presentation of the data, 348
library
  hazard, 331
  hazker, 75
  hazreg, 169, 214
  metrics, 272
Longitudinal data analysis with linear regression, 29
  application, 40
  computing fixed and random-effect models, 37
  fixed and random-effect linear regression, 38
  fixed-effect model, 32
  random effects model, 36

metrics library, 272

Nonparametric functional chemometric analysis, 245
  bandwidth choice, 256
  functional nonparametric regression, 252
  introduction to spectrometric data, 246
  nonparametric curves discrimination, 257
  nonparametric statistics for curves, 248
  prediction of fat percentage from continuous spectrum, 254, 260
  proximity between curves, 249

Ozone pollution forecasting, 221
  application to ozone prediction, 235
  data description, 222
  functional linear model, 226
  functional linear regression for conditional quantiles, 231
  functional prinicipal component analysis, 225
  multiple conditional quantiles, 234
  multiple functional linear model, 229
  prediction of the conditional mean, 236
  prediction of the conditional median, 236
  principal component analysis, 224
  selection of the parameters, 228

Partially linear models, 87
  definition, 87
  heteroscedastic cases, 97
  kernel regression, 89
  least square spline, 96
  local polynomial, 90

piecewise polynomial, 93
real data applications, 100
pines data, 297

Semiparametric reference curves es-
    timation, 181
    asymptotic property, 192
    case study on biophysical prop-
        erties of the skin, 195
    dimension reduction, 187
    estimation procedure, 191
    kernel estimation, 184
    methodological procedure, 197
    reference intervals in clinical
        and medical practice, 181
    results and interpretation, 198
    simulated example, 193
    sliced inverse regression, 187
Spatial statistics, 285
    analysis of geostatistical data,
        287
    correlogram and variogram, 292
    kringing, 290
    spatial point process analysis,
        297
    trend surfaces, 288
Statistical analysis of seismicity, 329
    Galicia earthquakes data, 337
    kernel estimation of hazard func-
        tion, 330
    occurence process of eathquakes,
        336
    real data application, 336
Survival analysis, 207
    Cox's regression, 215
    data sets, 208
    Kaplan-Meier estimate, 208
    log-rank test, 210
Survival trees, 167
    example, 175
    impurity based criteria, 170
    log-rank statistic criterion, 172

methodology, 170
pruning, 173
splitting criteria, 170

topo data, 287

Variable selection in PCA, 265
    backward elimination, 270
    backward-forward stepwise se-
        lection, 270
    examples, 273, 279
    methods and criteria, 267
    modified PCA, 268
    selection procedures, 269

Printing: Krips bv, Meppel
Binding: Stürtz, Würzburg